Child Health
and the
Environment

Child Health and the Environment

DONALD T. WIGLE, MD, PhD, MPH
*R. Samuel McLaughlin Centre for Population
Health Risk Assessment
Institute of Population Health
University of Ottawa
Ottawa, Canada*

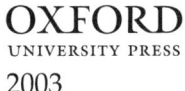

OXFORD
UNIVERSITY PRESS
2003

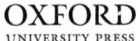

OXFORD
UNIVERSITY PRESS

Oxford   New York
Auckland   Bangkok   Buenos Aires   Cape Town   Chennai
Dar es Salaam   Delhi   Hong Kong   Istanbul   Karachi   Kolkata
Kuala Lumpur   Madrid   Melbourne   Mexico City   Mumbai
Nairobi   São Paulo   Shanghai   Taipei   Tokyo   Toronto

Copyright © 2003 by Oxford University Press, Inc.

Published by Oxford University Press, Inc.
198 Madison Avenue, New York, New York, 10016
http://www.oup-usa.org

Oxford is a registered trademark of Oxford University Press

Library of Congress Cataloging-in-Publication Data
Wigle, D. T.
Child health and the environment / Donald T. Wigle.
p. cm.
Includes bibliographical references and index.
ISBN 0-19-513559-8
1. Pediatric toxicology.   2. Environmentally induced diseases in children.
3. Children—Health risk assessment.   I. Title.
RA1225.W545 2003
615.9'0083—dc21   2002026944

9 8 7 6 5 4 3 2 1

Printed in the United States of America
on acid-free paper

To Beth,
children everywhere,
and Garreth,
who bravely fought non-Hodgkin's lymphoma
from age 10 to 19 years.

Acknowledgments

I thank all who contributed to this book including the anonymous reviewers. In particular, I thank John Last for his encouragement from the time this book was just an idea, and Jeffrey House for his many helpful suggestions, support, and patience. Special thanks go to colleagues who reviewed chapters and provided many helpful suggestions: Tye Arbuckle, Rick Burnett, Bob Dales, Eric Dewailly, Warren Foster, Rick Gallagher, Howard Morrison, Dieter Riedel, Pat Rasmussen, Will Robertson, Bob Spasoff, Paul Villeneuve, Slavica Vlahovich, and Mike Wade. I also thank Edith Barry, Lynda Crawford, and other Oxford staff for their help in improving the manuscript.

Preface

The public health goal of collectively assuring the conditions in which people can be healthy[1] is particularly relevant to children as they are vulnerable to environmental hazards but have little or no control over their environmental conditions. Children differ profoundly from adults with respect to physiology, metabolism, growth, development, and behavior. By interfering with child growth and development during critical time periods, environmental hazards may cause structural and functional deficits and lifelong disability. The long life expectancy of children carries the potential for relatively high cumulative exposures and time to develop delayed adverse health outcomes; for instance, intense sun exposure during childhood is a major determinant of adult melanoma risk.

This book explores potential health outcomes of prenatal and childhood exposure to environmental hazards, particularly anthropogenic contaminants. Among the overarching themes are the susceptibility of the rapidly developing fetus and infant to early-life toxic exposures and the importance of modifying factors (e.g., poverty, genetic traits, nutrition) and timely intervention. Public health policy development in this field

[1]National Academy of Sciences. 1988. The future of public health. Washington, D.C.: National Academy Press.

must respond to high public concern about the safety and well-being of children but is complicated by the multiplicity of environmental contaminants, major knowledge gaps, the limitations of toxicologic and epidemiologic studies, and a lack of scientific consensus on causal relationships. Under the precautionary principle, lack of full scientific certainty does not justify postponement of cost-effective measures to prevent significant potential public health risks. This book documents several historic examples of environment-related child health disasters resulting from failures to apply the precautionary principle.

Chapters 1 to 3 present overviews of key children's environmental health issues and the role of environmental epidemiology and risk assessment in child health protection. Chapter 1 shows that international, national, and other bodies have identified asthma, air pollution (indoor and outdoor), lead, pesticides, water contaminants (chemical and microbial), climate change, hormonally active agents, and environmental tobacco smoke as important environmental health issues for children. Epidemiologic studies have identified adverse health effects during gestation, childhood, and adulthood arising from early-life exposure to diverse environmental toxicants such as ionizing radiation, lead, methylmercury, polychlorinated biphenyls (PCBs), environmental tobacco smoke, and outdoor air pollutants. Nevertheless, knowledge about the proportions of prenatal, childhood, and adult adverse health outcomes that are attributable to prenatal and childhood environmental exposures is very limited. Chapter 2 illustrates epidemiologic strengths with published examples and discusses their limitations such as problems in quantifying exposures, assessing delayed effects, and limited ability to detect relatively small risks.

When there is evidence that a particular environmental factor poses a threat to human health, regulatory authorities face the challenge of deciding how much population exposure should be permitted. Chapter 3 describes the role of the U.S. National Academy of Sciences risk assessment framework in quantifying health risks for the purpose of setting exposure limits protective of human health. Among the issues covered are processes used by national and international agencies to assess causal relationships, the assessment of dose–response relationships, uncertainties surrounding recommended exposure limits, and the need for improved premarket testing of commercial chemicals for early-life toxicity. The chapter also addresses key issues related to risk assessments of carcinogens, reproductive toxicants, developmental toxicants, and neurotoxins.

Lead and mercury are potent neurotoxins and the developing fetus and infant are especially sensitive to their effects. The role of social factors (especially poverty) in childhood lead exposure; the importance of physiologic, nutritional, and developmental factors unique to childhood; possible developmental effects of prenatal parental lead exposure; the apparent absence of a blood lead threshold for hearing and cognitive deficits; and the persistent effects of childhood lead exposure on adolescent and adult cognitive performance are all discussed in Chapters 4 and 5. Major issues include controversies surrounding the efficacy of blood lead screening and lead abatement interventions, the possible neurotoxic effects of relatively low-level dietary methylmercury, and the need to further reduce the levels of population exposure to these toxicants. Sources and potential health effects of inorganic mercury, elemental mercury, arsenic, cadmium, and manganese are also discussed.

The disastrous health effects (intrauterine growth retardation, developmental delays, cognitive deficits, and chloracne) among infants of women highly exposed to PCBs are discussed in Chapter 6. Also covered are the possible health effects of early-life exposure to background levels of PCBs and related organochlorine compounds that share a common mechanism of toxicity, that is, activation of the aryl hydrocarbon receptor. This chapter documents the global dispersion and bioaccumulation of organochlorine compounds in aquatic and terrestrial food chains, and it flags such issues as uncertainties around the potential neurotoxic effects of relatively low-level lactational exposure to PCBs and related compounds, and the need to reduce human exposures.

About 3 million tons of conventional pesticide active ingredient chemicals are used annually worldwide, inevitably exposing the developing fetus and child to at least trace levels of currently used and persistent agents (e.g., DDT). Chapter 7 examines the known and potential health effects of pesticides, including acute poisonings, developmental effects, reproductive effects, neurotoxicity, and cancer. It addresses their potential to disrupt fetal and childhood growth and developmental processes and the inadequacy of premarket toxicity testing, as well as the potential role of pesticides in childhood cancer and the need to monitor population exposure levels.

Human experience with the drug diethylstilbestrol (DES) showed that prenatal exposure to this potent synthetic estrogen could cause reproductive tract abnormalities and vaginal cancer in offspring. Several environmental contaminants modulate endocrine function in experimental animals but their possible roles in human fetal and child development and health are unknown as very few epidemiologic studies have addressed these issues, and almost none have measured internal doses. Chapter 8 covers the potential roles of hormonally active environmental contaminants in the apparent trends toward reduced average age at menarche, reduced sperm quality, increased male reproductive tract birth defects, and increased cancer incidence rates. The importance of monitoring population exposures to hormonally active contaminants and tiered toxicity testing of high-production volume chemicals for hormonal activity are noted.

Children prenatally exposed to atomic bomb radiation had substantially increased risks of microcephaly and severe mental retardation while those exposed as young children during the 1986 Chernobyl nuclear accident had increased thyroid cancer risks. Relatively low-level prenatal exposure to medical X-rays appears to increase the risk of childhood leukemia but the possible role of low-level environmental radiation in adverse developmental outcomes (birth defects, intrauterine growth retardation) and childhood cancer is poorly understood. These issues and those related to other types of electromagnetic radiation are presented in Chapter 9. After describing the mixed evidence of a link between power-frequency magnetic fields and childhood cancer, this chapter notes widespread exposures and uncertainties, and calls for precautionary measures such as minimizing exposure during pregnancy and childhood. This chapter documents the role of intense childhood sun exposure in malignant melanoma and its possible links to cataracts and immune suppression. Also addressed are uncertainties related to the efficacy of sunscreen use in preventing melanoma, the importance of multiple interventions in protecting children from intense sun exposure, and the need to monitor their exposures and sun-protective behaviors (including those of their guardians).

Environmental tobacco smoke (ETS) is a major indoor air contaminant with known adverse effects on child health, notably respiratory and middle ear infections, lung function deficits, and asthma. In addition, ETS appears to cause sudden infant death syndrome and is a possible cause of childhood and adult cancers. Biologic agents, toxic gases, and volatile organic carbons (VOCs) comprise the other indoor air pollutants reviewed in Chapter 10. The chapter addresses the roles of house-dust mite antigens and other aeroallergens in the onset or exacerbation of asthma, carbon monoxide poisoning from indoor combustion sources, the possible role of VOCs and nitrogen dioxide in childhood respiratory disease and cancer, and the virtual absence of national comprehensive prevention programs for indoor air health hazards.

Children are vulnerable to outdoor air pollution because they often engage in physical activities or play outdoors; also, they have relatively high air intake compared to adults. Chapter 11 describes the role of major outdoor air pollutants in adverse developmental outcomes (intrauterine growth retardation, preterm birth), respiratory tract inflammation and hyperreactivity, lung function deficits, and respiratory illnesses such as incident asthma. The need to minimize exposure of children and pregnant women to ambient air pollutant levels from major sources, especially motor vehicles and industry is noted. Evaluation of progress in this field requires monitoring personal exposures and prevalence/incidence rates of potential respiratory health effects.

An adequate supply of safe drinking water is an elusive goal in economically disadvantaged regions globally. Chapter 12 addresses waterborne microbial and chemical hazards, the latter including chlorination disinfection by-products (DBPs) and toxic chemical contaminants from hazardous waste disposal and other sources. Emerging evidence of developmental effects (spontaneous abortions, stillbirths, intrauterine growth retardation, and certain birth defects) related to first trimester maternal DBP exposure, the susceptibility of surface waters to high DBP levels, and economic barriers to DBP abatement, particularly in small water systems, are discussed. Hazardous waste disposal and storage often contaminate groundwater but the few existing epidemiologic studies preclude an adequate assessment of this child health hazard. Needs to protect source waters, reduce DBP levels, control hazardous waste disposal, and monitor water quality are noted.

Children develop enteric infections by ingesting fecally contaminated water and other substances (e.g., formula mixed with contaminated water) and by engaging in hand-mouth behavior. Although such infections are a leading cause of childhood deaths in economically disadvantaged countries globally, Chapter 12 focuses mainly on microbial threats in developed countries. *Escherichia coli 0157:H7*, a major cause of acute renal failure in children, can be transmitted through contaminated drinking water. Water appears to be a source of *Helicobacter pylori* infection during childhood; this organism causes chronic gastrointestinal infection and increased risks of peptic ulcers and stomach cancer during adulthood. The need to address both microbial and disinfection by-product hazards is a major risk management challenge.

This book will interest professionals and graduate students in the fields of public health, pediatrics, environmental health, epidemiology, and toxicology. The introductory and concluding segments of each chapter should interest a wider audience including health policy analysts in voluntary and governmental agencies. The final chapter summarizes the associations between environmental exposures and child health outcomes described in the previous chapters and calls for measures to create the evidence needed to enable public health decisions protective of child health. The five tables in this chapter are unique in that they summarize available information on the burden of child health adverse outcomes and the potential role of environmental hazards together with the level of epidemiologic evidence.

Contents

Child Health
and the
Environment

1

Environmental Threats to Child Health: Overview

Control of childhood infections through sanitation, immunization, improved nutrition and housing, and antibiotics during the twentieth century greatly increased life expectancy at birth and dramatically changed patterns of childhood illnesses in developed countries. But there is growing evidence that global changes in atmosphere, terrestrial ecosystems, and climate, driven by population increase and consumption, pose threats to current and future human health. Children are especially vulnerable because they have no control over their prenatal and postnatal environments, including the quality of the air they breathe, the water they drink, the food they eat, and their place of residence. Exposure to environmental toxicants during prenatal and early childhood periods can disrupt developmental processes, causing structural and functional abnormalities that range from subtle to obvious, immediate to delayed, and transient to permanent. The leading health conditions that result in illness, disability, and death among children now include asthma, unintentional injuries, cancer, low birth weight, neurodevelopmental deficits, and birth defects. Apart from injuries, the proportions of these conditions attributable to environmental hazards are uncertain or unknown. By using a Delphi process and other sources to estimate attributable risks and economic impacts, a recent study concluded that 100% of lead poisoning, 30% of asthma, 5% of cancer, and 10% of neurobehavioral disorders among children in United States are caused by environmental pollutants and impose an economic burden of about $55 billion annually (Landrigan et al., 2002).

Enteric and related infections caused by use of fecally contaminated water and respiratory conditions related to indoor and outdoor air pollution cause about 13% of all disability-adjusted life years (DALYs) lost globally, with considerably higher proportions in economically disadvantaged regions. Indigenous groups dependent on traditional foods may have increased risks of exposure to environmental hazards such as methylmercury in fish, organochlorine compounds in whale blubber, and lead in waterfowl. Even in developed countries, children in disadvantaged groups have higher levels of exposure to environmental hazards such as lead, environmental tobacco smoke (ETS), cockroach antigen, and outdoor air pollution and lower access to protective interventions such as sunscreens.

This book addresses the impacts of chemical, radiologic, and biologic environmental contaminants on child health and development from conception to early adulthood. Chapters 2 and 3, respectively, describe the roles of epidemiology and environmental risk assessment in providing an evidence base for public health policy and program decisions. Succeeding chapters review current evidence on major environmental hazards including lead, mercury and other heavy metals, dioxins, polychlorinated biphenyls, pesticides, radiation, hormonally active agents, indoor air, outdoor air, and drinking water. The final chapter summarizes known and suspected environmental threats to child health and policy issues arising from knowledge gaps. The present chapter deals with important issues related to child health, environmental hazards, vulnerabilities of the developing fetus and child, and the prevention and control of environmental hazards.

Environmental Health Concerns About Children

Leading Adverse Child Health Outcomes

Major pregnancy and child health outcomes (events per year in the United States) and their known or suspected environmental links are presented in Table 1–1. The very large annual number of fetal deaths (almost 1 million recognized events) and low-birth-weight infants (about 300,000) indicate the major impact of these conditions on population health. The reported number of fetal deaths is likely to have been substantially underestimated; longitudinal studies of women using biomarkers to detect

TABLE 1–1. Adverse Fetal, Infant, and Child Health Outcomes, United States

(a) Adverse pregnancy outcomes

Outcome	Number of Events
Fetal deaths[a]	983,000
Low birth weight[b]	
<1,500 g	57,477
1500–2499 g	243,706
Total	301,183

(b) Childhood diseases

	Deaths[c,d]			Hospital-izations[e]
	Age <1 Yr	*Age 1–14 Yr*	*Age <15 Yr*	*Age <15 Yr*
Perinatal conditions (low birth weight, complications of pregnancy, other)	14,084	135	14,219	170,000
Birth defects	5,473	977	6,450	130,000
SIDS	2,648	—	2,648	—
Respiratory disease—total	687	644	1,331	741,000
(asthma)	(5)	(153)	(158)	(190,000)
Cardiovascular diseases	667	591	1,258	25,000
Gastrointestinal diseases	500	249	749	221,000
Cancer and other neoplasms	126	1,594	1,720	36,000
Nervous system diseases	441	877	1,318	89,000
Certain infectious diseases	562	493	1,055	173,000
Injuries (including poisonings)	1,285	6,163	7,448	228,000
Other	1,464	1,121	2,585	645,000
Total	27,937	12,844	40,781	2,458,000

[a]Miscarriages and stillbirths, USA, 1996. Source: Ventura et al. (1999).

[b]USA, 1999. Ventura et al. (2001).

[c]USA, 1999. Hoyert et al. (2001).

[d]USA, 1999. Anderson (2001).

[e]USA, 1999. Popovic (2001).

early pregnancy have shown that 20%–40% of conceptions end in fetal death before 20 weeks' gestation but only a quarter to a half are clinically recognized. Among human early fetal deaths, about 10%–20% have autosomal chromosome aneuploidy and 10%–20% have congenital heart defects.

Leading causes of infant deaths include perinatal conditions (e.g., conditions related to complications of pregnancy, labor, or delivery, preterm birth, intrauterine growth retardation, birth trauma, or respiratory distress), birth defects, and sudden infant death syndrome (SIDS). Among older children, the main fatal conditions are injuries, cancer, and birth defects. The main causes of childhood hospitalization are respiratory diseases (infections, asthma), injuries, and gastrointestinal conditions (infections, other). All of these conditions have known or suspected environmental links. Reported increases of birth defects and cancers among children and young adults and their known or suspected links to preconceptual, prenatal, and childhood exposures have raised public concern.

During the period from 1974 to about 1984 in Canada, incidence rates of overall childhood cancer increased by about 15%; since then, incidence rates of total and specific childhood cancers (leukemia, brain cancer, Hodgkin's disease, and non-Hodgkin's lymphoma) have been relatively constant. Childhood leukemia incidence rates increased in the United States during 1974–1991 but appear to have decreased slightly thereafter. Childhood brain cancer incidence rate increases have been reported in several countries; the U.S. increases occurred mainly during 1983–1986, possibly due to improved detection of low-grade cerebral and brainstem gliomas after the introduction of magnetic resonance imaging (MRI) (Smith et al., 1998). In sum, there is little convincing evidence of childhood cancer incidence rate increases since the late 1980s.

Incidence rates for several types of cancer have increased among young adults in Canada and some other countries during recent decades: melanoma, thyroid cancer (especially among females), testicular cancer, and non-Hodgkin's lymphoma. Intense sun exposure during childhood appears to explain most of the increase in melanoma. Some of the increase in non-Hodgkin's lymphoma among men was likely caused by human immunodeficiency virus (HIV) infection, but this cannot explain the striking global increases in this cancer across gender and age groups and beginning before the HIV epidemic. Infection with simian virus 40 was recently identified as a possible cause of non-Hodgkin's lymphoma among persons who received contaminated polio vaccines during 1955–1963 (Shivapurkar et al., 2002; Vilchez et al., 2002). Exposure to medical X-rays during childhood and youth may partially explain the increased thyroid cancer rates. Unexplained are testicular cancer incidence rates that increased twofold or more during the past three or four decades in several geographic regions, especially among more recent birth cohorts (see, e.g., Liu et al., 1999).

Recognized Children's Environmental Health Issues

There is considerable consistency in the children's environmental health issues identified as important by international and national agencies (Table 1–2). Six or more of the ten agencies acknowledged asthma, air (indoor and outdoor), lead, pesticides, and water contaminants (chemical

TABLE 1–2. Children's Environmental Health Issues Identified by International, National, and Other Organizations

Issue	Number of Agencies	Issue	Number of Agencies
Air—outdoor	9	Other metals (mercury, cadmium)	3
Water—infectious agents	9		
Lead	8	Persistent organic pollutants	3
Asthma	7	Acute respiratory infections	2
Air—indoor	7	Developmental disabilities (cerebral palsy, autism, learning disabilities, hearing loss)	2
Pesticides	7		
Water—chemical contaminants	6		
Environmental tobacco smoke	5		
Poverty	4	Injuries	2
Hormonally active agents	4	Radiation (ionizing)	2
Hazardous waste sites	4	Acute poisonings	1
Radiation (sunlight/ ultraviolet radiation)	4	Diarrheal diseases	1
		Food—contaminants	1
Birth defects	3	Genetically modified organisms	1
Cancer	3		
Climate change	3	Vectors of parasitic diseases (malaria)	1

Sources: World Health Organization (2001), European Centre for Environment and Health (1999), Lvovsky (2001) (note—the survey was not targeted to children, but the issues identified are strongly linked to child health), Pan American Center for Sanitary Engineering and Environmental Science (2001), G8 countries (1998), Commission for Environmental Cooperation (2000), U.S. Environmental Protection Agency (1996), Centers for Disease Control and Prevention (2000), U.S. Department of Health and Human Services (2000) (note: these are objectives for the entire U.S. population but relate directly to children's health), Council of State and Territorial Epidemiologists (2001) (note: these are objectives for the entire U.S. population but relate directly to children's health).

and microbial) as important issues directly relevant to children. The World Health Organization (WHO) Europe and the G8 nations (Canada, France, Germany, Italy, Japan, Russia, United Kingdom, United States of America) added three other issues—climate change, hormonally active agents (HAAs), and environmental tobacco smoke. An Environmental Protection Agency (EPA) advisory committee noted five areas where children's needs were not adequately addressed by existing EPA regulations: mercury emissions, farm worker protection, triazine pesticides (atrazine in drinking water), organophosphate and carbamate insecticides (neurotoxicity), and indoor and outdoor air quality and asthma.

Knowledge of Environmental Threats to Child Health

The relative importance of children's environmental health issues could be approached by measuring the frequency of adverse health conditions among children, identifying their causal factors, measuring exposure to causal factors, and estimating attributable risks. In practice, this is only partially feasible because of major gaps in understanding the relationships between prenatal and childhood environmental exposures and adverse health outcomes. On the one hand, up to 60% of SIDS deaths may be caused by prenatal and postnatal tobacco smoke exposure. On the other hand, several epidemiologic studies have shown associations between childhood cancer and pesticide exposure indices, but causality is uncertain because of the lack of strong epidemiologic evidence, positive or negative.

Cancer incidence patterns among identical and nonidentical twins indicate that about 80% of cancers that occur commonly during childhood are attributable to environmental factors or gene–environment interactions, but these remain largely unknown. The U.S. National Academy of Sciences estimated that toxic chemical and physical agents cause about 3% of all developmental disorders and that a combination of genetic and nongenetic factors (including infections, tobacco, alcohol, and environmental hazards) may cause about 25% of these disorders (National Academy of Sciences, 2000). It is important to recognize that very few epidemiologic studies of adverse developmental outcomes with large sample sizes and rigorous exposure assessment have been conducted. It seems likely that future studies will reveal higher attributable risks of environmental factors than current estimates indicate. Although the impacts of environmental toxicants on child health have not been quantified systematically, succeeding chapters describe many important known links.

Some environmental hazards have been assessed in a least a few high-quality epidemiologic studies (e.g., childhood leukemia and power-frequency magnetic field exposures), but uncertainties related to exposure indices, mixed exposures, low frequency of highly exposed subjects, and inconsistent findings have complicated the interpretation of study results. Although there have been many studies of pesticides and childhood cancer, few have had strong statistical power and exposure assessment. Despite extensive research on the exacerbation of asthma by environmental exposures, there have been relatively few studies of causal factors for incident asthma. In addition to adverse health outcomes during childhood and youth, early-life exposure to environmental hazards may cause cancer and other adverse health effects during adulthood.

The childhood equivalent of the Framingham Heart Study or the U.S. Nurses' Health Study would be large longitudinal studies with intensive environmental exposure assessments beginning before conception or during early pregnancy with prolonged follow-up to identify health outcomes during pregnancy, infancy, childhood, adolescence, and adulthood. Such studies, initiated in Europe and at the planning stage in the United States, promise to provide much needed information on a wide variety of potential health outcome and environmental exposure relationships (Golding et al., 2001; National Institute of Child Health and Human Development 2001).

CHILDREN'S VULNERABILITIES

The genome controls prenatal and postnatal growth and function but, as documented throughout this book, genes and the many molecular processes they control can be disrupted by environmental hazards. Inherited mutations and a wide range of social, behavioral, or other factors that increase exposure to environmental hazards can all increase a child's vulnerability. Sociodemographic subgroups of children may have both higher exposures related to older or deficient housing, residence in areas with high outdoor air pollution, dependence on contaminated drinking water, consumption of traditional foods, and the presence of household smokers and increased vulnerability because of maternal and childhood dietary deficiency and other risk factors.

The National Research Council report *Pesticides in the Diets of Infants and Children* documented age-related population heterogeneity with respect to exposure levels and toxicity (National Academy of Sciences, 1993). This report noted several unique aspects of children: (1) rapid body growth and development—the underlying molecular and cellular processes are vulnerable to disruption by toxicants, causing irreversible adverse effects on body structure (birth defects, reduced growth rates) and function, (2) the potential for relatively high exposures related to children's diet, behavior, and physiologic/metabolic differences from adults, (3) immature detoxification systems, and (4) inadequate toxicity testing of chemicals for developmental, neurobehavioral, immunologic, and reproductive system effects of perinatal exposures.

Disruption of Growth and Developmental Processes

Development has been described as evolution's foremost accomplishment in gene regulation, involving a complex orchestration of genes activated in specific cells at specific times (National Academy of Sciences, 2000). The cascades of genetically controlled molecular processes that underlie growth and development from fertilized egg to mature youth create periods during which toxic exposures can cause irreversible structural and/or functional abnormalities. Periods of vulnerability for adverse developmental outcomes depend on the mechanism of action of a given toxicant, the dose of toxicant taken up by the target tissue, the developmental timetable of the target tissue, and the age at evaluation of outcomes.

Birth Defects

Although there are known risk factors for birth defects (e.g., maternal smoking and alcohol consumption during pregnancy, relative folic acid deficiency, and use of certain pharmaceuticals), the attributable risks are generally low and the causes of most birth defects remain unknown. Research in this field is complicated by the fact that spontaneous abortion during the first trimester is quite common (20%–40% of all conceptions and about 10% of recognized pregnancies), and a high proportion of affected fetuses have birth defects and/or chromosomal abnormalities. Studies of birth defects among infants therefore include only a fraction of incident cases, that is, those prevalent at birth. Although molecular mechanisms of teratogens are poorly understood, rodent models indicate that many embryotoxins are proteratogens that are activated in vivo by enzymes including P450 cytochromes and peroxidases to electrophiles or free radicals that may damage DNA directly or indirectly through the formation of reactive oxygen species such as hydroxyl radicals. The embryo may be vulnerable to reactive intermediates because of immature detoxification systems. See later chapters for further discussion of potential environmental causes of birth defects.

Nervous System

The adult brain, a complex network of about 10^{11} neurons and 10^{14} synaptic connections, has a high metabolic rate, consumes about a fifth of the body's oxygen uptake, and is almost entirely dependent on glucose for energy. The development of the nervous system from the embryonic through the adolescent periods depends on genes and chemical messengers that guide a complex series of processes that occur at specific points in time and space. Development proceeds faster in some brain regions than others; for example, the growth rates of the human diencephalon and cerebellum, respectively, peak at birth and age 7 months. Although the neuronal population is complete by age 2 years, synapse formation and apoptosis continue until about age 5 years, and myelination continues through childhood and adolescence.

Periods of vulnerability during nervous system development include (Rice and Barone, 2000)

- Neural tube closure during early gestation
- Neuron proliferation, migration, synaptogenesis, gliogenesis, myelinogenesis, and apoptosis during gestation and infancy
- Brain remodeling during adolescence

The vulnerability of the developing brain to neurotoxins depends on access of the active agent to the nervous system and the timing of exposure in relation to developmental changes. The so-called blood–brain barrier is not fully developed until about age 6 months and, even then, it only partially protects the brain from environmental toxicants, especially lipid-soluble agents. Perinatal exposure to neurotoxins can disrupt subsequent cascades of developmental processes, greatly amplifying adverse effects, but later exposures may have little or no effect. Radiotherapy of brain tumors before age 4 years disrupts neuron proliferation and synapse formation and causes substantial cognitive deficits; treatment at age 4 to 7 years or later, respectively, causes mild or no detectable cognitive deficits.

Until the 1970s, concern about the impact of neurotoxins such as lead, mercury, and alcohol was almost entirely limited to adults. Frank mercury poisoning among infants ("pink disease" or acrodynia) was once thought to be an infectious disease; use of mercurous chloride in teething powder was not recognized as the actual cause until 1947, partly because the clinical signs differed from those of adult mercury poisoning. Perinatal exposure to methylmercury in Iraq and Japan during the 1950s and 1960s caused severe neurobehavioral deficits and deaths among offspring at exposure levels that caused minimal or no maternal toxicity. The use of lead in gasoline, paint, and other products caused widespread exposure of children and adverse effects ranging from subtle neurobehavioral deficits to severe and occasionally fatal childhood poisonings during much of the twentieth century. During the 1950s and 1960s, many newborn infants were washed daily with a 3% suspension of hexachlorophene; this practice was discontinued after discovery of a link to vacuolar encephalopathy of the brainstem reticular formation in preterm infants. Preterm human infants and young rats are far more susceptible than adults are to myelin degeneration caused by dermally absorbed hexachlorophene, a lipid-soluble substance with a very high affinity for myelin.

Animal studies have identified neurotoxic mechanisms relevant to humans. Ethanol and certain drugs (e.g., barbiturates) interfere with neurotransmitter activity at N-methyl-D-aspartate (NMDA) and γ-aminobutyric acid type A ($GABA_A$) receptors, the most ubiquitous receptor systems in the developing brain; exposure of rodents to such neurotoxicants during the neonatal brain growth spurt period causes widespread apoptosis of developing neurons. Neonatal exposure of rodents to pesticides that target neurotransmitter systems (e.g., chlorpyrifos) also disrupts brain development processes and triggers apoptosis (see Chapter 7, Pesticides). Further research is needed to assess the known and hypothesized links of environmental neurotoxins to schizophrenia, dyslexia, epilepsy, autism, mental retardation, attention deficit hyperactivity disorder (ADHD), learning disorders, and adult neurologic diseases.

Immune System

Known or suspected environmental immunosuppressants in humans include ultraviolet light (inhibits natural killer cell activity and contact hypersensitivity in adults), high-dose ionizing radiation, and 2,3,7,8-tetrachlorodibenzo-*p*-dioxin (TCDD). Rodent studies have shown that immune system development can be disrupted by perinatal exposure to relatively low doses of various toxicants (e.g., dioxin or dioxin-like organochlorines, polycyclic aromatic hydrocarbons, certain pesticides, heavy metals), with resultant persistent immunosuppression (Holladay and Smialowicz, 2000). These toxicants may interfere with hematopoietic cell proliferation, differentiation, and migration, expansion of lineage-committed stem cells, colonization of postnatal lymphopoietic compartments, cell–cell interactions, and maturation to immunocompetence. There is limited evidence that perinatal exposure of genetically predisposed rodents to immunotoxicants increases the risk of hypersensitivity responses and autoimmune diseases but little evidence from human studies. Adult humans exposed to contaminants in cooking oil and tryptophan supplements developed autoimmune connective tissue disorders, but the role of perinatal environmental toxicant exposures in autoimmune disease in humans is unknown.

Respiratory System

Development of the human respiratory system involves the differentiation, proliferation, and organization of multiple cell types into a complex system with over 300 million alveoli, the terminal gas exchange sacs (Pinkerton and Joad, 2000). Lung development begins at about 4 weeks' gestation, but alveolarization does not occur until the third trimester and the number of alveoli in a newborn's lungs is only 20% that of adults. Airway outgrowth, branching, and alveolarization continue until about age 18–20 years under the control of substances such as epidermal growth factor, transforming growth factor-α, and retinoic acid. Factors contributing to the susceptibility of the developing human respiratory system to environmental toxicants include the following:

- Several lung enzyme systems responsible for detoxification of xenobiotics are not fully developed at birth.
- Postnatal lung growth and development continues from birth until late adolescence, a period of 16–18 years during which children are exposed to airborne toxicants and aeroallergens.
- Polymorphisms in any of several candidate genes may increase susceptibility to asthma.

Perinatal exposure to ETS is associated with lung function growth deficits and incident asthma. The infant lung appears to be susceptible to idiopathic pulmonary hemosiderosis caused by combined exposure to the toxicogenic fungus *Stachybotrys chartarum* and ETS. Spores of *S. chartarum* are respirable and slowly release toxins that cause capillary fragility and suppress immune function; the ability of fungal toxins to inhibit protein synthesis in rapidly growing lungs may partially explain the susceptibility of infants to this disease.

Reproductive System
Experimental animal studies revealed vulnerable periods of exposure during reproductive system development including

- Spermatogenesis—preconceptual exposure of males to genotoxins can damage sperm DNA and cause early embryo death and birth defects
- Male reproductive development
  - Prenatal exposure of the male rat to androgen receptor antagonists (e.g., the pesticides vinclozolin, procymidone, linuron, and dichloro-diphenyltrichloroethane [DDT]) causes reduced anogenital distance and induces areolas at relatively low doses, hypospadias, agenesis of reproductive accessory tissues, and retained nipples at intermediate doses, and undescended testes and epididymal agenesis at high doses.
  - Immature and pubertal rats appear to be more sensitive than adults to testicular toxicity of phthalate esters and the pesticide, 1,2-dibromo-3-chloropropane.
- Ovarian development—neonatal exposure of female rats to androgens causes delayed puberty, irregular ovarian cycles, lower numbers of ovarian follicles, and premature cessation of ovulation.
- Puberty—exposure of experimental animals to certain neurotoxins (heavy metals, solvents, or pesticides) may accelerate or delay puberty.

Exposure

Behavior and Diet
Breast milk is a potentially important source of polychlorinated biphenyls (PCBs) and other fat-soluble contaminants for infants, especially those whose mothers consumed large amounts of contaminated fish or other foods. Infants and toddlers frequently mouthe or lick objects or surfaces; young children showed about 10 hand–mouth contacts per hour when videotaped while playing. Children often sit on floors or grass/soil while watching television, playing, or eating snacks, thus being exposed to tox-

icants in house dust, carpets, and soil via skin contact, ingestion, or inhalation. Compared to adults, 1-year-old infants consume (per unit body weight per day) twice as much tap water, total vegetables, and total citrus fruits and 10–20 times as many pears, apples, and total dairy products (Table 1–3); children aged 3–5 years consume 2–3 times as much tap water, total vegetables, and total citrus fruits and 7–8 times as many apples and total dairy products. These habits increase the risk of exposure to pesticide residues on citrus fruits and vegetables and to fat-soluble organochlorine compounds in dairy products.

Genetic Characteristics

Certain genetic traits interact with infectious, chemical, physical, nutritional, and other factors to cause adverse health effects. Diseases caused by single gene mutations may be aggravated by environmental contaminants; for example, cystic fibrosis is exacerbated by ETS. Genetic factors are also important in relatively common childhood conditions and diseases including birth defects, cancer, and asthma. Polymorphisms involve two or more distinct alleles at one genetic locus at stable frequencies in the population too large (usually defined as ≥1%) to be explained solely by recurrent mutation—the average heterozygosity per nucleotide site in humans is about 1:1000. Although persons with polymorphisms usually have no obvious health problems, they may be more susceptible to environmental and other hazards (see the examples in succeeding chapters). As the function of the human genome becomes better understood, the

TABLE 1–3. Ratio of Childhood to Adult Intakes (Amounts per Kilogram of Body Weight per Day) of Air, Water, and Selected Foods

Substance	Age <1 Year	Age 3–5 Years
Total tap water	2.1	2.4
Air—inhalation rates at rest	3.4	2.8
Total vegetables	1.8	1.9
Citrus fruits	2.2	3.0
Apples	14.2	8.4
Bananas	6.0	2.1
Peaches	9.5	3.1
Pears	20.7	2.3
Peas	3.5	2.4
Tomatoes	1.7	2.5
Total meats	1.7	2.3
Total dairy products	20.3	6.8

Source: U.S. Environmental Protection Agency (1997).

role of polymorphisms in susceptibility to environmental hazards will likely have major implications for disease prevention and control policies and programs. Existing environmental standards invoke uncertainty factors intended to protect susceptible subgroups; improved knowledge may show that current standards are inadequately protective of susceptible subgroups.

Physiology

Certain physiologic and metabolic characteristics during prenatal and postnatal development may increase the risk of adverse health effects from environmental toxicants. Compared to an adult, an infant has about twice the surface area per unit body weight and a correspondingly higher metabolic rate, a threefold higher intake of air per unit body weight per day, and an immature blood–brain barrier. The term *blood–brain barrier* encompasses multiple mechanisms that control access of blood components to the brain; fetal and neonatal blood–brain barriers are relatively impermeable to protein but are more permeable than adult barriers to small lipophilic molecules such as unconjugated bilirubin.

Metabolism

To varying degrees, toxicants absorbed into the body are detoxified in the liver, kidneys, and other tissues by xenobiotic[1] metabolizing systems. The metabolism of many lipophilic xenobiotics involves two phases: phase I— mainly oxidative reactions and phase II—conjugation with water-soluble moieties, a step that facilitates excretion. Phase I involves mixed-function oxidases (P450 cytochromes) that can (1) inactivate xenobiotics to less toxic derivatives amenable to conjugation and excretion or (2) activate them to strong electrophiles or unstable compounds that generate highly reactive free radicals. Phase I products may be conjugated during phase II with glucuronide, sulfate, acetate, glutathione, or other conjugating agents, reactions catalyzed by specific enzymes (e.g., glucuronyl transferase, N-acetyltransferase, glutathione S-transferase). Glutathione also scavenges electrophilic xenobiotics, thus protecting RNA, DNA, and other potential targets.

Humans display wide variations in susceptibility to xenobiotics, in part due to genetic polymorphisms in P450 cytochromes and other phase I and II enzymes. The genes that encode cytochromes are divided into

[1] A xenobiotic is any chemical not produced in vivo.

families and subfamilies, each with some degree of specificity for certain xenobiotics, including (1) CYP1—the CYP1A subfamily includes CYP1A1 (encodes a cytochrome active in metabolism of benzo(a)pyrene; occurs in the liver, lung, and kidney), CYP1A2 (encodes a cytochrome that metabolizes acetanilide; found mainly in the liver) and (2) CYP2, which includes several subfamilies—CYP2A1 and CYP2A2 encode cytochromes that are active in metabolism of sex steroids (testosterone, progesterone, and androstenedione) and xenobiotics; CYP2E1 is restricted to mammals and appears to encode a cytochrome that activates benzene, nitrosamines, and certain other xenobiotics, thereby contributing to their carcinogenicity. Children with polymorphisms for CYP1A1, CYP2E1, and other xenobiotic metabolizing enzymes appear to have an increased risk of developing acute lymphoblastic leukemia (Infante-Rivard et al., 1999; Krajinovic et al., 2002).

Immature Detoxification Systems

Pharmacokinetic studies of drugs used to treat newborn infants indicate that they can metabolize xenobiotics, but clearance is generally slow (Gow et al., 2001). Liver enzymes develop at different rates postnatally; for example, levels of glycine N-acyltransferase, involved in detoxification of drugs and other xenobiotics, are very low at birth and do not reach adult levels until about age 18 months. In a population exposed to air pollution, levels of polycyclic aromatic hydrocarbon (PAH)-DNA adducts, total aromatic-DNA adducts, and cotinine in cord blood were higher than those in maternal blood, suggesting reduced fetal detoxification capacity (especially since maternal exposure to PAHs exceeds fetal exposure) (Whyatt et al., 2001).

RISK MANAGEMENT ISSUES

Historical Perspective

The former belief that the placenta protects the fetus from toxic chemicals was shattered by repeated events during the mid-twentieth century involving serious and sometimes fatal effects of prenatal maternal exposures including ionizing radiation, methylmercury, diethylstilbestrol (DES), and thalidomide. Thalidomide, an antinausea drug once widely prescribed during pregnancy, caused severe birth defects in about 7000 infants during 1958–1962. This experience stimulated developmental toxicity testing of new commercial chemicals and birth defect monitoring in many countries, and it showed that:

- A chemical that was virtually nontoxic in mice and adult humans caused a markedly increased risk of severe birth defects when consumed during pregnancy.
- New commercial chemicals should be adequately screened for developmental toxicity in diverse experimental animals before humans are exposed (e.g., thalidomide is teratogenic in rabbits and primates, but rodents are generally resistant).
- International premarketing regulatory practices varied widely. The drug was available across the counter in Germany, the country with the highest number of affected infants; because of case reports of peripheral neuropathy in adult users, the U.S. Food and Drug Administration (FDA) restricted its use to clinical trials, saving many infants from devastating birth defects

Human Exposure Assessment

Children may be exposed to environmental contaminants in air, water, soil, dust, and food by ingestion, inhalation, or dermal contact. The potential anthropogenic sources of environmental contaminants include fossil fuel combustion, manufacturing processes, various uses of commercial products (pesticides, building materials, solvents), human activities (e.g., smoking indoors), waste disposal (hazardous waste disposal sites, incineration), and accidents. One of the major drivers is the vast and rapidly growing number of commercial chemicals. Over 70,000 commercial chemicals are registered for use in the United States, and the EPA receives about 1500 petitions annually to approve new chemicals or new uses of existing chemicals (U.S. Environmental Protection Agency, 2001a).

Few countries have assessed children's exposures to environmental contaminants through population-based biomonitoring. The United States has included children in the U.S. National Health and Nutrition Examination Survey (NHANES) surveys over the past 25 years and has assessed their exposure to contaminants including lead, other metals, ETS, phthalates, and organophosphate pesticides. The German Environmental Survey has been conducted three times since 1985–1986 and has included analyses of blood, urine, and scalp hair samples from children aged 6–14 years and environmental samples (house dust, drinking water, indoor and personal air, food) for metals, volatile organic chemicals (VOCs), and organochlorine compounds.

Recent Progress

Although much remains to be done to reduce children's exposures to known environmental hazards and to define the links between environmental factors and child health, there have been significant achievements:

- Blood lead levels declined sharply among children in all sex, age, ethnic, and income subgroups immediately after the introduction of lead-free gasoline in 1976.
- Population exposure to ETS has been reduced; median serum cotinine levels among nonsmokers in the United States decreased from 0.2 to 0.05 ng/mL between 1988–1991 and 1999.
- The U.S. 1996 Food Quality Protection Act requires that the unique exposures and susceptibilities of children be considered in pesticide risk assessment.
- Some countries have banned or restricted uses of a few pesticides mainly to protect children, such as daminozide and chlorpyrifos.
- Breast milk concentrations of PCBs, DDT/DDE (dichlorodiphenyldichloroethylene), and several other organochlorine compounds have decreased to varying degrees during recent decades.

Not all of these actions were targeted solely to children; the conversion to lead-free gasoline followed the introduction of catalytic converters by car manufacturers to reduce emissions under the 1970 Clean Air Act; lead inactivated the platinum catalyst in catalytic converters, necessitating the use of lead-free fuel.

Toxicity Testing of Commercial Chemicals

Volume. Regulatory agencies rely mainly on industry to conduct toxicity tests of new commercial chemicals. Extensive testing of pharmaceuticals, including clinical trials, has been required for many years and has shown that children's reactions often vary quantitatively and/or qualitatively from those of adults. The EPA estimated that up to a quarter of the approximately 70,000 commercial chemicals have neurotoxic potential, but only about 10% (excluding pharmaceuticals) have been tested for neurotoxicity. Most high production volume (HPV) chemicals (those produced in or imported into the United States in amounts of at least 500 tons per year) have not been subjected to the six basic toxicity screening tests prescribed by the Organization for Economic Cooperation and Development (OECD) for its 30 member countries. The U.S. National Toxicology Program, established in 1978 to coordinate toxicity testing on behalf of federal agencies, biomedical science communities, and the public, is probably the largest chemical toxicity testing program in the world, but even it can provide complete toxicologic evaluations on only 10–20 chemicals per year.

Developmental toxicity. In addition to the sheer number of commercial chemicals, routinely required toxicity tests may not detect important developmental effects. Relatively little toxicity testing has been directed to early embryogenesis, that is, the period between fertilization and gastrulation. In experimental animals, the effects of mutagens vary during early embryogenesis (Rutledge, 1997):

- Germ cells and early multipotential embryonic cells—mutagens affect many cells and organ systems, causing pre- and peri-implantation deaths, balanced chromosomal translocations (causing sterility or reduced fertility of offspring), growth retardation, and moderately increased rates of structural anomalies (mainly anencephaly, cleft palate, and skeletal anomalies).
- Zygote—exposure to mutagens at this stage causes early, middle, and late gestation deaths, as well as high rates of a restricted range of structural anomalies associated with chromosomal breaks and other cytogenetic abnormalities (mainly skeletal, eye, and abdominal wall closure defects, but no increase in anencephaly, spina bifida, or heart or urinary tract malformations).
- Preimplantation conceptus—mutagens cause growth deficits, high rates of structural anomalies (anencephaly, skeletal abnormalities, cleft palate), and late fetal death.

Nonmutagenic teratogens produce a spectrum of structural anomalies specific to time periods as brief as 1–2 days. In a review of the mechanisms of developmental defects, the U.S. National Academy of Sciences concluded that (National Academy of Sciences, 2000) (1) the mechanism of developmental toxicity is partially understood for a few toxicants (e.g., retinoic acid, diethylstilbestrol, and TCDD) but is not completely known for any compound; (2) testing should be done across the entire developmental period, including early fetal loss; and (3) there is potential to rapidly and inexpensively screen many chemicals for the ability to disrupt signaling pathways central to normal development.

Neurotoxicity. The EPA-designated toxicants that require developmental neurotoxicity testing include (in descending order) central nervous system teratogens and their structural analogues, adult neurotoxins, adult neuroactive agents, hormonally active compounds, and developmental toxicants. Much of the baseline evidence for triggers assumes that developmental and reproductive toxicity studies have been done, but the latter are required by the EPA only for registration of food-use pesticides and not for other pesticides or commercial chemicals (Claudio et al., 2000). Most of the 140 pesticides considered to be neurotoxic by the EPA have not been tested for developmental neurotoxicity, indicating that historic practices generally failed to trigger neurodevelopmental toxicity testing of known adult neurotoxins. An EPA advisory group recommended routine developmental neurotoxicity testing for registration of all food-use pesticides. Recommendations for neurotoxicity testing that address the need to protect child health include (International Programme on Chemical Safety, 2001) the following:

- Develop standardized test methods and norms to evaluate neurotoxicity in infants and children.
- Increase testing in animals involving perinatal exposure to chemicals and/or mixtures of chemicals to define the relative sensitivity of the developing nervous system to neurotoxic injury.
- Develop and validate efficient animal tests for developmental neurotoxicity for use in international collaborative studies.

Carcinogenicity testing. The Carcinogenic Potency Database contains the results of over 5000 carcinogenic bioassays on about 1300 chemical entities (Gold, 2001); in other words, only a fraction of the commercial chemicals have been tested for carcinogenicity in animals. An EPA review of animal carcinogenesis bioassay studies relevant to the issue of perinatal exposures found that lifelong exposure of animals beginning neonatally often produces a higher incidence of tumors with shorter latencies but seldom produces types of tumors not found in the standard bioassay; perinatal exposure alone to three known carcinogens did not consistently cause an increased incidence of cancer. The EPA review concluded that there is insufficient evidence to justify routine inclusion of a perinatal exposure component in the standard carcinogenesis bioassay, a conclusion endorsed by the EPA Scientific Advisory Panel. Notwithstanding this decision, carcinogens that are more potent or that cause unique types of cancer in rodents after perinatal exposure include cycasin (brain and jejunal tumors), DES (vaginal cancer and uterine adenocarcinomas in exposed females and testicular tumors among exposed males and the male offspring of perinatally exposed females), genistein (a natural phytoestrogen present in soy—uterine adenocarcinomas), and N-ethyl-N-nitrosourea (nephroblastoma and brain gliomas).

Toxicity testing priorities. The EPA Scientific Advisory Panel recommended that priorities for testing commercial chemicals for child health hazards should be based on criteria such as potential for children's exposures to exceed those of adults and should include those chemicals to which children are uniquely exposed or for which children have unique susceptibility rather than production volume alone. After excluding low-volume chemicals (less than 5 tons/yr) and high molecular weight, poorly absorbable polymers, there were about 15,000 chemicals produced or imported at levels above 5 tons/yr, including about 2800 HPV commercial chemicals. Since 1979, about 540 of the chemicals in the 15,000 chemical subset above have been tested within the EPA's Existing Chemicals Testing Program; these were mainly HPV chemicals. In 1990, the EPA developed a Master Testing List of over 500 existing chemicals (i.e., already used commercially) based on toxicity testing priorities of U.S. federal agencies and the OECD; as of 2001, testing actions were underway for almost 300 entities.

Despite this progress, only about 7% of HPV chemicals have been adequately tested; the remainder are missing one or more of the OECD Screening Information Data Set (SIDS) tests, and 43% are missing all SIDS tests (U.S. Environmental Protection Agency, 1998). Although the EPA is pursuing toxicity testing of HPV chemicals through voluntary agreements, it can require chemical manufacturers and processors to test existing chemicals that pose unreasonable risks to human health or the environment. Among the 491 HPV commercial chemicals to which children are likely exposed, only 25% have been adequately tested (U.S. Environmental Protection Agency, 2000). Under a voluntary EPA program, companies that manufacture or import 23 targeted chemicals are asked to sponsor a three-tier toxicity-testing program.

Strengthening Prevention

The Precautionary Principle

Modern use of the precautionary principle in environmental health can be traced to the 1992 United Nations Conference on Environment and Development that promulgated the Rio Declaration. Principle 15 of the Declaration states, "In order to protect the environment, the precautionary approach shall be widely applied by States according to their capabilities. Where there are threats of serious or irreversible damage, lack of full scientific certainty shall not be used as a reason for postponing cost-effective measures to prevent environmental degradation" (United Nations, 1992). Concern about the slow pace of efforts to address climate change, ecosystem degradation, and resource depletion was a major driver of the Rio Declaration.

Policymakers generally encounter a high level of uncertainty about children's environmental health risks because of knowledge gaps concerning relevant exposures and dose–response relationships for individual toxicants and mixtures. In the face of such uncertainty, a requirement for scientific consensus on causality is not necessarily appropriate for management of children's environmental health risks. As stated elsewhere, "If exposure is widespread and the consequences [are] serious, a need for primary prevention may suggest that even a moderate degree of evidence justifies regulatory action. On the other hand, if the probability of human exposure is low and the adverse health effects [are] uncertain, then the best policy may be collection of improved data" (Hertz-Picciotto, 1995). Scientific uncertainty about child health and the environment relates to several factors:

- Absent or inadequate evidence—gaps in knowledge of the toxicology and epidemiology of potential environmental hazards
- Inconsistent results of toxicologic studies—use of different test animal species or strains, differences in purity, dose, and route of exposure of the test substance, small sample size
- Inconsistent results of epidemiologic studies—limited statistical power, inadequate exposure estimates, uncontrolled confounders
- Uncertainty about the shape of the dose–response curve at doses below those observed
- Doubt about the adequacy of uncertainty factors used in quantitative risk assessments to compensate for knowledge gaps including extrapolation of results from animal studies to humans and the distribution of exposures and susceptibility factors among children in the general population

To obtain an improved evidence base for future policy and program development in this field, current efforts in two areas require strengthening: (1) research to better define environmental hazards, susceptible populations, and dose–response relationships and (2) tracking systems to monitor population exposure levels. The EPA and the National Institute of Environmental Health Sciences (NIEHS) have funded 12 children's environmental health research centers to address priority issues including child health effects of various toxicants (lead, mercury, PCBs, pesticides) and the role of environmental exposures in cognitive deficits, autism, learning disabilities, ADHD, and asthma (U.S. Environmental Protection Agency 2002).

Tracking Systems

Systems that track the occurrence of health conditions and their determinants have greatly aided prioritization, planning, and evaluation of disease control and prevention programs in specific fields (infectious diseases, unintentional injuries, disability, occupation-related diseases) and in nationwide health objectives (see, e.g., Thacker and Stroup, 1994). A framework for environmental tracking systems might include hazards, exposures, health outcomes, and children's environmental health policies. Tracking systems for child-related aspects of outdoor air pollution, for instance, might address hazard occurrence (e.g., concentrations of priority contaminants in outdoor air), exposure levels (e.g., proportion of children exposed to ambient air contaminant levels above current air quality standards), health outcomes (e.g., incidence of emergency room visits for childhood asthma), and health policies (e.g., clean air policies, standards, guidelines). It appears that no jurisdiction has implemented comprehensive tracking systems to monitor needs and progress related to children's environmental health, but some elements exist:

- Hazards
  - Outdoor air—many developed countries have national and/or regional monitoring networks to measure ambient air contaminants including particulate matter and ozone.
  - Drinking water—drinking water facilities in developed countries generally monitor microbial contaminants and may monitor chemical contaminants such as chlorination disinfection by-products (total trihalomethanes) and lead.
  - Indoor air—some national health surveys and many occasional surveys have included questions on the smoking habits of household members; census data may include information on housing characteristics such as fuels used for cooking and heating.
  - Food contaminants—some countries have conducted limited sampling of foods for pesticide residues and other contaminants; the enormous variety and volume of foods and the practice of testing batches rather than individual portions preclude detection of low-frequency, high-pesticide residue levels before distribution and consumption. This issue is further complicated by sparse or absent data on food consumption patterns within narrow age ranges among children (needed because of the large variation in diet as an infant or child ages).
- Exposures and doses—*exposure* generally refers to the level of a contaminant in environmental media (air, water, food, soil) to which a person is directly exposed, while the *internal dose* is the amount of con-

taminant taken up by an individual from all sources and is usually estimated by measuring contaminant levels in body tissues or fluids. Tracking systems relevant to estimation of children's environmental hazard exposures or doses include

- ○ Surveys of children and other household members including activities, smoking habits, pesticide use, and diet
- ○ Biomonitoring—surveys of children and mothers that collect biologic samples such as blood, urine, breast milk, and hair and analyze selected contaminant levels
- There have been few population surveys of children's diet and very limited tracking of children's doses of environmental contaminants, the recent effort of the U.S. Centers for Disease Control and Prevention being a notable exception (Centers for Disease Control and Prevention, 2001). Although a few countries have conducted breast milk contaminant monitoring for over 20 years, most monitoring has been confined to sporadic small samples of convenience (Hooper, 1999).
- Health outcomes—developed countries generally collect data on vital statistics (stillbirths, low birth weight, birth defects), hospitalizations/physician services (e.g., spontaneous abortion, birth defects, asthma, acute respiratory infections, gastrointestinal infections), and health status (e.g., health surveys that include items on parent-reported child health conditions such as physician-diagnosed asthma).
- Children's environmental health policies—some nongovernmental organizations track policies relevant to children's environmental health, but little organized information is published in the scientific literature. This is a promising area for coordinated, ongoing tracking and communications to better inform the public about unmet needs.

CONCLUSION

Children's environmental health is increasingly recognized as a global public health issue of great importance. International, national, and other bodies have identified asthma, air pollution (indoor and outdoor), lead, pesticides, water contaminants (chemical and microbial), climate change, HAAs, and ETS as important children's environmental health issues. Given our current limited knowledge, assumptions about thresholds for noncarcinogenic effects of certain perinatal toxicant exposures may prove inappropriate; for example, the apparent threshold for lead toxicity has decreased substantially during recent decades because of improved research methods. Knowledge is also very limited concerning the proportions of adverse health outcomes during pregnancy, childhood, and adulthood that are attributable to prenatal and childhood environmental exposures. Answers to this question will require substantial targeted epidemiologic and toxicologic research to measure relative risks and track environmental contaminant exposures.

The developing fetus and child are unusually susceptible to environmental hazards because of unique growth and developmental processes, immature metabolic systems, physiology, and behaviors. In developed countries, regulatory agencies have recently begun to adjust their risk assessment processes to better protect children. Children remain, however, continually exposed to multiple low-level environmental contaminants beginning in utero. The recent nascent efforts to undertake large longitudinal research studies of children with a major focus on assessment of exposures beginning in early gestation and detection of neurobehavioral and other adverse health outcomes should be encouraged and expanded.

The reader is referred to these selected websites for further information on children's environmental health:

- World Health Organization, The Gateway to Children's Environmental Health. Available at http://www.who.int/peh/ceh/index.htm
- U.S. Environmental Protection Agency, Office of Children's Health Protection. Available at http://yosemite.epa.gov/ochp/ochpweb.nsf/homepage
- U.S. National Institute of Child Health and Development, The Longitudinal Cohort Study of Environmental Effects on Child Health and Development. Available at http://nationalchildrensstudy.gov/

REFERENCES

Anderson RN. (2001). Deaths: Leading causes for 1999. National Vital Statistics Reports 49:88 pp.

Centers for Disease Control and Prevention. (2000). Strategic plan 1999–2003. Atlanta: Centers for Disease Control and Prevention.

Centers for Disease Control and Prevention. (2001). National report on human exposure to environmental chemicals. Atlanta: Centers for Disease Control and Prevention.

Claudio L, Kwa WC, Russell AL, Wallinga D. (2000). Testing methods for developmental neurotoxicity of environmental chemicals. Toxicol Appl Pharmacol 164:1–14.

Commission for Environmental Cooperation. (2000). Background paper for the Symposium on North American Children's Health and the Environment, Toronto, Canada, 10 May 2000. Montreal: Commission for Environmental Cooperation.

Council of State and Territorial Epidemiologists. (2001). Development of environmental public health indicators. Located at http://www.cste.org/ps/2001/2001-env-02.htm.

European Centre for Environment and Health, WHO. (1999). Children's health and the environment (EUR/ICP/EHCO 02 02 05/16). Rome: European Centre for Environment and Health.

G8 countries. (1998). 1997 Declaration of the environment leaders of the Eight on children's environmental health. Can J Public Health 89(Suppl 1):S5–S8.

Gold LS. (2001). The carcinogenic potency project. Located at http://potency.berkeley.edu/cpdb.html.

Golding J, Pembrey M, Jones R. (2001). ALSPAC—the Avon Longitudinal Study of Parents and Children. I. Study methodology. Paediatr Perinat Epidemiol 15:74–87.

Gow PJ, Ghabrial H, Smallwood RA, Morgan DJ, Ching MS. (2001). Neonatal hepatic drug elimination. Pharmacol Toxicol 88:3–15.

Hertz-Picciotto I. (1995). Epidemiology and quantitative risk assessment: a bridge from science to policy. Am J Public Health 85:484–91.

Holladay SD, Smialowicz RJ. (2000). Development of the murine and human immune system: differential effects of immunotoxicants depend on time of exposure. Environ Health Perspect 108(Suppl 3):463–73.

Hooper K. (1999). Breast milk monitoring programs (BMMPs): world-wide early warning system for polyhalogenated POPs and for targeting studies in children's environmental health. Environ Health Perspect 107:429–30.

Hoyert DL, Arias E, Smith BL, Murphy SL, Kochanek KD. (2001). Deaths: final data for 1999. National Vital Statistics Rep 49:114 pp.

Infante-Rivard C, Labuda D, Krajinovic M, Sinnett D. (1999). Risk of childhood leukemia associated with exposure to pesticides and with gene polymorphisms. Epidemiology 10:481–7.

International Programme on Chemical Safety. (2001). Environmental health criteria No. 223. Integrated approach to the assessment of neurotoxicity of chemicals. Geneva: International Programme on Chemical Safety.

Krajinovic M, Sinnett H, Richer C, Labuda D, Sinnett D. (2002). Role of NQO1, MPO and CYP2E1 genetic polymorphisms in the susceptibility to childhood acute lymphoblastic leukemia. Int J Cancer 97:230–6.

Landrigan PJ, Schechter CB, Lipton JM, Fahs MC, Schwartz J. (2002). Environmental pollutants and disease in American children: estimates of morbidity, mortality, and costs for lead poisoning, asthma, cancer, and developmental disabilities. Environ Health Perspect 110:721–8.

Liu S, Wen SW, Mao Y, Mery L, Rouleau J. (1999). Birth cohort effects underlying the increasing testicular cancer incidence in Canada. Can J Public Health 90: 176–80.

Lvovsky K. (2001). Environment strategy papers, No. 1. Health and environment. Washington, D.C.: The World Bank.

National Academy of Sciences. (1993). Pesticides in the diets of infants and children. Washington, D.C.: National Academy Press.

National Academy of Sciences. (2000). Scientific frontiers in developmental toxicology and risk assessment. Washington, D.C.: National Academy Press.

National Institute of Child Health and Human Development. (2002). The National Children's Study. Located at http://nationalchildrensstudy.gov/about/042002.cfm.

Pan American Center for Sanitary Engineering and Environmental Science. (2001). Children's health and the environment. Main themes. Located at http://www.cepis.ops-oms.org/indexeng.html.

Pinkerton KE, Joad JP. (2000). The mammalian respiratory system and critical windows of exposure for children's health. Environ Health Perspect 108(Suppl 3): 457–62.

Popovic JR. (2001). 1999 national hospital discharge survey: annual summary with detailed diagnosis and procedure data. Vital Health Stat 13:214 pp.

Rice D, Barone S Jr. (2000). Critical periods of vulnerability for the developing nervous system: evidence from humans and animal models. Environ Health Perspect 108(Suppl 3):511–33.

Rutledge JC. (1997). Developmental toxicity induced during early stages of mammalian embryogenesis. Mutat Res 396:113–27.

Shivapurkar N, Harada K, Reddy J, Scheuermann RH, Xu Y, McKenna RW, Milchgrub S, Kroft SH, Feng Z, Gazdar AF. (2002). Presence of simian virus 40 DNA sequences in human lymphomas. Lancet 359:851–2.

Smith MA, Freidlin B, Ries LA, Simon R. (1998). Trends in reported incidence of primary malignant brain tumors in children in the United States. J Natl Cancer Inst 90:1269–77.

Thacker SB, Stroup DF. (1994). Future directions for comprehensive public health surveillance and health information systems in the United States. Am J Epidemiol 140:383–97.

United Nations. (1992). Report of the United Nations Conference on Environment and Development, Rio de Janeiro, 1992, Annex 1. Rio declaration on environment and development. New York: United Nations.

U.S. Department of Health and Human Services. (2000). Healthy people 2010 (S/N 017-001-00547-9). Washington, D.C.: U.S. Government Printing Office.

U.S. Environmental Protection Agency. (1996). Environmental health threats to children (EPA 175-F-96-001). Washington, D.C.

U.S. Environmental Protection Agency. (1997). Exposure factors handbook (EPA/600/P-95/002Fa). Washington, D.C.

U.S. Environmental Protection Agency. (1998). Chemical hazard data availability study. Located at http://www.epa.gov/opptintr/chemtest/hazchem.pdf.

U.S. Environmental Protection Agency. (2000). Voluntary children's chemical evaluation program. Located at http://www.epa.gov/chemrtk/vccep/childhlt.htm.

U.S. Environmental Protection Agency. (2001a). Chemical testing and information home page. Located at http://www.epa.gov/opptintr/chemtest/index.htm.

U.S. Environmental Protection Agency. (2002). Centers for Children's Environmental Health and Disease Prevention Research. Located at http://es.epa.gov/ncer/centers/cecehdpr/01/.

Ventura SJ, Martin JA, Curtin SC, Menacker F, Hamilton BE. (2001). National Vital Statistics Reports 49:99 pp.

Ventura SJ, Mosher WD, Curtin SC, Abma JC, Henshaw S. (1999). Highlights of trends in pregnancies and pregnancy rates by outcome: estimates for the United States, 1976–96. Natl Vital Stat Rep 47:1–9.

Vilchez RA, Madden CR, Kozinetz CA, Halvorson SJ, White ZS, Jorgensen JL, Finch CJ, Butel JS. (2002). Association between simian virus 40 and non-Hodgkin lymphoma. Lancet 359:817–23.

Whyatt RM, Jedrychowski W, Hemminki K, Santella RM, Tsai WY, Yang K, Perera FP. (2001). Biomarkers of polycyclic aromatic hydrocarbon-DNA damage and cigarette smoke exposures in paired maternal and newborn blood samples as a measure of differential susceptibility. Cancer Epidemiol Biomarkers Prev 10:581–8.

World Health Organization. (2001). The gateway to children's environmental health. Setting priorities. Located at http://www.who.int/peh/ceh/taskforce.htm.

2

Environmental Epidemiology

Epidemiology is the study of the distribution and determinants of health conditions in human populations as a basis for preventive and other interventions. Unique to environmental epidemiology is its focus on environmental factors to which humans are unwittingly exposed. The scope of environmental epidemiology addressed in this book includes studies of adverse health outcomes in human populations and their relationship to prenatal and childhood exposures to environmental hazards. The purpose of this chapter is to describe the types of environmental epidemiologic studies, their strengths and weaknesses, their role in describing population distributions of exposures and health outcomes, and their use to generate and test hypotheses about environmental threats to child health. The discussion includes important issues underlying the limited ability of epidemiologic studies to identify hazards when population exposures are low and health outcomes are subtle or delayed.

EPIDEMIOLOGY

Strengths

The major strength of epidemiologic studies is their ability to assess relationships between environmental exposures and health outcomes directly in humans under real-life conditions. This avoids uncertainties related to extrapolations between species and from the high doses used in animal studies to the generally lower doses observed in humans. Other strengths include the ability to

- Evaluate risks in large populations with diverse exposures and genetic traits
- Exploit administrative databases with high-quality diagnostic information on many adverse health outcomes
- Assess interactions between environmental exposures and other factors unique to humans, such as alcohol, ETS, and genetic factors

Limitations

Timeliness
Epidemiologic studies can identify hazards only after humans have already been exposed and have developed adverse health effects. Toxicants that cause delayed health effects such as cancer may be recognized only after populations have been exposed for many years.

Nonexperimental Design
Environmental epidemiology usually involves observational studies of humans inadvertently exposed to environmental toxicants (see the exceptions noted below). Observational studies are susceptible to biases related to selection of subjects, inadequate control of potential confounders, and measurement of exposures and health outcomes. Scientific consensus on the significance of observational study results may be elusive and may delay decisions to act on potential environmental hazards, especially if the biologic mechanisms are unknown (see discussion of the precautionary principle near the end of Chapter 1).

Exposure Assessment
Exposure assessment is as a major obstacle in environmental epidemiologic studies, and the absence of quantitative exposure data is the main reason for not using epidemiologic studies in quantitative risk assessments (Rothman, 1993). Exposure indices used in epidemiologic studies must be practical, affordable, and able to capture information on exposures that occur at low average levels but may fluctuate substantially over time. Potential components of exposure indices include dose (intensity, pattern), timing (frequency, relationship to critical developmental periods, duration, time since first exposure), and exposure route (inhaled, ingested, dermal). When the biologic mechanism of an exposure–risk relationship is not understood, there is considerable uncertainty concerning

the exposure index most likely to increase the risk of a given health outcome. This is an issue, for instance, in epidemiologic studies of power-frequency magnetic fields and childhood cancer (see Chapter 9, Radiation). In such studies, exposure assessments have included time-weighted average exposures above a threshold value, cumulative exposures, personal or residential exposure levels, proximity to power lines, and electric appliance use, but there is no biologic basis to define the best exposure indices.

Precision and Validity

Precision is the inverse of the variance of an estimate arising from random measurement error, and increasing the sample size is the main method used to improve precision. *Measurement validity* is the degree to which a measurement method actually measures a given characteristic (e.g., how well does motor vehicle traffic density reflect differences in ambient carbon monoxide exposure?). *Internal* and *external validity*, respectively, reflect the degree to which inferences about the study population and general populations are valid (Rothman and Greenland, 1998). Internal validity implies accurate effect estimates (apart from random errors) within a study; three main types of bias may reduce internal validity: selection, confounding, and information bias.

Selection bias. The relation between exposure and health outcome varies between study participants and persons in the base population[1] and may arise, for instance, through self-selection or diagnostic bias.

Confounding. The apparent relationship between an exposure and a health outcome actually results from two or more effects, including the exposure of interest. A confounder is a variable that can cause or prevent the outcome of interest, is not an intermediate variable, and is associated with the factor of interest in the base population. Methods used in epidemiologic studies to avoid or adjust for confounders include stratified and multivariate analyses.

Information bias. This arises from misclassification, that is, errors in measurement of exposures, other individual characteristics, or health outcomes. Differential misclassification occurs when measurement errors depend on the exposure or health outcome of interest; for example, in a case-control study of childhood cancer, the mothers of cases may put more effort into recalling past exposures than the mothers of healthy controls,

---

[1] *Base population* refers to the population sampling frame from which the study sample was drawn.

thereby creating spurious associations. Nondifferential misclassification happens when measurement error is independent of exposure or health outcome status. When nondifferential misclassification of a dichotomous exposure occurs independent of other errors, the effect estimate is biased toward the null, that is, the true association will be underestimated. Epidemiologic studies occasionally include direct estimates of misclassification; for example, parental recall bias for information on proximity to power lines and exposure to prenatal X-rays was assessed in a case-control study of childhood leukemia (Infante-Rivard and Jacques, 2000). There are circumstances under which nondifferential misclassification can bias the effect estimate away from the null. For information on this and other sources of bias, the reader is referred to other sources (Rothman, 2002; Rothman and Greenland, 1998).

Extrapolation of Dose–Response Relationships
Neither epidemiologic nor experimental animal studies can readily measure lifetime excess risks of interest to regulators, that is, 10^{-5} or 10^{-6}. Results in the observed exposure range must be extrapolated to substantially lower exposures with no direct evidence of the shape of the dose–response curve at such levels. The degree to which exposure metrics used in epidemiologic studies correlate with actual doses is usually unknown, contributing uncertainty to dose–response relationships and their extrapolation. In humans or animals, exposure to high doses of a toxicant may cause health outcomes that mask low-dose effects; for example, high doses of ionizing radiation can kill cells, while lower doses can cause cell transformation leading to cancer.

Other Issues
Ethical, cultural, privacy, response-burden, and related issues constrain the design and conduct of epidemiologic investigations. Study protocols are generally assessed for adherence to ethical principles including autonomy (respecting individual rights and freedoms), beneficence (doing good), and nonmaleficence (doing no harm). In some cases, the ethics principle of justice (fair and equitable distribution of resources) may be assessed, for example, ensuring that high-risk disadvantaged groups are included in a cohort or intervention study. Ethical issues increase with the sensitivity of information collected and can arise at various points in etiologic epidemiologic studies including:

- Study design and conduct—selection of the study population, protocol development, subject recruitment, solicitation of informed consent, and adequacy of quality control and follow-up procedures

- Interpretation and communication of results to individual participants and others, including health authorities and the public
- Banked biologic specimens—stewardship issues include secure storage, controlled access, and use for unanticipated research objectives not communicated to subjects at the time informed consent is obtained

The increasing opportunity for epidemiologists to conduct research involving the linkage of computerized databases is countered by public concern about privacy. Study protocols must include methods to protect privacy and provide evidence of potential benefits of the proposed research. The American College of Epidemiology noted deficiencies in existing ethics guidelines for epidemiologists in the areas of education, policy, and advocacy and called for dynamic guidelines that emphasize core values, obligations, and virtues (Weed and Coughlin, 1999). Although the risk to child health is minimal in observational epidemiologic studies, the age at which children can give truly informed consent is not well defined; for example, longitudinal studies need parent/guardian consent when the child is young but may require shared or direct consent as the child ages.

Exposure Assessment

Epidemiologists assess exposure to environmental hazards by several methods including (1) self-reported information captured with the aid of standardized questionnaires, (2) proximity to sources of contaminants, (3) environmental contaminant measurements coupled with information on residential history or activities, and (4) biomarkers of the internal dose. It is important to note that there may be relatively strong or very weak correlations between contaminant levels in environmental media (air, water, soil, dust, foods) and the dose actually taken up by a child or parent. The biologically relevant dose is generally the concentration of a contaminant or its biologically active derivative in target tissues, but peak or cumulated doses over time may be etiologically important for delayed health effects. Although some tissue contaminant levels can be measured (e.g., lead in deciduous teeth), they provide only limited information on exposure patterns, especially over long time periods; for instance, concentrations of organophosphate pesticide urinary metabolites reflect recent exposure.

    Accurate assessment of exposure to environmental and other factors, including potential confounders, is essential for detecting health effects of low-level environmental contaminants. Bias can arise not only from misclassification of the exposure of interest, but also from misclassification of confounders, potentially biasing the effect estimates toward or away from the null (Greenland, 1980). Validated exposure methods, whether questionnaire, administrative record, or laboratory based, help reduce misclassification of exposure. Other challenges include evaluation of complex exposures (e.g., mixtures of toxicants with variable compositions and toxicity) and assessment of exposures during critical perinatal time periods when susceptibility to developmental, reproductive, and neurotoxic effects is high.

Estimation of Past Exposures
Epidemiologic studies dependent on recall of exposures are susceptible to misclassified exposure status, thereby reducing statistical power and increasing the likelihood of biased risk estimates. Valid exposure recall is facilitated when exposure factors are well defined and relatively stable over time (e.g., self-reported information on smoking habits, occupation, and place of residence). Historic administrative records documenting information on environmental contaminant levels are not subject to recall bias, but older data may be limited by subsequent changes in the scope, methods, and sensitivity of contaminant analyses. For instance, chlorinated disinfection by-products in drinking water were not routinely measured until recent decades; even today, historic data are usually limited to total trihalomethanes, compounds that represent only a few of the several hundred disinfection by-products and only a fraction of the total mutagenic activity in chlorinated water. Similarly, historic ambient air pollution data are generally limited to a few major contaminants; ambient air VOCs, for instance, have been excluded from routine monitoring in the United States except in certain centers with major summer ozone pollution problems.

Some epidemiologic studies have collected information on individual exposure for certain factors (e.g., ETS, residential history) but have used geographically based data to assess exposure to environmental contaminants (e.g., data on ambient air quality and drinking water quality). Individual exposure levels tend to be misclassified when group-based exposure indices are used because of individual differences in activity patterns, exposure rates, metabolism, and excretion (Hatch and Thomas, 1993). Personal dosimetry studies, for instance, have shown that ambient environmental contaminant data explain only 2%–25% of personal exposures for most toxic and carcinogenic VOCs and pesticides (Wallace, 1993).

Environmental Contaminant Level and Internal Dose Estimation
Methods for assessing environmental exposures of children and parents range from simple questionnaires to personal monitoring devices and lab-

oratory analyses of contaminants in blood and other biologic samples. Potential methods and information sources include:

Environmental contaminant levels
- Administrative records
  - Occupation—exposure information on workplace records may be limited to job title but may include environmental exposure levels, for example, for persons exposed to airborne toxicants in underground mines.
  - Air and water quality—government agencies may collect data on air and water quality; such data are generally limited to larger population centers even in economically advantaged countries.
- Self-reported information
  - Young children—information may be collected from parents with the aid of standardized questions on parental, child, and home characteristics; in panel studies, parents may keep daily diaries of children's activities.
  - Older children—these children may complete questionnaires and/or keep a daily diary of activities.
- Contaminant measurements
  - Environmental contaminants may be measured in samples of media including air, water, house dust, soil, and food, such as, house dust mite antigens in dust samples from a child's mattress.
  - Personal sampling—children may be monitored using devices attached to the clothing to measure air contaminant levels, magnetic field strength, and ultraviolet light intensity as the child moves through various microenvironments over the course of a few hours, a day, or several days.
- Models
  - Environmental contaminant levels may be estimated by modeling of contaminant emission data and supplementary information.
  - Internal doses may be estimated by modeling of data on contaminant levels in environmental media, consumption rates (air, water, food, soil, dust), and activity patterns (e.g., percentage of time spent indoors).

Biomonitoring. Biomarkers of internal doses include contaminant levels (e.g., heavy metals, dioxins, PCBs) in blood, breast milk, urine, hair, tissue, or other samples from children and/or their mothers. Certain molecular or cellular effects of toxicants are proxies for the internal dose, such as, 4-aminodiphenyl hemoglobin adducts (tobacco smoke) and persistent chromosome translocations in peripheral lymphocytes (ionizing

radiation). For infants and young children, in particular, minimally invasive samples and microanalytic techniques are essential (e.g., to enable
multiple contaminant analyses on finger prick or heel prick blood samples). Biomarkers of exposure and susceptibility will become more important in epidemiologic studies to the extent that they represent the biologically relevant dose and reduce misclassification of exposure status.
At present, however, many biomarkers reflect only recent exposures (e.g.,
urinary levels of organophosphate insecticide metabolites), a serious limitation for investigation of health outcomes with latent periods substantially longer than the tissue half-life of the toxicant(s) of interest.

Study Power

Power, defined as the likelihood that an epidemiologic study will demonstrate an association if one exists, depends on several factors including
the strength of the association, the observed number of health outcomes,
and the range and distribution of exposures in the study sample (Prentice and Thomas, 1993). Inadequate power is a major source of inconsistency between epidemiologic studies, especially when point estimates of
risk are compared. Random exposure measurement error and low exposure levels can greatly reduce study power. Differences between studies
in distribution of exposure levels can outweigh other factors as a cause
of heterogeneous effect measures of the same association; small studies
with high exposures may be more powerful than larger studies with lower
exposures (Hertz-Picciotto and Neutra, 1994).

Interactions between environmental and other factors are potentially
of great public health importance, but the power of epidemiologic studies to detect interactions is generally an order of magnitude less than their
power to detect main effects (Greenland, 1993). Constraints related to
power are not limited to epidemiologic studies; animal experiments compensate for small sample sizes by exposing animals to very high doses of
toxicants, raising uncertainty about exposure–risk relationships at low
doses. For a more complete coverage of design issues, the reader is referred to other sources (Elwood, 1998; Gordis, 2000; Rothman and Greenland, 1998).

STUDY TYPES

Research on environmental threats to child health has included case reports and ecologic, cross-sectional, case-control, cohort, and experimental epidemiologic studies.

Descriptive Studies

Descriptive epidemiologic studies illustrate the population-based variation in the risk of health outcomes by person, place, and time by generating age-specific and age-standardized incidence, prevalence, or mortality rates by sex, health outcome, geographic area, and time period. When the number of health outcome events in the study population is small, analyses may include indirect age-standardized ratios of observed to expected events. Descriptive data serve to (1) assess needs for and progress in disease prevention and control, (2) generate etiologic hypotheses, (3) assess time trends, (4) identify emerging health problems, (5) raise awareness of the burden of various health conditions, and (6) provide a baseline for forecasting future disease burdens.

Many governmental and voluntary agencies produce and disseminate the results of descriptive studies and promote their use in development and evaluation of disease prevention and control policies and programs. For examples, the reader can access websites for surveillance of birth defects (International Clearinghouse for Birth Defects 2002) and cancer (American Cancer Society 2002; Health Canada 2002). Other sources for additional details on descriptive epidemiologic studies include Stroup and Teutsch (1998) and Teutsch and Churchill (2000).

Acute effects such as pesticide poisonings may be attributed to a causal agent based on well-documented physician reports of one or a few cases. Children poisoned by organophosphate or carbamate insecticides, for instance, can be diagnosed through clinical signs and symptoms and reduced plasma butyrylcholinesterase or red blood cell acetylcholinesterase levels. Systematic reporting of such events through surveillance systems serves to assess preventive programs.

Although case reports alone rarely provide evidence of cause–effect relationships for delayed health effects, they are valuable for generating hypotheses and stimulating investigations that are more definitive. The causal role of soot in scrotal cancer among young chimney sweeps was suspected 150 years before the identification of benzo(a)pyrene and other carcinogens in soot (Pott, 1775). During the late nineteenth century, a physician attributed childhood lead poisoning cases to hand–mouth behavior and residence in homes with lead-based paint (Gibson, 1892).

Cluster Investigation

A *cluster* is defined as an aggregation of relatively uncommon events in space and/or time in amounts believed or perceived to be greater than expected by chance. Generally, a cluster is reported to public health authorities when concerned persons perceive an apparently excessive incidence of conditions such as birth defects or childhood cancer in their residential area. There have been many reported clusters of childhood leukemia with hypothesized links to environmental hazards including ionizing radiation and hazardous waste sites. The Centers for Disease Control and Prevention (CDC) investigated 108 cancer clusters between 1961 and 1990 and did not find a clear cause for any of them (Caldwell, 1990). Although the likelihood of identifying a causal agent from investigation of a cluster is very low, timely investigation helps to reassure the public that reasonable measures have been taken to detect potential causes. Investigators generally confront a poorly defined base population from which the cases arose, however, increasing the chance of overestimating the disease rate through *boundary shrinkage* (Olsen et al., 1996). There is also potential for recall bias related to heightened awareness of potential causes among case families.

Proposed criteria for identifying clusters where investigation is more likely to be fruitful include (Neutra, 1990)

- Cases—there are at least five cases of a disease that has known causes, or the cluster is an acute condition or an endemic condition (i.e., persistent high occurrence).
- Exposure—the suspected causal agent persists in the environment or in vivo and can be measured, exposure levels vary in the target population or there is the potential to study several exposed and unexposed communities, people can recall their exposure accurately, or it can be reconstructed from records
- Other—high relative risk exists, and obvious artifacts have been eliminated.

In view of the low likelihood of detecting causes of clusters and limited public health resources, the CDC recommended a four-phase approach comprising the initial response, assessment, a major feasibility study, and an etiologic investigation (Centers for Disease Control and Prevention, 1990). The protocol includes communications with regional authorities and the public, study design and methods, criteria for confirmed and probable cases, questionnaires for systematic information collection, specified samples and laboratory tests for diagnostic and exposure indicators, and report format.

The first evidence of the extreme toxicity of in utero methylmercury exposure to the developing fetus came from an investigation of a cluster of a strange polio-like disease among inhabitants of Minimata, a small fishing village in Japan; ultimately, over 2000 patients were diagnosed including 40 infants who generally appeared normal at birth but exhibited severe neurotoxicity within a few months. This and related events are described in more detail in Chapter 5 (Metals—Mercury, Arsenic, Cadmium, and Manganese).

Ecologic Studies

In pure ecologic studies, the unit of observation is a group of people and analyses assess the relation between group exposures (e.g., an average level or prevalence rate of a given factor) and health outcomes (e.g., a disease incidence or mortality rate) (Morgenstern and Thomas, 1993). Because this design does not capture information on exposures and health outcomes at the individual level, there are major uncertainties in the interpretation of risk estimates (see below). Further discussion uses a recent categorization of ecologic studies (Rothman and Greenland, 1998).

Multiple-Group Designs

Exploratory study: compares disease rates among population subgroups during the same time period, without measurement of environmental exposures at the individual or group level; analyses assess the degree of spatial autocorrelation or clustering suggestive of environmental effects.

Analytic study: assesses the association between average exposure levels and disease rates among multiple population subgroups; analyses include ordinary least squares and linear or exponential relative rate models.

Time-Trend Designs

Exploratory study: compares disease rates over time in a defined population and may be used to forecast future trends; analyses range from simple graphical displays to autoregressive integrated moving averages (ARIMA) and age-period-cohort models.

Analytic study: assesses the association between average exposure levels and disease rates over time; analyses are as noted above.

Mixed Designs

Exploratory study. This study combines multiple-group and time-trend features; analyses include ARIMA and age-period-cohort models.

Analytic study. This study examines the association between differences in average exposure levels and disease rates over time and between multiple population subgroups.

Reasons for choosing an ecologic study design include low cost, convenience, impracticality of measuring individual exposures for many individuals, uniform exposures within regions necessitating comparison of several regions, and simplicity of analyses and presentation (Rothman and Greenland, 1998). Ecologic studies generally take advantage of routinely available information and provide relatively rapid results that may justify more definitive investigations. Because they are based on information about groups, privacy and confidentiality issues are minimal or nonexistent. Ecologic studies are appropriate for assessing the association between relatively rapid changes in illness rates and average exposure levels, such as daily emergency room visits for asthma and daily (or more frequent) air pollution levels, applying variable lag periods to allow time for adverse health outcomes to occur.

The major weakness of ecologic studies is their reliance on data for groups rather than individuals; associations between exposures and health outcomes at the group level may not reflect those at the individual level (Morgenstern, 1982; Morgenstern and Thomas, 1993). Given the absence of information on disease risks among exposed and unexposed individuals, such studies cannot directly estimate exposure effects. This weakness is exacerbated when the disease of interest occurs only after long or highly variable latent periods; under such conditions, a time-trend analytic study assesses disease rates for a population of constantly changing individuals as persons enter or leave the base population over time. Ecologic studies are also subject to biases related to confounder misclassification, multicolinearity of risk factors, and temporal ambiguity of cause and effect. See other sources for more detailed discussion of these and other limitations of ecologic studies (Morgenstern and Thomas, 1993).

Examples
- A multiple-group analytic study in Sweden revealed a substantially higher risk of acute lymphatic leukemia among children living in areas with medium or high average radon levels (Kohli et al., 2000)
- A time-trend analytic study showed that daily hospital admissions of infants for respiratory diseases during the summer high-ozone season were associated with daily 1-hour maximum ozone levels independent of other ambient air pollutants and climatic conditions (Burnett et al., 2001)

Hypothesis-Testing Studies

Cross-Sectional Studies
A cross-sectional study for investigating disease etiology generally surveys a population (or a sample of a population) at a point in time and

captures exposure information using standardized questionnaires, sometimes supplemented by other measures (physical examination, functional tests, collection and analysis of blood, urine, or other biologic samples). Certain demographic characteristics (e.g., age, sex, ethnicity, education), environmental exposures (e.g., presence of pets or smokers in the home), and health outcomes (e.g., physician-diagnosed childhood asthma) can be assessed reliably using self- or parent-administered questionnaires, enabling the use of large sample sizes at relatively low cost. National health surveys conducted for general health planning and policy purposes have been used occasionally to capture environment-related exposure and health outcome information; as documented below and in later chapters, NHANES is a noteworthy example.

Although such studies can identify the prevalent cases in a population at a given point in time, they cannot identify the base population from which the cases arose. Studies of health conditions with long latent periods that only collect point-in-time information are prone to temporal ambiguity, that is, current exposures may not reflect those during the etiologically relevant period. Parents of an asthmatic child, for example, may have modified their smoking habits, pet ownership status, or home environment since onset of the disease. Cross-sectional studies are also subject to length-biased sampling, that is, overrepresentation of cases with long-duration diseases and underrepresentation of those with short-duration diseases. Nevertheless, cross-sectional studies that collect accurate information on exposures during etiologically relevant time periods can provide valid exposure-specific risk estimates.

Examples. A cross-sectional study of children provided the first strong evidence of neurotoxicity from moderate lead exposure of children. Lead levels in tooth dentine were measured; these reflect cumulated lead exposure since birth, thus avoiding the need to rely on current exposure status or recall of past exposures (Needleman et al., 1979). The NHANES has been used repeatedly to assess important child health and environmental issues including

- Blood lead levels in relation to declining use of leaded gasoline in the late 1970s (Annest et al., 1983), long-term blood lead concentration trends (Centers for Disease Control and Prevention, 2000), and the relation between lead exposure and cognitive function (Lanphear et al., 2000)
- Lung function and outdoor air pollution (Schwartz, 1989)
- Risk factors for childhood asthma (Lanphear et al., 2001)

Case-Control Studies

Well-conducted population-based case-control studies are generally relatively inexpensive, produce reasonable risk estimates, are very appropriate for identification of environmental or other hazards, and are often the only practical design for investigation of rare diseases such as childhood cancer or the less common birth defects. Case-control studies generally include samples of cases (persons with a specific health condition) and controls (healthy persons or persons with other health conditions believed to be unrelated to the exposure of interest). Increasingly, researchers try to recruit samples representative of a defined population, usually defined by geographic area of residence; this is not always possible, and some studies use other samples (e.g., hospital-based). Most studies of childhood cancer have recruited newly diagnosed (i.e., incident) cases, while investigations of birth defects and asthma have usually included prevalent cases.

Selection of controls representative of the base population from which the cases developed is a major challenge. Equally demanding is the collection of unbiased retrospective exposure information, especially for delayed health outcomes; cases and controls may differentially recall their exposures. Similar to cross-sectional studies, case-control investigations of prevalent cases may identify associations with factors that influence survival or severity rather than etiology. Unless the sampling fractions are known (as in nested case-control studies), case-control assessments can estimate relative risk but not absolute risk among exposed subjects. Case-control studies are inefficient for studies of rare exposures unless they are conducted within a high-exposure cohort. See other sources for further information about case-control studies (Gordis, 2000; Rothman and Greenland, 1998).

Examples. The role of environmental factors in spontaneous abortion, stillbirths, birth defects, SIDS, childhood cancer, and other health outcomes has been assessed in numerous case-control studies. For instance:

- A nested case-control study of childhood cancer within a cohort of over 32,000 twins born in Connecticut during 1930–1969 demonstrated an association between leukemia and in utero exposure to X-rays (Harvey et al., 1985)
- The Baltimore-Washington Infant Study showed that a specific congenital heart defect (transposition of the great arteries) was associated with maternal first trimester exposure to pesticides (Loffredo et al., 2001)

Cohort Studies

A cohort study generally begins with a group of healthy persons with heterogeneous exposures, or with two or more groups of healthy persons with contrasting exposures, and follows them over time to detect adverse health outcomes. Information may be collected prospectively, retrospectively, or both. In countries with computerized population-based health care and/or vital statistics records, follow-up of cohorts may be achieved through computerized record linkage (see, e.g., Fair et al., 2000). Cohort studies have several strengths including:

- Avoidance of temporal ambiguity, that is, virtual certainty that exposure precedes the health outcome of interest
- Lack of selection bias related to disease status, that is, subjects are recruited while healthy
- Ability to assess the relation between exposures of interest and multiple health outcomes including specific diseases and overall survival
- Ability to assess risks of rare exposures, such as the future risk of adult cancers among a cohort of children exposed to high-dose ionizing radiation

Potential weaknesses of cohort studies include loss of subjects during follow-up (if substantial, this can cause loss of statistical power and introduction of bias), inefficiency for investigation of rare health outcomes, reliance on baseline exposure assessment, and high cost. Exposure status may change for persons followed for long periods to detect delayed health effects; in principle, this problem can be addressed by repeat exposure assessments, but prospective cohorts are generally expensive, especially if they require large samples and extensive exposure measurements.

Examples
- A record-based cohort study of over 140,000 births showed that women who consumed chlorinated dark water had a twofold increased risk of giving birth to children with urinary tract defects (note: certain dark surface waters are high in humic acids and generate high levels of chlorinated by-products when chlorinated) (Magnus et al., 1999)
- A longitudinal study of over 7000 pregnancies showed an association between paternal gonadal exposure to diagnostic X-rays during the year before conception and reduced birth weight, independent of maternal smoking and other potential confounders (Shea and Little, 1997)

Experimental Studies
The simplest experimental study design involves random assignment of individuals or groups to receive or not receive an intervention and follow-up to detect health outcomes. Children are unable to give informed consent, and their participation in experimental studies is almost always limited to potentially beneficial interventions. Older children have occa-

sionally been included in experimental studies of air pollutants, for example, to test the effect of short controlled exposures to ozone on respiratory function and symptoms. The main advantage of experiments is the greatly increased chance that observed differences between subjects exposed or not exposed to the intervention are not caused by unknown or uncontrolled confounders. The relatively high cost of most experimental intervention studies usually limits them to relatively small samples sizes and limited statistical power. Randomization at the group level reduces statistical power and precision because of within-group dependence of the outcome variable (Donner et al., 1981). Nonrandom loss of subjects to follow-up can introduce bias, and noncompliance with the intervention can cause underestimation of the true effect.

Examples. Examples of the relatively few experimental studies that have been done include field trials of sunscreen use to prevent benign nevi in children (Gallagher et al., 2000), house dust mite antigen reduction to reduce childhood asthma severity (Weeks et al., 1995), and house dust control to reduce childhood lead levels (Lanphear et al., 1996).

CONCLUSION

Epidemiologic studies provide valuable information on the relationships between environmental exposures and the risk of adverse health outcomes in humans under real-life conditions. They have identified adverse health effects during gestation, childhood, and adulthood arising from early life exposure to diverse environmental toxicants including ionizing radiation, lead, methylmercury, PCBs, ETS, and outdoor air pollutants. In addition, epidemiologic studies have revealed limited evidence of health effects from environmental factors including pesticides, chlorinated disinfection by-products in drinking water, and extremely low frequency electromagnetic fields. Their major limitation is their post hoc nature, that is, they can detect hazards only after humans have been exposed and developed adverse health effects. Proposed criteria for selecting epidemiologic studies appropriate for quantitative risk assessments are shown in Table 2–1 (Hertz-Picciotto, 1995). Epidemiologic studies of many children's environmental health issues conducted to date failed to satisfy all five criteria because:

• Most children have low exposures to many environmental contaminants; any associations with adverse health effects are likely to be weak unless sufficient numbers of children across a range of exposures are available to assess dose–response relationships.

TABLE 2–1. Criteria for Selecting Epidemiologic Studies for Risk Assessments

Criteria	Necessity of Criterion Being Met To:		
	Serve as a Basis for Dose–Response Extrapolation	Check Plausibility of an Animal-Based Risk Assessment	Contribute to the Weight of Evidence for a Suspected Health Hazard
1. Moderate to strong positive association	Necessary	Not necessary; often this criterion is not met	If met, adds to weight of evidence for a hazard
2. Strong biases ruled out or unlikely	Necessary	Should be met, at least partially	If met, strengthens evidence that agent is or is not a hazard
3. Confounding controlled, or likely to be limited	Necessary	Should be met, at least partially, or limits on confounding should be estimated	If met, strengthens evidence that agent is or is not a hazard
4. Quantification of exposures linked to individuals	Necessary	Some quantification of exposures is needed, even if based on data external to study site	Usually not met
5. Montonic dose–response relationship	Not necessary but adds certainty to risk estimates	Not necessary	May or may not be met
Summary of requirements	Criteria 1–4 should be met	Two of criteria 1–3 should be met	All other studies

Source: Hertz-Picciotto (1995).

- Quantification of environmental exposures is generally difficult, especially when only individual recall information is available; even if appropriate exposure biomarkers exist, there may be problems including access to adequate biologic specimens (e.g., blood), reliance on indices that can only measure recent exposures (e.g., organophosphate pesticide metabolites in urine), and the high cost of laboratory analyses.
- Monotonic dose–response relationships are more likely to be observed when the true association is moderate or strong and in studies with good exposure data and power; these conditions have been met in some but not most epidemiologic studies.

REFERENCES

American Cancer Society. (2002). Facts and figures 2002. Located at http://www.cancer.org

Annest JL, Pirkle JL, Makuc D, Neese JW, Bayse DD, Kovar MG. (1983). Chronological trend in blood lead levels between 1976 and 1980. N Engl J Med 308: 1373–7.

Burnett RT, Smith-Doiron M, Stieb D, Raizenne ME, Brook JR, Dales RE, Leech JA, Cakmak S, Krewski D. (2001). Association between ozone and hospitalization for acute respiratory diseases in children less than 2 years of age. Am J Epidemiol 153:444–52.

Caldwell GG. (1990). Twenty-two years of cancer cluster investigations at the Centers for Disease Control. Am J Epidemiol 132:S43–7.

Centers for Disease Control and Prevention. (1990). Guidelines for investigating clusters of health events. MMWR 39:1–23.

Centers for Disease Control and Prevention. (2000). Blood lead levels in young children—United States and selected states, 1996–1999. MMWR 49:1133–7.

Donner A, Birkett N, Buck C. (1981). Randomization by cluster. Sample size requirements and analysis. Am J Epidemiol 114:906–14.

Elwood JM. (1998). Critical appraisal of epidemiological studies and clinical trials. New York: Oxford University Press.

Fair M, Cyr M, Allen AC, Wen SW, Guyon G, MacDonald RC. (2000). An assessment of the validity of a computer system for probabilistic record linkage of birth and infant death records in Canada. The Fetal and Infant Health Study Group. Chronic Dis Can 21:8–13.

Gallagher RP, Rivers JK, Lee TK, Bajdik CD, McLean DI, Coldman AJ. (2000). Broad-spectrum sunscreen use and the development of new nevi in white children: A randomized controlled trial. JAMA 283:2955–60.

Gibson JL. (1892). Notes on lead-poisoning as observed among children in Brisbane. Proc Intercolonial Med Congr Aust 3:76–83.

Gordis L. (2000). Epidemiology. Philadelphia: W.B. Saunders Company.

Greenland S. (1980). The effect of misclassification in the presence of covariates. Am J Epidemiol 112:564–9.

Greenland S. (1993). Basic problems in interaction assessment. Environ Health Perspect 101(Suppl 4):59–66.

Harvey EB, Boice JD, Honeyman M, Flannery JT. (1985). Prenatal x-ray exposure and childhood cancer in twins. N Engl J Med 312:541–5.

Hatch M, Thomas D. 1993. Measurement issues in environmental epidemiology. Environ Health Perspect 101(Suppl 4):49–57.

Health Canada. (2002). Cancer surveillance on-line. Located at http://cythera. ic.gc.ca/dsol/cancer/.

Hertz-Picciotto I. (1995). Epidemiology and quantitative risk assessment: a bridge from science to policy. Am J Public Health 85:484–91.

Hertz-Picciotto I, Neutra RR. (1994). Resolving discrepancies among studies: the influence of dose on effect size. Epidemiology 5:156–63.

Infante-Rivard C, Jacques L. (2000). Empirical study of parental recall bias. Am J Epidemiol 152:480–6.

International Clearinghouse for Birth Defects. (2002). International Clearinghouse for Birth Defect monitoring systems. Located at http://www.icbd.org/index.html.

Kohli S, Noorlind Brage H, Lofman O. (2000). Childhood leukaemia in areas with different radon levels: a spatial and temporal analysis using GIS. J Epidemiol Commun Health 54:822–6.

Lanphear BP, Aligne CA, Auinger P, Weitzman M, Byrd RS. (2001). Residential exposures associated with asthma in US children. Pediatrics 107:505–11.

Lanphear BP, Dietrich K, Auinger P, Cox C. (2000). Cognitive deficits associated with blood lead concentrations <10 microg/dL in U.S. children and adolescents. Public Health Rep 115:521–9.

Lanphear BP, Winter NL, Apetz L, Eberly S, Weitzman M. (1996). A randomized trial of the effect of dust control on children's blood lead levels. Pediatrics 98:35–40.

Loffredo CA, Silbergeld EK, Ferencz C, Zhang J. (2001). Association of transposition of the great arteries in infants with maternal exposures to herbicides and rodenticides. Am J Epidemiol 153:529–36.

Magnus P, Jaakkola JJ, Skrondal A, Alexander J, Becher G, Krogh T, Dybing E. (1999). Water chlorination and birth defects. Epidemiology 10:513–7.

Morgenstern H. (1982). Uses of ecologic analysis in epidemiologic research. Am J Public Health 72:1336–44.

Morgenstern H, Thomas D. (1993). Principles of study design in environmental epidemiology. Environ Health Perspect 101(Suppl 4):23–38.

Needleman HL, Gunnoe C, Leviton A, Reed R, Peresie H, Maher C, Barrett P. (1979). Deficits in psychologic and classroom performance of children with elevated dentine lead levels. N Engl J Med 300:689–95.

Neutra RR. (1990). Counterpoint from a cluster buster. Am J Epidemiol 132:1–8.

Olsen SF, Martuzzi M, Elliott P. (1996). Cluster analysis and disease mapping— why, when, and how? A step by step guide. BMJ 313:863–6.

Pott P. (1775). Cancer scroti. In Chirurgical observations relative to the cataract, the polypus of the nose, the cancer of the scrotum, the different kinds of ruptures, and the mortification of the toes and feet, pp. 63–68. London: T.J. Carnegy.

Prentice RL, Thomas D. (1993). Methodologic research needs in environmental epidemiology: data analysis. Environ Health Perspect 101(Suppl 4):39–48.

Rothman KJ. (1993). Methodologic frontiers in environmental epidemiology. Environ Health Perspect 101(Suppl 4):19–21.

Rothman KJ. (2002). Epidemiology: an introduction. New York: Oxford University Press.

Rothman KJ, Greenland S. (1998). Modern epidemiology. Philadelphia: Lippincott-Raven.

Schwartz J. (1989). Lung function and chronic exposure to air pollution: a cross-sectional analysis of NHANES II. Environ Res 50:309–21.

Shea KM, Little RE. (1997). Is there an association between preconception paternal x-ray exposure and birth outcome? The ALSPAC Study Team. Avon Longitudinal Study of Pregnancy and Childhood. Am J Epidemiol 145:546–51.

Stroup DF, Teutsch SM. (1998). Statistics in public health: quantitative approaches to public health problems. New York: Oxford University Press.

Teutsch SM, Churchill RE. (2000). Principles and practice of public health surveillance. New York: Oxford University Press.

Wallace L. (1993). A decade of studies of human exposure: what have we learned? Risk Anal 13:135–9.

Weed DL, Coughlin SS. (1999). New ethics guidelines for epidemiology: background and rationale. Ann Epidemiol 9:277–80.

Weeks J, Oliver J, Birmingham K, Crewes A, Carswell F. (1995). A combined approach to reduce mite allergen in the bedroom. Clin Exp Allergy 25:1179–83.

3
Risk Assessment

Risk assessment has been described as a bridge between science and policy (Hertz-Picciotto, 1995). More formally, it is the use of a factual base to define the health effects of exposure of individuals or populations to hazardous materials and situations (National Academy of Sciences, 1983). The goal is to provide an evidence base for decisions on policies and programs to protect the public from identified health hazards. The process involves the synthesis of epidemiologic, toxicologic, and related research findings and judgments on causal relationships and exposure–risk relationships. This chapter discusses general issues related to hazard identification, dose–response assessment, and risk characterization. Topics include processes used by national and international agencies to identify causal relationships and health-protective exposure limits followed by discussion of key issues related to risk assessments of carcinogens, reproductive toxicants, developmental toxicants, and neurotoxins.

Risk Assessment Framework

The model most frequently used for quantitative risk assessment is that proposed by the U.S. National Academy of Sciences in its 1983 landmark report on risk assessment (National Academy of Sciences, 1983):

- Hazard identification—determination of whether a particular chemical is a causal factor[1] for particular health outcomes
- Dose–response assessment—quantification of the relationship between the dose (or exposure) and the probability of adverse health outcomes
- Exposure assessment—quantification of the extent of human exposure before or after application of regulatory controls
- Risk characterization—description of the nature and magnitude of the human risk including attendant uncertainty

The National Academy of Sciences report defined risk assessment as a scientific process distinct from socioeconomic and other political considerations. The sparseness and uncertainty of relevant scientific knowledge were the main problems identified for assessment. In a departure from that 1983 report, the recently revised U.S. risk assessment framework emphasized economic costs (The Presidential/Congressional Commission on Risk Assessment and Risk Management, 1997a, 1997b). It also recommended early and active stakeholder involvement, testing of chemical mixtures, inclusion of microbiologic and radiation hazards (in addition to chemicals), comparable risk metrics for carcinogens and other hazards, increased use of mode of action information, and realistic exposure scenarios. After comparing chemical risk assessment procedures, assumptions, and policies across four federal agencies, the U.S General Accounting Office concluded that incomplete scientific information on human health effects and exposure to hazards continues to be a major source of uncertainty (U.S. General Accounting Office, 2001).

Hazard Identification

Hazard identification is the determination of whether a particular agent is or is not causally linked to particular health effects (National Academy of Sciences, 1983). Toxicologic and epidemiologic studies provide essential information for hazard identification and dose–response assessment. Only animal studies can identify new hazards before human exposure occurs, and only epidemiologic studies can directly demonstrate human health risks related to existing environmental hazards.

Reasonable evidence of causality is a prerequisite for a meaningful risk assessment. In assessing the impact of tobacco use on human health, the 1964 U.S. Surgeon General's report grouped the available scientific evidence into two main categories (U.S. Surgeon General, 1964): (1) ex-

---

[1] A *causal factor* of an event has been defined as a factor whose operation increases the frequency of the event (Elwood, 1998).

perimental studies of animals exposed to tobacco smoke, tars, and specific chemical components—these showed that tobacco smoke contains several carcinogens, promoters, and toxic gases that cause adverse health effects in tissues and cells similar to those in heavy smokers—and (2) clinical and epidemiologic studies of humans—these demonstrated multiple pathologic effects in cells and tissues of smokers and strong associations between smoking and lung cancer, heart disease, emphysema, and several other diseases. The Surgeon General's report used the criteria illustrated below for lung cancer to evaluate the causal significance of associations between smoking and health effects:

- Consistency—all 36 reasonably designed epidemiologic studies found associations between smoking and lung cancer.
- Strength—the 16 studies that measured relative risk all found similar high values (9–10 for average smokers, 20 or higher for heavy smokers).
- Specificity—although smoking causes more than one adverse health outcome, tobacco smoke is a complex mixture capable of causing more than one disease and even single toxicants can cause multiple health effects.
- Temporal relationship—the reported age at onset of smoking occurred well before any detectable health effects.
- Coherence—a causal association was consistent with evidence of increasing lung cancer death rates, dose–response relations, anatomic site of cancer, and death rate differentials between men and women, urban and rural populations, and socioeconomic subgroups.

Hill (1965) concluded that none of the Surgeon General's criteria provide indisputable evidence for or against causality. The absence of appropriate temporality, however, would be strong evidence against causality, assuming no ambiguity about time relations (Rothman and Greenland, 1998). Hill stated that strong associations are more likely to be causal because a potential confounder would have to be even more closely associated with the health outcome and likely to be already evident. A strong association, however, is neither necessary nor sufficient to prove causality and only rules out modest effects from confounders or other sources of bias (Rothman and Greenland, 1998).

Studies may produce inconsistent evidence if some populations lack factors required for the effect of a putative causal factor; thus, one can assess consistency only when a causal mechanism is understood in detail. Other factors contributing to inconsistency include random variation in small-sample studies and measurement errors. Specificity is not a discriminating criterion; as stated succinctly elsewhere, "there is no biological justification for specificity and it is useless and misleading" (Rothman and Greenland, 1998).

Hill noted the importance of a monotonic dose–response relationship; this appears to be true for some hazards (e.g., genotoxic carcinogens), but others have apparent thresholds. Because biologic plausibility and coherence of evidence must be judged within the context of current knowledge, violation of these criteria may simply reflect knowledge gaps. Positive biologic plausibility—for example, evidence from experimental animal studies—may be supportive of causality, but negative experimental evidence can be misleading if it arises from a weak intervention or low statistical power. Given these limitations of causal criteria, researchers could adopt causal *values* to encourage debate on uncertainty and scientific values (Kaufman and Poole, 2000).

Dose–Response Assessment

This phase of risk assessment determines the relation between exposure magnitude and the probability of particular health effects using two main approaches, one for carcinogens and the other for noncarcinogens. The main difference is the default assumption for carcinogens of low-dose linearity with no threshold, compared to an assumption of low-dose nonlinearity with a threshold for noncarcinogens. Regulatory agencies have used lifetime excess cancer risks of 10^{-6} to 10^{-5} as minimal risk targets[2] in setting exposure limits for the general population to carcinogens and certain other toxicants with no apparent threshold. Dose–response relationships observed in animal or human subjects are generally based on exposures that cause far higher lifetime risks; for example, 50% or more of the animals in the highest dose category of carcinogenesis bioassays may develop cancer.

The challenge is to use observed dose–response data to estimate risks at exposures several orders of magnitude below the observed range. Ideally, epidemiologic estimates of disease incidence rates by sex, age, and exposure level should be available to support low-dose extrapolations and other risk estimates. Toxicants may have linear, sigmoidal, U-shaped, or inverted U-shaped dose–response relationships. If the observed data do not include the full range necessary to detect a true non-linear dose–response relationship, low-dose extrapolation could be quite misleading. Simulation modeling indicates that point estimates of low-dose risks may differ from the actual risks by three orders of magnitude or more, depending

---

[2]An excess risk of 10^{-6} means that among 1 million persons exposed for a lifetime at the exposure limit level, one extra cancer would occur.

on the statistical model used and the effects of competing risks, background response, latency, and experimental design (Krewski et al., 1983).

Exposure Assessment

This phase of risk assessment estimates the extent of human exposure under various intervention scenarios. Data on the prevalence of exposure by intensity, sex, and age (together with the related risk data mentioned above) greatly facilitate risk estimates for various exposure scenarios. The main environmental exposure indices are measures of environmental contaminant concentrations and internal dose levels. Population-based data on internal dose levels are rarely available and, in their absence, risk assessors often rely on modeled estimates dependent on external contaminant levels (air, water, food, and soil), human behavior (consumption data, activities), bioavailability, and route-specific absorption factors (inhalation, oral, dermal). Given the uncertainties surrounding these factors, recent efforts to develop population-based estimates of internal dose promise to provide more precise exposure estimates, at least for those hazards for which valid biomarkers of internal dose exist. Biomarkers of internal dose reflect exposures from all sources and pathways over times that vary by the in vivo half-lives of contaminants.

The 1996 Food Quality Protection Act (FQPA) mandated the U.S. EPA to consider aggregate risks (from total exposure to a single agent via multiple sources and pathways) and cumulative risks (from exposure to two or more distinct chemicals sharing a common mode of action) of pesticides. Aggregate risk assessment requires information on pesticide levels in all relevant environmental media, bioavailability, route-specific absorption factors, and human exposure factors (air, food, and water consumption) specific for sex and age. The CDC's recent biomonitoring activities have generated data on urinary organophosphate insecticide metabolite levels for children and adults (Centers for Disease Control and Prevention, 2001); this type of biomonitoring promises to improve exposure estimates used in risk assessments.

Risk Characterization

This phase of risk assessment describes the nature and magnitude of the risk to human health related to a particular hazard and the attendant uncertainties. Outputs include (1) an evaluation of the nature and magnitude of potential adverse health effects based on synthesis of information from hazard identification, dose–response assessment, and human exposure assessment, (2) quantitative estimates of exposures that cause minimal risk (for apparent nonthreshold toxicants) or exposures that likely cause no excess risk (for toxicants with apparent thresholds), and (3) a summary of the risk assessment process including reasons for selecting key studies, critical effects and their relevance to humans, limitations of available data, data gaps, areas of uncertainty, and level of scientific confidence in the risk assessment results.

Threshold Toxicants

The reference dose (RfD) or concentration (RfC) of a toxicant is the estimated amount that is assumed to be without an appreciable risk of noncancer adverse health outcomes over a lifetime of exposure (including the noncancer toxic effects of carcinogens such as arsenic). Derivation of a RfD or RfC includes

- Estimation of the no observed adverse effect level (NOAEL), the lowest observed adverse effect level (LOAEL), or the benchmark dose for the adverse health effect most sensitive to the toxicant of interest (or the most sensitive mammalian species)
- Division of the NOAEL, LOAEL, or benchmark dose by factors (often referred to as *uncertainty* or *safety factors*) of up to 10 each to compensate for the uncertainties discussed below

The National Academy of Sciences has identified five uncertainty and modifying factors for potential use in developmental risk assessments: (1) extrapolation from animals to humans, (2) human chronic exposures compared to subchronic exposures in animals, (3) variation in susceptibility within genetically diverse human populations, (4) incomplete toxicity databases, and (5) susceptibility of human developing systems (National Academy of Sciences, 2000). The last two criteria may be invoked for pesticides used on foods under the FQPA, that is, an additional factor of up to 10 may be applied if children are thought to have increased exposures or susceptibility or if supporting data are incomplete. The OECD concluded that the product of uncertainty factors would normally range from 100 to 500 for NOAELs for repeat dose toxicity and up to 5000 for severe or irreversible developmental effects that occur at exposure levels below those inducing well-defined parental toxicity.

Most RfDs and RfCs are based on studies of experimental animals or adult humans (Table 3–1). Uncertainty factors are substantially larger for assessments dependent on animal compared to human data (e.g., 10 for methylmercury based on developmental neurotoxicity in humans versus 1400 for tetrachloroethylene based on hepatotoxicity and weight gain in rats). The EPA has not developed an RfD for lead because of uncertainty

TABLE 3–1. Low-Dose Risk Estimates for Noncancer Health Effects from Chronic Exposure to Selected Toxicants

Substance	RfD or RfC[a]	Uncertainty Factor[b]	Critical Effect
Arsenic (inorganic)	3×10^{-4} mg/kg/day	3	Oral (water)—hyperpigmentation and keratosis of skin, possible vascular complications (humans)
Cadmium	5×10^{-4} mg/kg/day	10	Oral (water, food)—significant proteinuria (humans)
Mercury (elemental)	3×10^{-4} mg/m^3	30	Inhalation—hand tremor, memory disturbances, slight autonomic dysfunction (humans)
Methylmercury	1×10^{-4} mg/kg/day	10	Oral (food)—developmental neurotoxicity (humans)
Bromodichloromethane	0.02 mg/kg/day	1000	Oral (oral/gavage)—renal cytomegaly (mice)
Tetrachloroethylene	0.01 mg/kg/day	1000	Oral—hepatotoxicity in mice, weight gain in rats
PCBs (Arochlor-1016)	7×10^{-5} mg/kg/day	100	Oral—reduced birth weight (monkeys)
PCBs (Arochlor-1254)	2×10^{-5} mg/kg/day	300	Oral—inflamed Meibomian glands, distorted nails, decreased IgG and IgM response to sheep red blood cells (monkeys)
Alachlor	0.01 mg/kg/day	100	Oral—hemosiderosis, hemolytic anemia (dogs)
Chlorpyrifos	0.003 mg/kg/day	10	Oral—decreased plasma cholinesterase activity after 9 days (humans)
Permethrin	0.05 mg/kg/day	100	Oral—increased liver weights (rats)

Source: U.S. Environmental Protection Agency (2000b).

[a]RfD = mg/kg/day (diet) or mg/L (water); RfC = mg/m^3 (inhalation).

[b]NOAEL or LOAEL divided by RfD or RfC.

about a threshold for lead toxicity; evidence indicates effects on certain blood enzymes and auditory and cognitive functions at very low blood lead levels (see also Chapter 4, Lead).

Although the EPA has set a maximum contaminant level for dioxin in public drinking water of 3×10^{-8} mg/L, it recently concluded that dioxin is a human carcinogen and that current population exposure levels may increase the lifetime excess probability of cancer by up to 10^{-3} to 10^{-2} (U.S. Environmental Protection Agency, 2000a). Because this risk is much higher than that usually considered acceptable for general population exposure, the EPA did not recommend an RfD for dioxin (under its traditional approach, the EPA would have had to assign an RfD that is two to three orders of magnitude lower than current background exposure levels). A review panel has recommended that the EPA augment its RfDs and RfCs for chronic exposures with those for acute, short-term, and longer-term exposures to better address children and other sensitive subpopulations.

The U.S. Agency for Toxic Substances and Disease Registry (ATSDR) estimates virtually safe exposure limits for noncarcinogens by the process described above but refers to them as *minimal risk levels* (MRLs). The ATSDR uses MRLs as screening levels to identify hazardous waste site contaminants and potential health effects that may be of concern. Minimal risk levels have been derived for acute (<15 days), intermediate (15–364 days), and chronic (≥1 year) exposure durations and for oral and inhalation routes (see selected examples in Table 3–2). Comparison of Tables 3.1 and 3.2 indicates that the EPA and the ATSDR occasionally produce different risk levels for the same toxicant; for example, the EPA RfD for chronic oral exposure to cadmium is 5×10^{-4} mg/kg/day, while the ATSDR MRL for the same exposure is 2×10^{-4} mg/kg/day. Such differences may arise from reviews conducted at different times, that is, with differing sets of evidence. The ATSDR has defined an MRL of 10^{-9} mg/kg/day for chronic oral dioxin exposure based on neurotoxicity in monkeys.

The use of uncertainty factors is illustrated by the derivation of the EPA's RfD for methylmercury that was based on:

- A benchmark dose (BMD)[3] from two epidemiologic studies of neurologic abnormalities among prenatally exposed infants.

---

[3]A BMD may be defined as the dose (or its 95% lower confidence limit) of a toxicant that produces a specified increased incidence of a response, for example, 1% or 5% of the maximum toxic response, based on data within the observed dose range (International Programme on Chemical Safety, 1999).

TABLE 3–2. Minimum Risk Levels for Selected Toxicants by Duration of Exposure

Substance	Duration and Route	MRL	Uncertainty Factors	Health Effects
Arsenic	Acute oral	0.005 mg/kg/day	10	Gastrointestinal effects and facial edema (humans)
	Chronic oral	3×10^{-4} mg/kg/day	3	Hyperpigmentation and keratosis of skin (humans)
Benzene	Acute inhalation	0.05 ppm	300	LOAEL for immunologic effects (mice)
	Intermediate inhalation	0.004 ppm	90	LOAEL for neurologic effects (mice)
Cadmium	Chronic oral	2×10^{-4} mg/kg/day	10	Renal effects (humans)
Chlorpyrifos	Acute or intermediate oral	0.003 mg/kg/day	10	NOAEL for AChE inhibition in human adult males orally exposed to chlorpyrifos
	Chronic oral	0.001 mg/kg/day	100	NOAEL for AChE inhibition in orally exposed rats
Hexachlorobenzene	Acute oral	0.008 mg/kg/day	300	LOAEL for hyperactivity in offspring of prenatally exposed rats
	Intermediate oral	10^{-4} mg/kg/day	90	Degenerative changes in ovaries of orally exposed monkeys
	Chronic oral	2×10^{-5} mg/kg/day	1000	LOAEL for peribiliary lymphocytosis and fibrosis of the liver in orally exposed adult male rats
Mercury (elemental)	Chronic inhalation	2×10^{-4} mg/m^3	30	Hand tremor in industrially exposed men
Mercury (inorganic)	Acute oral	0.007 mg/kg/day	100	NOAEL for increased absolute and relative kidney weights in rats
	Intermediate oral	0.002 mg/kg/day	100	NOAEL for increased absolute and relative kidney weights in rats
Methylmercury	Chronic oral	3×10^{-4} mg/kg/day	4	Neurodevelopmental effects in Seychelles Islands children exposed to methylmercury from fish prenatally and postnatally
PCBs	Intermediate oral	3×10^{-5} mg/kg/day	300	LOAEL for neurobehavioral effects in infant monkeys exposed from birth to a PCB congener mixture similar to that in human breast milk
	Chronic oral	2×10^{-5} mg/kg/day	300	LOAEL for immunologic effects in adult monkeys exposed to Aroclor 1254
Dioxin (2,3,7,8-TCDD)	Acute oral	2×10^{-7} mg/kg/day	21	Reduced serum total hemolytic complement activity in mice
	Intermediate oral	2×10^{-8} mg/kg/day	30	Decreased thymus weight in guinea pigs
	Chronic oral	10^{-9} mg/kg/day	90	Altered social interactions in monkeys exposed perinatally

Source: (Agency for Toxic Substances and Disease Registry (2002).

- A threefold uncertainty factor for variable susceptibility in human populations. The EPA used this instead of a tenfold factor because the BMD was based on effects in a sensitive subpopulation: developing fetuses.
- A threefold uncertainty factor for missing data. There was no two-generation animal study, and there were no epidemiologic data on exposure duration in relation to developmental effects and adult peripheral neuropathy.

Nonthreshold Toxicants

There is no consensus on a method for risk assessment of chemicals suspected to have nonthreshold critical effects, such as genotoxic carcinogens and germ cell mutagens; existing approaches are based largely on characterization of dose–response relationships. For carcinogens, the EPA estimates unit risks and slope factors; see, for instance, those for arsenic, cadmium, and bromodichloromethane (Table 3–3). Note that the RfD for chronic oral exposure to bromodichloromethane is 20 μg/kg/day based on noncancer risks (Table 3–1). Based on a cancer slope factor of 6.2×10^{-5} per μg/kg/day in male mice (Table 3–3), chronic exposure at the RfD would cause an estimated lifetime excess cancer risk of $20 \times 6.2 \times 10^{-5}$ or about 1.2×10^{-3}; this is two to three orders of magnitude higher than the commonly used definitions of acceptable risk for the general population, but the RfD incorporates an uncertainty factor of 1000. See further discussion below under "Carcinogens."

Aggregate and Cumulative Risks

Methods for cumulative risk assessment of chemicals with a common mode of action include estimation of toxic equivalents or a combined margin of exposure index. These methods require toxicity data for multiple chemicals tested in the same animal species, and they assume that effects of each chemical are additive and have similar dose–response relationships. The toxic equivalents method has been widely applied to dioxins and related organochlorines that bind to the AhR receptor (see Chapter 6, PCBs, Dioxins, and Related Compounds). Potential problems in assessing aggregate or cumulative pesticide risks are illustrated by consideration of anticholinesterase (AchE) inhibitors (Wilkinson et al., 2000). In addition to organophosphorus and carbamate insecticides, many drugs and food constituents inhibit AChE to some degree. Aggregate or cumulative exposure estimates for AchE inhibitors would require many datasets that do not exist (not all AChE inhibitors have undergone toxicity testing, especially testing involving perinatal exposures) and numerous assumptions concerning dose–response relationships and additivity of effects. Even if modeling methods are developed, much research will be

TABLE 3–3. Low-Dose Risk Estimates for Cancer from Chronic Exposure to Selected Toxicants

	Cancer	Unit Risk[a]	Slope Factor[b]
Arsenic (inorganic)	Skin (humans exposed orally to water)	5×10^{-5} per $\mu g/L$ (water)	1.5×10^{-3} per $\mu g/kg/day$
Cadmium	Lung (men occupationally exposed by inhalation)	1.8×10^{-3} per $\mu g/m^3$ (air)	na
Bromodichloromethane	Kidney (orally exposed male mice)	1.8×10^{-6} per $\mu g/L$ (water)	6.2×10^{-5} per $\mu g/kg/day$

Source: U.S. Environmental Protection Agency (2000b).

[a]The upper-bound excess lifetime cancer risk from continuous exposure to an agent at 1 $\mu g/L$ in water or 1 $\mu g/m^3$ in air; for example, if the unit risk = 1.5×10^{-6} $\mu g/L$, up to 1.5 excess tumors are expected to develop per 1 million people exposed for a lifetime to the chemical at a level of 1 $\mu g/L$ in water or 1 $\mu g/m^3$ in air.

[b]Upper 95% confidence limit on excess cancer risk from lifetime exposure to an agent, usually expressed as a proportion of a population affected per mg/kg/day; generally reserved for use in the low-dose region, that is, exposures corresponding to risks less than 1 in 100.

needed to generate the data needed to test model assumptions and support aggregate and cumulative risk assessments.

SELECTED RISK ASSESSMENT PRACTICES

This section addresses those aspects of selected risk assessments that relate to child health protection. Approaches to assigning level of evidence for carcinogenicity are particularly well developed and are discussed in some depth.

Carcinogens

Hazard Identification
This section describes identification of carcinogens by the World Health Organization's International Agency for Research on Cancer (IARC) and variations adopted by the U.S. EPA. To evaluate a given substance, the IARC convenes an expert panel to assess the quality of relevant toxicologic and epidemiologic studies using standardized criteria. After assessing and summarizing the quality and results of studies, IARC panels judge the weight of evidence that the agent in question is carcinogenic for humans using these criteria:

- Strength of association—although moderate associations do not imply lack of causality, stronger associations are more likely to indicate causality.
- Consistency—associations replicated using different study designs and under different circumstances of exposure are more likely to represent a causal relationship than findings from single studies.
- Dose–response relationship—a monotonic increase in the cancer risk with increasing exposure is considered a strong indication of causality; a decline in risk after cessation of exposure also suggests causality.
- Specificity—increased risk of a specific anatomic and/or histologic type of cancer supports causality, especially if limited to one histologic type within the same organ.

Based on the above considerations, the panel decides the level of evidence of carcinogenicity for humans and experimental animals (Table 3–4). Finally, the panel assesses the weight of evidence to decide the likelihood that an agent is a human carcinogen (Table 3–5). The IARC and the EPA have independently assessed the carcinogenicity of many substances; most differences in ratings relate to designation of probable human carcinogens. With few exceptions, the EPA requires sufficient evidence in an-

TABLE 3–4. Level of Evidence of Carcinogenicity in Humans and Animals

Level of Evidence	Epidemiologic Evidence	Animal Study Evidence
Sufficient	A positive relationship has been observed between the exposure and cancer in studies in which chance, bias, and confounding could be ruled out with reasonable confidence	Increased incidence of cancer or an appropriate combination of benign and malignant neoplasms in (1) two or more species of animals or (2) in two or more independent studies in one species; exceptionally, a single study in which malignancies occur with high incidence or unusual site/type of tumor, or early age at onset
Limited	A positive association has been observed between exposure and cancer for which a causal interpretation is considered to be credible, but chance, bias, or confounding could not be ruled out with reasonable confidence	Evidence is restricted to a single experiment, unresolved questions regarding the design, conduct, or interpretation of the study, or only benign neoplasms or lesions of uncertain neoplastic potential or neoplasms that commonly occur spontaneously
Inadequate	Available studies are of insufficient quality, consistency, or statistical power to decide the presence or absence of a causal association, or no data on cancer in humans are available	Available studies have major qualitative or quantitative limitations, or no data on cancer in experimental animals are available
Evidence suggesting lack of carcinogenicity	Several adequate studies covering the full range of known human exposure levels consistently do not show an increased risk of cancer at any exposure level; the studies should be methodologically sound and yield a pooled risk estimate near unity with a narrow confidence interval; no individual study nor the pooled results should show any sign of a dose–response relationship; this decision applies only to the tumor sites and levels of exposure studied	Adequate studies involving at least two species are available that show no evidence of carcinogenicity; this applies only to the species, tumor sites, and levels of exposure studied

Source: International Agency for Research on Cancer (1999).

Note: The IARC and the EPA both consider other evidence including data on preneoplastic lesions, tumor pathology; genotoxicity; structure–activity relationships; metabolism, pharmacokinetics, physicochemical parameters, analogous biologic agents, and mechanisms of carcinogenesis.

TABLE 3–5. Categorization of Overall Weight of Evidence for Human Carcinogenicity, IARC[a] and EPA[b]

Human Carcinogenicity	IARC	EPA
Human carcinogen	1. Sufficient evidence in humans or (occasionally) limited human and sufficient animal evidence plus strong evidence that carcinogenesis is mediated by a mechanism that also operates in humans	A. This group is used only when there is sufficient evidence from epidemiologic studies to support a causal association between exposure to the agents and cancer
Probable human carcinogen	2A. Limited human and sufficient animal evidence, or inadequate human and sufficient animal evidence plus strong evidence that carcinogenesis is mediated by a mechanism that also operates in humans, or (occasionally) limited human evidence	B1. Usually reserved for limited evidence of carcinogenicity from epidemiologic studies B2. Sufficient evidence from animal studies and inadequate or no evidence from epidemiologic studies
Possible human carcinogen	2B. Limited human and animal evidence, or inadequate human and sufficient animal evidence, or inadequate human, limited animal, and other supporting evidence	C. Limited evidence of carcinogenicity in animals and absent or inadequate human data; includes a variety of evidence such as a single well-conducted positive study, tumor responses of marginal statistical significance in studies having inadequate design or reporting, benign but not malignant tumors caused by a nonmutagen, and responses of marginal statistical significance in a tissue known to have a high or variable background rate
Not classifiable as to human carcinogenicity	3. Inadequate human and inadequate or limited animal evidence, or, inadequate human and sufficient animal evidence plus strong evidence that the mechanism of carcinogenicity in experimental animals does not operate in humans	D. Inadequate or no human and animal evidence
Evidence of non-carcinogenicity for humans	4. Evidence suggesting lack of carcinogenicity in humans and in animals, or (occasionally), inadequate human evidence but evidence suggesting lack of carcinogenicity in animals consistently and strongly supported by a broad range of other relevant data	E. No evidence of carcinogenicity in at least two adequate animal studies in different species or in both human and animal adequate studies; should not be interpreted as a definitive conclusion that the agent will not be a carcinogen under any circumstances

[a] Source: International Agency for Research on Cancer (1999).
[b] Source: U.S. Environmental Protection Agency (1986).

imals or limited human evidence, whereas the IARC requires both. Despite the uncertainties of cross-species extrapolations, the IARC concluded that "In the absence of adequate data on humans, it is biologically plausible and prudent to regard agents and mixtures for which there is sufficient evidence of carcinogenicity in experimental animals as if they presented a carcinogenic risk to humans" (International Agency for Research on Cancer, 1999). Agents identified as known or probable human carcinogens are candidates for the next steps of quantitative risk assessments.

Dose–Response and Exposure Assessment
Under its 1986 carcinogen risk assessment guideline, the EPA adopted the health protective position that, in the absence of knowledge of mode of action, a linear dose–response relationship should be assumed at exposure levels between zero and the lowest levels observed in human and animal studies. The guidelines indicated a preference for human dose–response data or, in their absence, data from animal species that respond most like humans.

The EPA recently adopted new carcinogen risk assessment guidelines (revised in 1999) but noted that they may be further revised, depending on evolving science or comments from peer reviewers, the public, or others; the guidelines include these specific provisions to better protect the fetus, infants, and children (U.S. Environmental Protection Agency, 1999, 2001): (1) risk assessors should evaluate the relevance and applicability to children of a postulated mode of action (e.g., based on age-related differences in uptake, metabolism, and excretion of an agent), (2) an RfD or RfC approach could be considered when there is sufficient evidence of a biologic threshold[4]; low-dose linearity, however, should be assumed for children if there is no strong evidence that children and adults are comparable with regard to a postulated mode of action, (3) the dose should be based on weight (not surface area)—this provides increased protection in extrapolations from animals to humans, and (4) dose–response assessment should include evaluation of risks by tumor type and the relevance of each tumor type to children and other sensitive subpopulations.

These provisions are justified by the known increased cancer risks of children after perinatal exposure to ionizing radiation and prenatal DES exposure. Supporting evidence comes from rodent studies showing that combined perinatal and adult carcinogen exposure often produces a higher tumor incidence and a shorter latent period than adult exposure alone.

---

[4]The EPA's Science Advisory Board recommended inclusion of criteria to evaluate if the evidence on mode of action is valid.

Risk Characterization

Risk characterization should summarize information from hazard identification, dose–response assessment, exposure assessment, and risk modeling. This includes toxicokinetics, genotoxicity, structure–activity relationships of chemicals and properties of microbial agents (e.g., genomic
integration) relevant to carcinogenicity, effects in model systems, and numerical risk estimates. The last, based on assumptions of low-dose linearity and constant lifetime exposure, should include (1) unit risk—the
excess lifetime cancer risk per unit dose of carcinogen, (2) dose at a given
risk level—carcinogen dose that corresponds to a given risk, and (3) population risk—the excess lifetime cancer risk at a specified carcinogen dose
in an exposed population.

   Important aspects of carcinogen risk characterization in the 1999 EPA
draft guidelines include the following:

- The assigned level of evidence should describe both the likelihood of
  human carcinogenicity and the conditions under which cancer risks
  would arise; for example, an agent could be rated as a likely carcinogen when inhaled but not when ingested.
- Increased weight should be given to an agent's properties, including mode
  of action and structure–activity relationships to known carcinogens.

These changes assume that increased knowledge of the mode of action at
cellular and subcellular levels, as well as toxicokinetic and metabolic processes, justifies inferences that go beyond available data on the relationships between exposures and risks of cancer in humans and animals. For
instance, it has been argued that chloroform is likely a threshold carcinogen; if this conclusion is accepted, the result could be less stringent
regulations for exposures related to occupation and drinking water.

Developmental Toxicants

Developmental toxicants are agents that cause preimplantation loss, early
fetal death (spontaneous abortion), late fetal death (stillbirth), impaired
growth, structural abnormalities (birth defects), and functional deficits
(e.g., mental retardation) (National Academy of Sciences, 2001). A wider
definition includes adverse effects detected at any point in the life span
of the organism caused by exposure of either parent (preconceptual), the
fetus (in utero), or the child until sexual maturity (International Programme on Chemical Safety, 2001; U.S. Environmental Protection Agency,
1991). About 3% of newborn infants have major developmental disorders
characterized as life-threatening, requiring major surgery, or presenting a
significant disability (National Academy of Sciences, 2000).

Epidemiologic studies have demonstrated associations and exposure–risk relationships between high-level exposures to environmental contaminants (e.g., methylmercury, PCBs contaminated by dioxins and furans, ionizing radiation) and adverse developmental effects. The proportions of adverse human developmental outcomes attributable to environmental hazards, however, are uncertain because of limited epidemiologic research in this field and the difficulty of demonstrating developmental effects of perinatal exposure at background contaminant levels. The fact that known human developmental toxicants generally cause similar effects in at least one experimental animal species tested indicates the relevance of animal models to human health. Experimental and epidemiologic studies have shown the importance of the timing of exposure during pregnancy; for example, exposure to toxicants during early gestation can cause birth defects.

The EPA guideline for developmental toxicity risk assessment provides for the use of available animal and human data and information from pharmacokinetic and structure–activity studies. The level of evidence is assessed using categories virtually identical to those shown in Table 3–6 for reproductive toxicity risk assessment (the difference being that minimum evidence of no hazard in animals requires data from studies in at least two species showing no developmental toxicity at doses that were minimally toxic to the adult). The assumption that a biologic

TABLE 3–6. EPA Categorization of Overall Weight of Evidence for Human Reproductive Hazards

Level of Evidence	Criteria
Sufficient human evidence of hazard	Convincing epidemiologic evidence; biologic plausibility
Sufficient animal and/or limited human evidence of hazard	Positive findings in animals in at least one well-executed study in one species (e.g., one that meets the EPA's guidelines for two-generation studies) and/or limited epidemiologic evidence
Insufficient evidence of hazard	Evidence ranges from nonexistent to animal or human studies that have a limited study design or conduct (e.g., low statistical power, limited array of adverse outcomes, inadequate dose selection or exposure information, uncontrolled confounders)
Sufficient evidence of no hazard	Minimum evidence of no hazard requires data on an adequate array of outcomes from more than one study with two species showing no adverse reproductive effects at doses that were minimally toxic; may be supplemented by human data showing no apparent hazard

Source: U.S. Environmental Protection Agency (1996).

dose–response threshold generally exists for developmental toxicants may not apply to all toxicants; for example, it may be appropriate to use a linear low-dose extrapolation for developmental toxicants that act through a genotoxic mechanism (Kimmel, 2001). Also, the spectrum of developmental abnormalities may vary with the dose because fetal death at high doses may preclude expression of effects seen at lower doses; this suggests that LOELSs from animal studies that do not include an adequate range of doses may be misleading.

Neurotoxins

Developmental neurotoxicity encompasses any adverse effects on nervous system structure or function caused by prenatal and early childhood exposure to a toxicant (Mileson and Ferenc, 2001). Potential developmental neurotoxic outcomes include adverse effects on autonomic, sensory, motor, and cognitive functions, social behaviors, and biologic rhythms; these effects may be accompanied by molecular and structural changes (Cory-Slechta et al., 2001). An estimated 3%–8% of liveborn infants have neurodevelopmental disabilities including dyslexia, ADHD, major cognitive deficits, and autism (U.S. Department of Health and Human Services, 1999; Weiss and Landrigan, 2000).

The nervous system differs from other organs and tissues by having the widest variety of specialized cell functions, a blood-brain barrier that modulates access of chemicals, and a severely limited ability to regenerate. The prefrontal cortex in humans has executive functions, including planning and control of impulses and emotions, and does not reach adult volume until about age 10 years; extensive remodeling of this region occurs during adolescence, including a 30%–40% reduction in synaptic density. Known developmental neurotoxins in humans and experimental animals include lead, methylmercury, ionizing radiation, and PCBs. Examples of nervous system developmental processes disrupted by one or more of these toxicants include differentiation, neuronal proliferation, neurotrophic signals, neuronal migration, synaptogenesis, gliogenesis and myelination, and apoptosis (Rice and Barone, 2000).

There are four approaches to detection of neurobehavioral effects in humans: clinical neurologic examination, self-report checklists, performance tests, and neuropsychologic tests. Performance and neuropsychologic test deficits may be detectable at exposure levels below the generally high levels required to cause clinically apparent signs. Performance tests have been developed to assess attention/vigilance, mathematical processing, verbal processing, spatial processing, memory, psychomotor skills (e.g., reaction time, manual dexterity), and multitasking. Performance tests and infants tests applied before age 1 year are markedly less affected by socioenvironmental influences than are IQ and school achievement tests. Standardized tests of neuropsychologic development during infancy, childhood, and adolescence include (Fiedler et al., 1996; Rice and Barone, 2000)

- Neonatal Behavioral Assessment Scale (NBAS)—tests young infants for neuromuscular and motor reflexes, muscle tone, activity level, reaction to sensory stimuli, and autonomic function. It is sensitive to effects of prenatal exposure to PCBs, opiates, and certain pharmaceuticals but is not predictive of neurobehavioral function during later childhood, and no norms exist.
- Bayley Scales of Infant Development—an apical test, that is, successful responses require the integrity of multiple elements of cognitive and fine motor function, attention to the task, and motivation to perform. The test is sensitive to the effects of prenatal exposure to alcohol, lead, PCBs, and methadone but is nonspecific (standardized norms are available).
- Fagan Test of Infant Intelligence (visual recognition memory test)— assesses the ability of infants to remember visual images and is moderately predictive of IQ measured later in childhood; it is sensitive to effects of prenatal exposure to PCBs, methylmercury, and alcohol.
- McCarthy Scales of Children's Abilities, Wechsler Preschool and Primary Scale of Intelligence—Revised, Wechsler Intelligence Scale for Children III, Stanford-Binet, and Kaufman Assessment Battery for Children—these tests assess older children's neurologic and cognitive development including psychomotor, memory, verbal, and perceptual functions. They are sensitive to the effects of perinatal exposure to lead, alcohol, and PCBs (standardized norms exist)

Until very recently, neurotoxicity testing required by regulatory agencies focused almost exclusively on obvious neurologic dysfunction in adult animals associated with general neuropathology, with little or no attention to neurobehavioral effects and developmental neurotoxicity. The EPA has obtained adequate developmental neurotoxicity testing data on only a few pesticides and industrial chemicals. Even for chemicals tested for neurotoxicity in adult animals, risk assessment is virtually limited to qualitative hazard identification and to the early stage of risk characterization because of insufficient data to support quantitative risk evaluations (Landrigan et al., 1994).

Problems arise in extrapolating the results of developmental neurotoxicity tests from animals to humans. The human brain has much more prenatal development than the rodent brain, important differences in the relative rates at which specific brain regions develop, a vastly larger and functionally more complex prefrontal cortex, and a much larger proportion of cortex devoted to vision including color discrimination, spatial resolution, and higher-order processing and integrating functions. The rodent brain devotes a much larger proportion of the cortex to olfactory functions.

Reproductive Toxicants

Reproductive toxicity includes adverse effects of substances on sexual maturation at puberty, gamete production and transport, the female reproductive cycle, sexual behavior, fertility, gestation, parturition, lactation, and reproductive senescence (International Programme on Chemical Safety, 2001; National Academy of Sciences, 2001). The EPA guideline for reproductive toxicity risk assessment specifies level of evidence categories to evaluate potential reproductive hazards (Table 3–6). Positive findings from a single study of high quality would generally provide sufficient animal evidence of reproductive hazard. Confidence in positive findings is increased if there is evidence of a dose–response relationship, biologic plausibility, consistent results from multiple studies, explanatory evidence for discordant results, appropriate exposures (route, level, duration, frequency), an adequate array of observed outcomes, and appropriate statistical power and analyses.

Although about 10% of human couples experience increased time to pregnancy or infertility, there has been relatively little epidemiologic research on early life environmental exposures and adverse reproductive effects. DES is the only known human reproductive toxicant that acts in utero. The few known environmental reproductive toxicants in humans were discovered from studies of occupationally exposed men and include lead, the pesticides 1,2-dibromo-3-chloropropane, chlordecone, and ethylene dibromide, and certain solvents (see later chapters for more details). Animal models may be insensitive indicators of hazards to human male fertility; the average number of sperm per ejaculate in human men is only about two to four times that associated with impaired fertility, while rodent sperm counts are up to 1000-fold those linked with maximum fertility. Nevertheless, existing evidence of hazards from perinatal exposures comes mainly from animal studies.

Reproductive toxicity dose–response assessments have generally used curve-fitting models that have biologic plausibility but do not incorporate the mode of action. The EPA guideline, however, calls for use of biologic information to assess the shape of the dose–response relationship below the observable range. For instance, a dose threshold for reproductive effects may be supported by evidence of host defense mechanisms such as the testicular Sertoli cell barrier. The RfDs or RfCs for reproductive toxicants are based on the NOAEL, LOAEL, or BMD for the adverse reproductive effect most sensitive to the toxicant of interest (or the most sensitive mammalian species) and application of uncertainty factors. The dose–response curves for the antiandrogenic effects from perinatal exposure of rodents to vinclozolin vary widely, with several showing antiandrogenic effects at doses well below the NOAEL observed in Tier I toxicity testing and no apparent threshold; such findings support alternatives to NOAELs such as a BMD.

CONCLUSION

The 1983 National Academy of Sciences report on risk assessment provided a useful framework for integrating toxicologic and epidemiologic data into quantitative estimates of human health risks at low exposure levels. Importantly, it recommended separating the scientific process of risk assessment from the political evaluation of its socioeconomic implications. The National Academy of Sciences report noted the pervasive uncertainties in risk assessments and attributed them mainly to knowledge gaps, a finding that remains true two decades later. There has been a tendency in recent years to include cost considerations in risk assessments and to give increased weight to the mode of action of toxicants, particularly carcinogens, as opposed to the results of animal bioassays. The 1983 report also stated that protection of public health would be better served if scientists improved their communication of risk assessment findings to decision makers and the public rather than factoring political considerations (such as costs) into risk assessments.

The four categories of risk assessment described in this chapter illustrate several issues and challenges: inadequate developmental toxicity and developmental neurotoxicity testing of commercial chemicals, uncertainties surrounding recommended exposure limits, and the important role of epidemiologic studies in carcinogen and neurotoxicity risk assessments but their weaker role in reproductive and developmental toxicity risk assessments (because of a dearth of epidemiologic research in the latter areas). These uncertainties argue for substantial strengthening of epidemiologic and toxicologic research, including postmarketing studies to ensure early detection of unexpected adverse health effects of existing and new products.

The reader is referred to further information on risk assessment from these national and international agencies:

- International Programme on Chemical Safety—established in 1980 by collaboration of the International Labour Office, the United Nations Environment Programme, and the World Health Organization to evaluate environmental chemical hazards to human health: http://www.who.int/pcs
- OECD. (2002). Located at http://www.oecd.org
- U.S. EPA: http://cfpub1.epa.gov/ncea/cfm/nceahome.cfm
- Agency for Toxic Substances and Disease Registry: http://www.atsdr.cdc.gov
- U.S. National Academy Press publications: http://www.nap.edu/

REFERENCES

Agency for Toxic Substances and Disease Registry. (2002). Minimal risk levels (MRLs) for hazardous substances. Located at http://www.atsdr.cdc.gov/mrls.html

Centers for Disease Control and Prevention. (2001). National report on human exposure to environmental chemicals. Atlanta: Centers for Disease Control and Prevention.

Cory-Slechta DA, Crofton KM, Foran JA, Ross JF, Sheets LP, Weiss B, Mileson B. (2001). Methods to identify and characterize developmental neurotoxicity for human health risk assessment. 1. Behavioral effects. Environ Health Perspect 109(Suppl 1):79–91.

Elwood JM. (1998). Critical appraisal of epidemiological studies and clinical trials. New York: Oxford University Press.

Fiedler N, Feldman RG, Jacobson J, Rahill A, Wetherell A. (1996). The assessment of neurobehavioral toxicity: SGOMSEC joint report. Environ Health Perspect 104(Suppl 2):179–91.

Hertz-Picciotto I. (1995). Epidemiology and quantitative risk assessment: a bridge from science to policy. Am J Public Health 85:484–91.

Hill AB. (1965). The environment and disease: association or causation? Proc R Soc Med 58:295–300.

International Agency for Research on Cancer. (1999). Preamble to the IARC monographs. Lyon: International Agency for Research on Cancer.

International Programme on Chemical Safety. (1999). Environmental health criteria 210: Principles for the assessment of risks to human health from exposure to chemicals. Geneva: International Programme on Chemical Safety.

International Programme on Chemical Safety. (2001). Environmental health criteria No. 225. Principles for evaluating health risks to reproduction associated with exposure to chemicals. Geneva: International Programme on Chemical Safety.

Kaufman JS, Poole C. (2000). Looking back on "causal thinking in the health sciences." Annu Rev Public Health 21:101–19.

Kimmel CA. (2001). 1999 Warkany lecture: improving the science for predicting risks to children's health. Teratology 63:202–9.

Krewski D, Crump KS, Farmer J, Gaylor DW, Howe R, Portier C, Salsburg D, Sielken RL, Van Ryzin J. (1983). A comparison of statistical methods for low dose extrapolation utilizing time-to-tumor data. Fundam Appl Toxicol 3: 140–60.

Landrigan PJ, Graham DG, Thomas RD. (1994). Environmental neurotoxic illness: research for prevention. Environ Health Perspect 102(Suppl 2):117–20.

Mileson BE, Ferenc SA. (2001). Methods to identify and characterize developmental neurotoxicity for human health risk assessment: overview. Environ Health Perspect 109(Suppl 1):77–8.

National Academy of Sciences. (1983). Risk assessment in the federal government: managing the process. Washington, D.C.: National Academy Press.

National Academy of Sciences. (2000). Scientific frontiers in developmental toxicology and risk assessment. Washington, D.C.: National Academy Press.

National Academy of Sciences. (2001). Evaluating chemical and other agent exposures for reproductive and developmental toxicity. Washington, DC: National Academy Press.

Rice D, Barone S Jr. (2000). Critical periods of vulnerability for the developing nervous system: evidence from humans and animal models. Environ Health Perspect 108(Suppl 3):511–33.

Rothman KJ, Greenland S. (1998). Modern epidemiology. Philadelphia: Lippincott-Raven.

The Presidential/Congressional Commission on Risk Assessment and Risk Management. (1997a). Framework for environmental health risk management, Volume I (stock number 055-000-00567-2). Washington, DC: Government Printing Office.

The Presidential/Congressional Commission on Risk Assessment and Risk Management. (1997b). Risk assessment and risk management in regulatory decision-making, Volume II (stock number 055-000-00568-1). Washington, DC: Government Printing Office.

U.S. Department of Health and Human Services. (1999). Mental health: a report of the surgeon general. Rockville, MD: U.S. Department of Health and Human Services.

U.S. Environmental Protection Agency. (1986). Guidelines for carcinogen risk assessment. Fed Reg 51:33992-4003.

U.S. Environmental Protection Agency. (1991). Guidelines for developmental toxicity risk assessment. Fed Reg 56:63798-826.

U.S. Environmental Protection Agency. (1996). Guidelines for reproductive toxicity risk assessment. Fed Reg 61:56274-322.

U.S. Environmental Protection Agency. (1999). Guidelines for carcinogen risk assessment (NCEA-F-0644). Washington, DC: U.S. Environmental Protection Agency.

U.S. Environmental Protection Agency. (2000a). Exposure and human health reassessment of 2,3,7,8-tetrachlorodibenzo-*p*-dioxin (TCDD) and related compounds. Washington, DC: U.S. Environmental Protection Agency.

U.S. Environmental Protection Agency. (2000b). Integrated risk information system. Washington, DC: U.S. Environmental Protection Agency.

U.S. Environmental Protection Agency. (2001). Notice of opportunity to provide additional information and comment. Fed Reg 66:59593-4.

U.S. General Accounting Office. (2001). Chemical risk assessment. Selected federal agencies' procedures, assumptions, and policies (GAO-01-810). Washington, DC: U.S. General Accounting Office.

U.S. Surgeon General. (1964). Smoking and health. (Public Health Service Publication No. 1103). Washington, DC: Public Health Service, U.S. Department of Health, Education, and Welfare.

Weiss B, Landrigan PJ. (2000). The developing brain and the environment: an introduction. Environ Health Perspect 108(Suppl 3):373–4.

Wilkinson CF, Christoph GR, Julien E, Kelley JM, Kronenberg J, McCarthy J, Reiss R. (2000). Assessing the risks of exposures to multiple chemicals with a common mechanism of toxicity: how to cumulate? Regul Toxicol Pharmacol 31: 30–43.

4
Metals—Lead

The twentieth century saw greatly expanded use and environmental dispersion of lead, a dense metal valued since antiquity because of its low melting point, pliability, and durability. Analysis of a Swiss peat bog showed that annual average lead deposition increased 1600-fold between 5000 B.C. and the maximum in 1979. Recognition of adult lead poisoning with abdominal colic can be traced to Hippocrates in about 370 B.C. (in metal workers) and Baker in 1767 (who linked Devonshire colic to consumption of lead-contaminated cider) (Table 4–1). Childhood lead poisoning was recognized as a distinct entity in 1892 and neurotoxicity in experimental animals by the 1920s. There has been substantial progress in reducing childhood lead exposure, but many children remain at risk.

The objective of this chapter is to illustrate how failure to apply the precautionary principle allowed inappropriate uses of lead, massive environmental contamination, and major adverse impacts on child health. The first section focuses mainly on the susceptibility of the developing human nervous system to adverse neurobehavioral effects from relatively low-level lead exposure, as evidenced by epidemiologic and toxicologic studies. The discussion includes environmental indices and biomarkers of lead exposure and toxicokinetics. The risk management section addresses lead sources (air, water, food, soil/dust) and interventions for preventing childhood lead exposure.

TABLE 4–1. Selective Chronology of Lead ($_{82}$Pb^{207})

370 B.C.	Hippocrates attributed abdominal colic in a metal worker to lead exposure
1767	Devonshire colic attributed to lead-contaminated cider (Sir George Baker, England)
1892	Childhood poisoning from lead-based paint reported in Australia
1909	France, Belgium, and Austria ban white lead interior paints
1923	First public sale of leaded gasoline (Dayton, Ohio)
1943	Lead poisoning shown to have persistent neurotoxic effects in children
1970	U.S. Clean Air Act establishes the EPA; "acceptable" blood lead level reduced from 60 to 40 μg/dL
1975	CDC investigation shows that lead emissions in air are a health hazard for children; first catalytic converters used to reduce motor vehicle emissions
1978	EPA bans lead-based paint and lead-based paint products; blood lead action level reduced from 40 to 30 μg/dL
1979	Deficits in psychologic and classroom performance linked to moderate lead levels in deciduous teeth
1976–80	NHANES II shows that mean blood lead declined by about 40% in all age, sex, and racial groups during this period in step with declining use of leaded gasoline
1986	EPA reduced drinking water lead standard from 50 to 5 μg/L and banned use of lead in plumbing solder and fixtures
1987	Elevated hearing threshold discovered at blood lead levels as low as 10 μg/dL
1991	Lead solder in food and beverage cans banned; action level for blood lead reduced to 10 μg/dL
1994	Meta-analyses showed IQ deficits in children with blood lead levels of 10–20 μg/dL; United Nations calls on governments to eliminate lead from gasoline worldwide
1991–4	NHANES III shows geometric mean blood lead level of 2.7 μg/dL (CI 2.5–3.0) and prevalence of levels of 10+ μg/dL of 4.4%, among children aged 1–5 years
1999	NHANES 1999 data show that geometric mean blood lead level of children aged 1–5 years was 2.0 μg/dL (CI 1.7–2.3)
2000	Neurobehavioral effects in children at blood lead levels below 5 μg/dL

HEALTH EFFECTS

Acute childhood lead poisoning is now rare in developed countries, but widespread low-level exposure continues. Low-level or moderate lead exposure during early childhood causes persistent adverse neurobehavioral effects including cognitive deficits. Relatively subtle neurobehavioral deficits occur at blood lead levels below 5 μg/dL (Lanphear et al., 2000) but clinically obvious symptoms occur only at levels exceeding about 50 μg/dL (Table 4–2). Encephalopathy with delirium, convulsions, paralysis, coma, and death may occur at blood lead levels above 80 μg/dL,

TABLE 4–2. Health Effects of Lead in Children by Blood Lead Level

Blood lead ($\mu g/dL$)	Health Effects
>125	Acute encephalopathy, death
>80	Encephalopathy, renal toxicity (aminoaciduria)
>60	Colic
>20	Anemia, peripheral neuropathy, reduced nerve conduction velocity
>15	Increased zinc protoporphyrin, impaired vitamin D activation
>10	Growth deficits
<10	IQ and hearing deficits, inhibition of ALAD and pyrimidine-5'-nucleotidase

Source: Agency for Toxic Substances and Disease Registry (1999).

indicating that the margin between blood lead levels sufficient to cause obvious symptoms and those that can cause massive brain damage or death is only about a factor of 2.

Toxic Mechanisms

Rapid development of the human brain before age 3 years involves a complex cascade of processes including cell division and migration, differentiation of neuroblasts to neurons with axons, dendrites, synapses, and neurotransmitter systems, and programmed cell death (apoptosis). This section describes some of the mechanisms through which lead can disrupt brain development.

Genetic Susceptibility

There is no clear evidence of genetic susceptibility to lead toxicity, but genetic polymorphisms may play a role. δ-Aminolevulinic acid dehydratase (ALAD), the vitamin D receptor gene (VDR), and the hemochromatosis gene (HFE—encodes the hereditary hemochromatosis protein), respectively, control heme synthesis, gastrointestinal calcium absorption, and iron transport. At low to moderate lead exposure levels, over 99% of lead in blood is firmly bound to red cell proteins, mainly ALAD. Environmentally exposed ALAD-2 homozygotes and heterozygotes have higher blood lead levels than ALAD-1 homozygotes (Shen et al., 2001), possibly because of a higher affinity of the ALAD-2 protein for lead. But no firm evidence exists for an association between ALAD genotype and susceptibility to lead toxicity at background exposure levels, precluding its use as a risk marker for lead screening programs. Calcitriol, the activated form of vitamin D, binds to nuclear vitamin D receptors in intestinal, kidney, and bone cells and activates transcription of genes that encode calcium-binding proteins; these include calbindin-D, an intestinal cell transport protein that promotes calcium and lead absorption. Among men occupationally exposed to lead, carriers of the B allele of VDR had higher blood and bone lead levels, suggesting that they had higher lead absorption capacity than noncarriers; there appear to be no reports on this relationship in children (Schwartz et al., 2000).

Normal HFE protein controls gastrointestinal iron absorption by binding to the transferrin receptor and reducing its affinity for iron-loaded transferrin. The net impact of HFE mutations is increased gastrointestinal iron absorption; lead absorption may also be increased, but direct evidence is lacking. The role of HFE polymorphisms in susceptibility to lead toxicity remains hypothetical but, given a prevalence of 4% in NHANES III, potentially important.

Lead–Protein Interactions
The mechanisms of lead neurotoxicity are incompletely understood, but its ability to compete with iron, zinc, and calcium at binding sites on proteins and disrupt their function may be fundamental. Even at low levels, lead binds almost irreversibly to zinc-dependent proteins including gene transcription factors, membrane ion-transport enzymes, intracellular signaling enzymes, and ALAD. By inhibiting ALAD, lead reduces production of heme and heme-dependent proteins (hemoglobin, cytochromes, myoglobin), causes accumulation of δ-aminolevulinic acid (δ-ALA, a neurotoxin at high levels), and impairs oxygen transport and storage, mitochondrial energy production, and P450 detoxification systems. Tissue-specific low molecular weight proteins bind lead, a property that may reduce lead neurotoxicity but may also facilitate lead uptake and carcinogenesis in kidney cells.

Synapse Formation and Function
In the absence of synapse formation, neurons fail to obtain adequate amounts of neurotrophins, antiapoptotic proteins produced by target tissues; approximately half of the neurons produced during development normally do not form synapses and undergo apoptosis. Lead reduces the likelihood of synapse formation by disrupting sialylation or desialylation of neuronal cell adhesion molecules (NCAMs), and functioning of NMDA receptors, protein kinase C, and calcium-dependent ion channels. The NCAMs are cell surface glycoproteins that mediate adhesion between neurons and between neurons and muscle cells. Glycosylation of NCAM by the enzyme sialyltransfererase (ST) soon after training periods appears to be a key mechanism for synapse formation and memory in rodents (Davey and Breen, 1998). Extremely low levels of lead induce ST activity in neu-

rons, causing inappropriate glycosylation of NCAM that may contribute to subsequent learning deficits in adult rats. Lead also inhibits dendrite formation and branching essential steps in synapse formation.

Neuronal plasticity, the ability of synaptic efficacy to change in response to neural activity, is a likely biologic mechanism for learning. Synaptic efficacy may undergo long-term depression (LTD) induced by low levels of synaptic activity or long-term potentiation (LTP) induced by the opposite conditions. Excitatory amino acids (glutamic and aspartic acids) and their NMDA receptors play major roles in activity-dependent synaptic plasticity and in the stabilization and elimination of synaptic connections during development. Lead interferes with the NMDA-type receptor and raises the threshold for LTP, a mechanism that may partially explain learning deficits from lead exposure (Guilarte, 1997).

By competing with calcium, lead disrupts calcium-dependent ion channels, intracellular signaling enzymes such as protein kinase C, and NMDA receptors and alters synaptic transmission. At picomolar levels, lead activates protein kinase C and diminishes the synaptic signal-to-noise ratio by stimulating spontaneous and inhibiting evoked presynaptic neurotransmitter release (Johnston and Goldstein, 1998). These low-dose effects may disrupt brain endothelial cell differentiation, blood-brain barrier development, learning, and memory.

Lead Absorption

Bioavailability of ingested lead varies by chemical form and amount of lead, diet (intake of calcium, iron, phosphate, vitamin D, and fat), age, and pregnancy status. Adults absorb 10%–15% of lead ingested with meals, but children and pregnant women can absorb up to 50%. Because lead absorption at intestinal calcium binding sites is inhibited by dietary calcium, children and pregnant women with low calcium intakes have increased lead absorption. Low calcium intake induces activation of vitamin D to 1,25-dihydroxyvitamin D in kidney and calcium-binding protein (calbindin-D) in intestinal cells, thus increasing absorption of calcium, lead, and other trace metals; lead, in turn, inhibits renal vitamin D activation. Iron deficiency also appears to increase duodenal lead absorption. Maternal bone lead appears to be mobilized during pregnancy and lactation, particularly among women who do not take calcium supplements (Gulson et al., 1998).

Neurotoxicity

Neurotoxicity of lead in children was first described in Australia (Gibson, 1892). This nineteenth-century study was remarkable for the use of postcard questionnaires sent to parents and the use of chemical analysis to measure lead concentrations in paint samples. Gibson concluded that the affected children lived in houses with paint that had oxidized to an easily removed powder containing high lead concentrations, had ingested sufficient lead to cause poisoning, and should be removed from their homes. Turner (1897) identified four clinical categories of moderate to severe childhood lead poisoning: (1) symmetrical paralysis of extensor muscles of the hands and feet, (2) abdominal colic, (3) epilepsy, and (4) ocular neuritis with paralysis of eye muscles. Current knowledge indicates that low to moderate childhood lead exposure can cause behavioral abnormalities and deficits in global intelligence, short-term memory, reading, spelling, hearing sensitivity, visuomotor performance, perception integration, and reaction time (Agency for Toxic Substances and Disease Registry, 1999; U.S. Environmental Protection Agency, 2001a).

Cognitive Function

As recently as 1972, the National Academy of Sciences stated that emissions of lead into air had no known harmful effects. In the same year, ironically, the (CDC) was investigating the health of persons living near a large lead smelter in El Paso, Texas. House dust and blood lead levels were strongly associated with proximity to the smelter. Among children living within 1.6 km of the smelter, 69% had blood lead levels of at least 40 μg/dL; this group had significant IQ deficits and reduced finger-wrist tapping speed compared to less exposed children (Landrigan et al., 1975a, 1975b). Subsequent studies of children living near other lead smelters produced similar findings.

A cross-sectional study of young children in Boston produced the first strong evidence of neurotoxicity from moderate lead exposure during childhood (Needleman et al., 1979). Cumulative exposure since birth was assessed by measuring the lead concentration in deciduous teeth, thus avoiding reliance on blood lead, an indicator of both recent and longer-term exposure. Children with high dentin lead levels had a mean full-scale IQ deficit of 4.5 points (compared to those with low dentin lead levels), with lower scores on verbal, auditory, speech, and attention subscales. When reassessed at age 18 years, the high-exposure group had greatly increased risks of reading disability and high school dropout (Needleman et al., 1996).

Several longitudinal and numerous cross-sectional studies have confirmed that low and moderate lead exposure during childhood causes adverse neurobehavioral outcomes. The evidence has been summarized in meta-analyses (Needleman and Gatsonis, 1990; Pocock et al., 1994; Schwartz, 1994) and literature reviews (Agency for Toxic Substances and

Disease Registry, 1999; Banks et al., 1997; Thacker et al., 1992; U.S. Environmental Protection Agency, 1998). Major conclusions from these reports include the following:

- A doubling of blood lead from 10 to 20 μg/dL, or of tooth lead from 5 to 10 μg/g, appears to cause an average full-scale IQ deficit of 1–3 points.
- Full-scale IQ deficits among school-age children were more consistently associated with blood lead levels at about age 2 years in cohort studies and tooth lead levels in cross-sectional studies, compared to current blood lead levels in cross-sectional studies

A reduction in average full-scale IQ of 5 points would reduce the proportion of very gifted people (IQ $\geq$ 130) in a population by a factor of about 2.5 and double the proportion of mentally retarded persons (IQ < 70) (Weiss, 1990). The predicted impact of a 10 μg/dL increment in blood lead at age 2 years in the Boston longitudinal study of middle-class children was an average full-scale IQ deficit at age 10 years of about 6 points, independent of potential confounders (Bellinger et al., 1992). In the Port Pirie smelter town longitudinal study, IQ at age 7 years was most closely associated with average blood lead levels from birth to any age between 15 months and 4 years; the predicted impact of an increase in average blood lead at ages 1–4 years from 10 to 30 μg/dL was a full-scale IQ deficit of 4–5 points (Baghurst et al., 1992). Of note was the particularly strong relationship between lead and WISC subscale deficits related to perceptual organization and synthesis, spatial visualization, nonverbal concept formation, and visuomotor coordination. Further follow-up of the Port Pirie cohort showed that (1) children in the highest tertile of blood lead at ages 2–4 years had cognitive deficits that persisted to at least age 11–13 years even though their blood lead levels had declined substantially, (2) there was a dose–response relation between lead and full-scale IQ, with no evidence of a threshold, and, (3) children with lifetime average blood lead levels above 15 μg/dL had an increased prevalence of problem behaviors (see, e.g., Burns et al., 1999).

The importance of lead exposure during early childhood and the peaking of blood lead levels at about age 2–3 years likely explain the greater consistency in cross-sectional studies of older children that used tooth lead rather than current blood lead to assess exposure. The cross-sectional study of almost 5000 children in NHANES III (1988–1994) is noteworthy in that performance scores for arithmetic, reading, nonverbal reasoning, and short-term/working memory were inversely related to blood lead levels even in the range below 10 μg/dL (Lanphear et al., 2000).

The belief that the neurotoxic effects of even high-level lead exposure were reversible was first challenged by a follow-up study of children previously treated for lead poisoning demonstrating persistent poor school performance, impulsive behavior, and short attention span (Byers and Lord, 1943). The authors hypothesized that persistent neurotoxicity was related to prolonged release of lead from stores in bone or to irreversible damage to the developing nervous system. A recent review of five longitudinal studies concluded that even low to moderate early childhood lead exposure is associated with neurobehavioral deficits that persist after exposure levels decline (Tong, 1998).

Other factors associated with poverty can cause IQ deficits: malnutrition, iron deficiency, certain infections, head injury, and inferior prenatal care. Several studies, however, were able to adjust for such potential confounders and still showed a lead effect. The biologic plausibility of neurotoxicity from low-level lead exposure is supported by experiments in rats and nonhuman primates; studies of monkeys exposed only prenatally or postnatally showed learning and memory deficits at blood lead levels as low as 10 μg/dL and learning and memory deficits that persisted years after exposure cessation (Rice, 1992).

Sensorimotor Effects
Children with blood lead levels less than 20 μg/dL exhibited visual-evoked potential abnormalities (Altmann et al., 1998), and those with levels below 10 μg/dL had elevated hearing thresholds (Osman et al., 1999). Lead causes retinal degeneration with apoptotic loss of rods and bipolar cells in both neonatal and adult rats at blood lead levels below 20 μg/dL. Moderate lead exposure during early childhood is associated with motor deficits including reduced finger-wrist tapping speed, motor nerve conduction velocity (with a possible threshold at blood lead levels of 20–30 μg/dL), and fine motor deficits (Schwartz et al., 1988).

Behavioral Problems
Children with high tooth lead levels are more likely to be distractible, dependent, hyperactive, easily frustrated, and unable to follow directions (Needleman et al., 1979). Prenatal and childhood lead exposure indices have been linked to delinquent and antisocial behaviors during adolescence in longitudinal studies (Burns et al., 1999; Dietrich et al., 2001).

Other Effects

Developmental Effects
A review of epidemiologic studies concluded that prenatal lead exposure likely increases the risk of preterm delivery and is inconsistently associated with reduced birth weight (Andrews et al., 1994). More recent stud-

ies have provided limited evidence that birth weight is inversely related to maternal lead exposure (Gonzalez-Cossio et al., 1997; Irgens et al., 1998) and possibly to paternal lead exposure (Lin et al., 1998). Stature and head circumference during early childhood appear to be inversely related to current blood lead levels in cross-sectional and longitudinal studies (see, e.g., Ballew et al., 1999; Rothenberg et al., 1999). There is also some evidence that lead exposure during early childhood may increase the risk of obesity during late adolescence (Kim et al., 1995).

Historic and modern studies of low/moderate and high-level paternal or maternal lead exposure have produced limited evidence of an association with spontaneous abortion (Hertz-Picciotto, 2000). Of note was the strong exposure–risk relationship extending to maternal first trimester blood lead levels below 15 μg/dL in a recent nested case-control study (Borja-Aburto et al., 1999). There is inadequate evidence that parental occupational lead exposure increases the risk of stillbirth. Limited evidence indicates associations between parental occupational or environmental lead exposure and oral cleft, neural tube, and cardiac defects (Aschengrau et al., 1993; Irgens et al., 1998; Kristensen et al., 1993; Vinceti et al., 2001).

Blood, Renal, and Immunologic Effects

Hemoglobin levels are reduced in young children with moderate or high lead exposure, independent of iron deficiency. Iron deficiency anemia facilitates gastrointestinal lead absorption; children from low-income families, therefore, are at increased risk of anemia from iron deficiency and both increased lead exposure and absorption. A recent review of lead nephrotoxicity concluded that low-level lead exposure is associated with increased urinary excretion of low molecular weight proteins and lysosomal enzymes, but the relation between these sensitive signs of renal tubular damage and the risk of renal disease is uncertain (Loghman-Adham, 1997). Children may be more susceptible to lead-induced urinary protein excretion than adults (Fels et al., 1998). There is inadequate evidence to assess whether lead exposure impairs immune function.

Exposures

Internal Dose Indicators

Available biomarkers of internal dose include lead concentrations in blood (including cord blood), urine, breast milk, hair, deciduous teeth, and other bones. Blood, urinary, and hair lead levels reflect exposures over the past several months, while bone (including teeth) lead concentrations indicate lifetime cumulative exposures in children. At low to moderate lead exposure levels, over 99% of lead in blood is firmly bound to red cell proteins, mainly ALAD; about 0.3%–0.7% is unbound and is the biologically active fraction. The half-life of lead in whole blood is about 30 days. Plasma lead is difficult to measure accurately because even slight hemolysis of red blood cells causes major artifactual increases. Whole blood lead levels are easily and reliably measured and have been used to assess lead exposure in most childhood blood lead screening programs and epidemiologic studies. Because lead cycles between blood and bone, blood lead levels in older children and adults reflect both recent and past exposures. Blood lead in infants and toddlers, however, reflects recent exposure because body lead stores (especially in bone) are still low. Among children in the general population, blood lead levels usually peak at age 2 years in parallel to exposure from soil and dust. Maternal blood lead levels peak during the first and third trimesters; older mothers had steeper increases in blood lead during the third trimester, consistent with mobilization from bone during late pregnancy (Hertz-Picciotto et al., 2000).

It was not until 1982 that the first population-based prevalence data were available in the United States using blood samples collected during NHANES II (Mahaffey et al., 1982). Among children aged 1–5 years, 98% of black and 85% of white children had blood lead levels of at least 10 μg/dL (Table 4–3). During the next decade, the percentage of children with elevated blood lead levels decreased to 21% among blacks and 5.5% among whites. Similar declines occurred in all subgroups defined by age, sex, race/ethnicity, income level, and urban status. Prevalence rates of elevated blood lead levels were associated with age of housing among all ethnic and income groups except the highest income category (Table 4–4). The geometric mean blood lead level of children declined from 15.0 μg/dL in 1976–1980 to 2.7 μg/dL in 1991–1994 and to 2.0 μg/dL in 1999 (Centers for Disease Control and Prevention, 2000; Pirkle et al., 1998). The

TABLE 4–3. Percentage of Children with Elevated Blood Lead Levels ($\geq$10 μg/dL), United States, NHANES II and III

	1976–80	1988–91
All persons aged 1–74 yr	77.8	4.3
All children aged 1–5 yr	88.2	8.9
All children aged 6–19 yr	71.7	2.6
Black children aged 1–5 yr	97.7	20.6
White children aged 1–5 yr	85.0	5.5

Source: Brody et al. (1994), Pirkle et al. (1994).

TABLE 4–4. Percentage of Children Aged 1–5 Years with Blood
Lead Levels 10+ µg/dL, United States, 1991–94

	Year Housing Was Built		
	Pre-1946	*1946–73*	*Post-1973*
Race/ethnicity			
Black, non-Hispanic	21.9	13.7	3.4
Mexican American	13.0	2.3	1.6
White, non-Hispanic	5.6	1.4	1.5
Family income level			
Low	16.4	7.3	4.3
Middle	4.1	2.0	0.4
High	0.9	2.7	NA
Urban status			
Pop. 1,000,000+	11.5	5.8	0.8
Pop. <1,000,000	5.8	3.1	2.5

NA, not available.

Source: Pirkle et al., 1998.

prevalence of elevated blood lead levels has likely decreased substantially among children in many other countries, but few have tracking systems to demonstrate this.

Bone, because of its mass and high affinity for lead, contains high proportions of the body lead burden in children (73%) and adults (94%) (Agency for Toxic Substances and Disease Registry, 1999). The bone lead concentration reflects long-term exposure and can be measured in deciduous teeth or by X-ray fluorescence of bones in vivo. The half-life of lead in bone ranges from years to decades, depending on bone type, metabolic state, and age; the half-life is shorter in children because of bone remodeling and high turnover rates during growth. Release of bone lead contributes to blood lead levels long after exposure ends.

Over the range 5–100+ µg/dL, lead progressively inhibits the red cell enzyme ALAD, increasing plasma δ-ALA levels, but such increases can also be caused by iron deficiency at low blood lead levels. Lead also blocks the action of the enzyme heme synthetase, leading to elevated blood levels of erythrocyte protoporphyrin. Neither heme precursor is a specific indicator of lead exposure. Because hair grows about 1 cm per month and lead levels in segments of hair reflect exposures at the time they were formed, segmental hair analysis provides information on lead exposures over time. Hair is subject, however, to external contamination and detects only 57% of children with elevated blood lead levels, precluding its use as a screening method. Urinary lead levels correlate weakly with total blood lead but strongly with plasma lead levels. Urinary lead excretion during the 24 hours after challenge with a chelating agent reflects body lead burden.

Modeled Exposure Estimates

The EPA developed the Integrated Exposure Uptake Biokinetic (IEUBK) model to estimate human lead uptake using data on lead concentrations in multiple media (air, dust, soil, paint, food, and water) and estimated average human consumption levels. This model assumes that lead from all sources is absorbed via the lungs and gastrointestinal tract and enters a blood plasma reservoir that equilibrates with lead in all tissues with age-specific parameters for each transfer process. Biokinetic models are subject to several uncertainties including the bioavailability of lead in various media and the prevalence and intensity of behavioral factors, particularly hand–mouth activity. Nevertheless, using environmental lead data for four communities, modeled geometric mean blood lead estimates for each community fell within 0.7 μg/dL of directly measured blood lead levels (Hogan et al., 1998).

RISK MANAGEMENT

Tetraethyl lead in gasoline and lead pigments in paint were the main sources of lead exposure for children in the twentieth century. Other important sources included foods in lead-soldered cans and drinking water contaminated by lead or lead alloy plumbing materials. During the mid-twentieth century, the Lead Industries Association (LIA) campaigned successfully against attempts to reduce or prohibit the use of lead in paint and plumbing materials and the use of lead arsenate on foods (Silbergeld, 1997).

Prevention

Childhood lead control policies that emphasize primary prevention of lead exposure will ultimately reduce or eliminate the need for screening at-risk children (Lanphear, 1998). Based on NHANES III (1991–1994), there were about 900,000 children in the United States with blood lead levels above the health-concern blood lead level ($\geq$10 μg/dL) set by the CDC compared to about 14 million children in 1978 (Table 4–5). The U.S. strate-

TABLE 4–5. Number of Children with Blood
Lead Levels of 10+ µg/dL, United States

Year	Number
1976–80[a]	14.2 million
1991–94[b]	0.9 million

[a]Age 6 months to 5 years. *Source:* Mahaffey et al. (1982).

[b]Age 1 to 5 years. *Source:* Pirkle et al. (1998).

gies for eliminating blood lead levels over 10 µg/dl among young children by the year 2010 include (1) controlling lead paint hazards in low-income housing, (2) expanding blood lead screening programs and follow-up services for at-risk children, (3) conducting intervention research, and (4) tracking progress and refining strategies (President's Task Force on Environmental Health Risks and Safety Risks to Children, 2000).

The United States appears to be the first country that banned lead from gasoline, paint, and plumbing. Denmark was the first European Union country to ban most uses of lead other than lead-acid car batteries (Danish Environmental Protection Agency 2001). The estimated future economic benefits from increased worker IQ and productivity attributable to reduced blood lead levels since 1976 among children are $110–$319 billion increased earnings over the lifetime of the U.S. cohort aged 2 years in 2000 (in 2000 dollars and assuming a 3% discount rate), with similar savings for each year's birth cohort (Grosse et al., 2002).

Air

Sources. In 1925, leading medical scientists, members of the U.S. Public Health Service, and industry representatives discussed the use of leaded gasoline. Alice Hamilton of Harvard Medical School noted that lead is a cumulative poison that usually does not produce easily recognized symptoms. A Standard Oil representative stated that industry could not respond to a remote probability of harm from a product that allegedly improved fuel economy. The U.S. government allowed continued use of tetraethyl lead after a committee appointed by the Surgeon General reported in early 1926 that lead from this source was not an acute hazard to the community. Subsequent exposure of virtually the entire populations of developed countries to lead from this source could have been avoided if the warnings of health authorities had been heeded (Needleman, 1997).

Annual lead emissions in the United States decreased from 221,000 tons in 1970 to less than 4000 tons in 1997 (Table 4–6); at peak use in the mid-1970s, combustion of leaded gasoline contributed about 90% of lead

TABLE 4–6. Lead Emissions into Air (tons), United States, 1970–1998

	1970	1980	1990	1998
On-road vehicles	171,961	60,501	421	19
Metal processing	24,224	3,026	2,170	2,098
Other	24,684	10,626	2,384	1,856
Total	220,869	74,153	4,975	3,973

Source: U.S. Environmental Protection Agency (2000a).

emissions. Such emissions contained water-soluble, inorganic lead in respirable particles from which lead was easily absorbed into blood. Evidence that leaded gasoline was the major determinant of lead exposure in the general population came from NHANES II (1976–1980), a population-based health survey of the United States (Annest et al., 1983). Average blood lead levels among persons age 6 months to 74 years declined by a remarkable 37% during the short period 1976–1980. Similar decreases occurred in each race, sex, and age subgroup and closely paralleled the declining sales of leaded gasoline and a 40% decline in ambient air lead concentrations during 1975–1980. For young children, there was a strong correlation ($r = 0.95$, $p < 0.001$) between blood lead levels and total lead used in gasoline for each 6-month period (see Fig. 4–1). Indoor air and umbilical cord blood lead levels in Boston during the period 1979–1981 correlated strongly with monthly leaded gasoline sales (Rabinowitz et al., 1984). Similar changes in airborne lead and childhood blood lead levels were observed in other countries after the introduction of lead-free gasoline.

Emissions from industrial sources, mainly lead smelters and battery manufacturers, have decreased by only 6% since 1988 and are now the major sources of airborne lead emissions. Upgrading of the El Paso lead smelter dramatically reduced lead exposure indices, but even after the smelter closed in 1985, soil and blood lead levels of children living close to the smelter were still elevated a decade later. Cross-sectional and longitudinal studies of children living in proximity to other lead smelters confirmed this child health threat.

Intervention. The approximately 40% decline in average blood lead levels in the United States during the late 1970s was mainly due to the 1970 Clean Air Act. Under this act, the EPA persuaded car manufacturers to add catalytic converters to new vehicles in 1975 to reduce exhaust emissions; lead-free gasoline was introduced in the same year (lead ren-

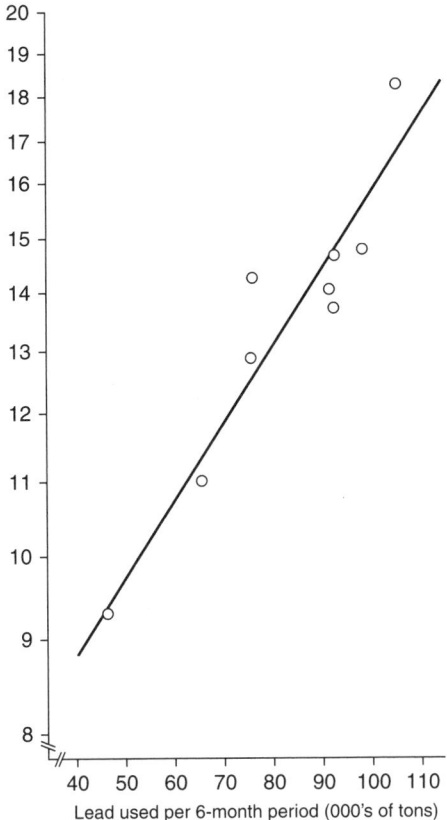

Lead used per 6-month period (000's of tons)

FIGURE 4–1. Average blood lead levels by 6-month periods of white children aged 6 months through 5 years and total lead used in gasoline production per 6 months during 1976–1980. The blood lead values used to compute these averages were preadjusted by regression analysis to account for the effects of sex, income, degree of urbanization, region of the country, and season (Annest et al., 1983). (Copyright © 1983, Massachusetts Medical Society. All Rights reserved.)

ders catalytic converters ineffective). The EPA set national ambient air quality standards (NAAQS) for lead in 1978 and banned the use of leaded gasoline in highway vehicles in 1995. Emissions from industrial sources caused all recent violations of the lead NAAQS.

In some developing countries weak environmental standards, rapidly increasing numbers of cars, use of leaded gasoline, and elevated blood lead levels still occur. The United Nations Commission on Sustainable Development in 1994 called for worldwide elimination of lead from gasoline. This action caused the World Bank, the OECD, and the United Nations Economic Commission for Europe to encourage and assist nations to phase out leaded gasoline. By 1997, 13 countries had eliminated leaded gasoline and 18 had initiated a phase-out. The member states of the United Nations Economic Commission for Europe agreed in 1998 to phase out the use of leaded gasoline by the beginning of 2005.

Soil, House Dust, and Paint

For many years, seasonal variations in childhood blood lead levels (highest in summer) were attributed to sun exposure and dermal activation of vitamin D, causing increased gastrointestinal lead absorption. Current evidence indicates that children are more exposed during summer because of increased house dust lead concentrations and longer outdoor play periods in areas with contaminated soil (Yiin et al., 2000). Hand–mouth behavior of young children, combined with play activities at floor or ground level, greatly increases the chance of exposure to lead-contaminated dust and soil (Lanphear and Roghmann, 1997).

Sources. In populated areas, soil lead levels tend to be highest in the urban core of large cities; soil lead levels of several hundred micrograms per gram are common in urban cores where high traffic volumes occurred for decades during the leaded gasoline era. Lead concentrations above 10,000 μg/g have been observed in soil samples below the drip line of buildings with exterior lead-based paint, but atmospheric deposition is the main source of lead in soil outside the drip line. Soil tracked into homes is a major source of house dust; lead isotope ratios of house dust are virtually identical to those of street dust and soil. In the early 1980s, about 95% of house dust lead in newer housing and at least 50% in older housing originated in leaded gasoline (Fergusson and Schroeder, 1985). Vinyl miniblinds containing lead as a plasticizer are an unusual but important source of lead-contaminated dust and have never been subjected to a product recall.

A pooled analysis of 12 cross-sectional studies indicated that the major source of lead exposure for young children with blood lead levels of 10–25 μg/dL was house dust (Lanphear et al., 1998). Blood lead levels of young children were most closely related to interior floor dust lead loading and handwipe lead level (Succop et al., 1998). Children who ingest soil while playing outdoors between meals may absorb a considerable fraction of the lead content because a much larger fraction of ingested lead is absorbed when fasting.

Houses built during 1920–1950 contained tens of pounds of paint lead (Table 4–7). Children can take up lead from paint by eating paint chips or by ingesting house dust or soil contaminated by the breakdown of old paint. Ingested lead-based paint chips were an important cause of substantial blood lead elevations, particularly among African American chil-

TABLE 4–7. White Lead Used in House Paint by Decade

Year	Total (000's of tons)	Amount per Housing Unit (lb.s)
1920–29	1,307	87
1930–39	737	42
1940–49	476	22
1950–59	196	7
1960–69	82	3
1970–79	29	1

Source: President's Task Force on Environmental Health Risks and Safety Risks to Children (2000).

dren living in deteriorating pre-1950 housing. Radiographic evidence of recent paint chip ingestion was found in about 25% of children with markedly elevated blood lead levels ($\geq$55 μg/dL) but rarely among those with lower levels (McElvaine et al., 1992). The marked and rapid decline of blood lead levels concurrent with decreased use of lead in gasoline during the late 1970s occurred despite the absence of any significant remediation of lead-based paint. If lead-based paint was the most important source of lead exposure for children, blood lead levels would likely peak in winter, when children tend to remain indoors. In sum, it appears that leaded gasoline caused high average background blood lead levels in the general population and that lead-based paint was mainly a problem in low-income population subgroups in older deteriorating housing. Since such housing was commonly found in the high-traffic core of large urban areas, affected populations must have often had major exposures from both sources.

Intervention. France, Belgium, and Austria banned the interior use of lead paint in 1909, but the United States and many other countries did not act until the 1970s or later; in 1978 the U.S. Consumer Product Safety Commission ruled that paint used for residences, toys, furniture, and public areas must contain no more than 0.06% lead by weight. About 26 million homes in the United States have significant lead-based paint hazards, including, deteriorated lead-based paint areas, floor or window sill dust lead loadings, or lead levels in bare soil above specified thresholds (U.S. Department of Housing and Urban Development, 2001).

An evaluation of 11 U.S. residential lead hazard control projects concluded that floor and window sill dust lead levels remained substantially lower over a 3-year follow-up period and children's geometric mean blood lead levels decreased from 11.0 μg/dL at baseline to 8.2 μg/dL 1 year postintervention (Galke et al., 2001). A systematic review of residential residential lead abatement randomized trials concluded that there was no impact on mean blood lead levels, but there was a significantly lower prevalence of blood lead levels of 15 μg/dL or greater in the intervention groups (6% vs. 14%) (Haynes et al., 2002).

The Residential Lead-Based Paint Hazard Reduction Act requires sellers and landlords of most housing built before 1978 to disclose known lead-based paint and related hazards to buyers or renters and provide printed information on how to protect their families from lead in the home. Given the need for much more intensive intervention, this act appears to provide little real protection for children whose parents cannot afford safer housing. The EPA developed new standards for lead in paint, dust, and soil in 2000 (Table 4–8). These standards govern properties receiving federal assistance and activities by certified lead services providers, and guide action by state and local health departments, property owners, contractors, lenders, and insurers. The U.S. Department of Housing and Urban Development (HUD) estimated that interim control of lead hazards in pre-1960 low-income housing will yield a net benefit

TABLE 4–8. Standards for Lead in Environmental Media

Medium	Standard	Agency
Ambient air	0.5 μg/m^3 annual average	WHO[a]
	1.5 μg/m^3 quarterly average	EPA[b]
Drinking water	10 μg/L	WHO[c]
	15 μg/L	EPA[d]
Floor dust	40 μg/sq ft	EPA[e]
Interior window sill dust	250 μg/sq ft	EPA[e]
Bare soil in play areas	400 μg/g	EPA[e]
Bare soil in rest of yard	1200 μg/g	EPA[e]
Food		
Children aged 0–6 yr	6 μg/day[f]	FDA[f]
Children aged ≥7 yr	15 μg/day	
Pregnant women	25 μg/day	

[a]World Health Organization (2000a).

[b]U.S. Environmental Protection Agency (2001b).

[c]World Health Organization (2000b).

[d]U.S. Environmental Protection Agency (2000b).

[e]U.S. Environmental Protection Agency (2001a).

[f]U.S. Food and Drug Administration (1993): provisional tolerable total intake level (level of daily intake likely to pose no risk of adverse effects to almost all individuals in the general population).

of $8.9 billion (at a 3% discount rate) over the next 10 years (President's Task Force on Environmental Health Risks and Safety Risks to Children, 2000). In 1999, Rhode Island became the first state to pursue legal action against the manufacturers of lead-based paints.

Water

Water can leach lead from materials used in water distribution systems, homes, or storage containers including lead pipes and solder. Lead pipes are still present in many older communities and can cause substantial contamination, especially when water is soft and acidic. Elevated lead intakes of infants occurred in areas of Germany and the United Kingdom where high-lead tap water was consumed as such or added to dehydrated infant formulas and cereals. Among a nationally representative sample of German children, blood lead levels were related to gender (male), age, lead level in drinking water, and outdoor dust fall (Seifert et al., 2000). Tap water lead in Glasgow decreased during 1981–1993 but remained the leading cause of elevated maternal blood lead levels; about 13% of infants were exposed to formula made from tap water containing lead above the European Community's limit value (10 μg/L) (Watt et al., 1996). Tap water lead levels above the EPA standard (15 μg/L) occurred in 5% of standing samples in a recent U.S. survey.

Food

Historically, food has been an important source of lead exposure, for example, foods stored in lead-soldered cans or lead-glazed ceramic containers. During the 1970s, over 90% of food cans were lead soldered, and the FDA asked the food processing industry to intervene voluntarily. Lead levels in infant foods and juices fell by 85% during 1973–1978 with the conversion to lead-free soldered cans of infant formula and glass jars for infant juices. Average daily dietary lead intake of a child aged 2 years in the United States declined from 30 μg/day in 1982 to 5 μg/day during 1986–1988 and to 1.3 μg/day in 1994–1996 (the FDA banned the use of lead-soldered cans in 1991). Reduced contamination of food crops by airborne lead and reduced use of lead-glazed cookware also helped reduce the dietary lead intake (Centers for Disease Control and Prevention, 1991). Exceptions include northern Quebec, where 26% of reproductive-age Inuit women had blood lead levels of at least 10 μg/dL, associated with consumption of waterfowl contaminated by lead shot (Dewailly et al., 2001). Lead-glazed pottery continues to be an important source of lead exposure in several countries; ceramics from Mexico, China, Korea, Italy, and Spain imported into the United States as recently as 1995 were found to release large amounts of lead into food and drink.

The Joint FAO/WHO Expert Committee on Food Additives reduced the Provisional Tolerable Weekly Intake for lead from all sources from 50 to 25 μg per kilogram body weight because of concern for children. During the 1980s, mean weekly dietary lead intake of infants and children was about 3 μg/kg in the United States, 15–20 μg/kg in Sweden and Canada, and 26–28 μg/kg in Poland, Germany, and Hungary. Diets high in calcium or calcium supplements have been linked to lower blood lead levels in pregnant women. Maternal wine consumption and cigarette smoking were associated with increased cord blood lead levels; wine and tobacco, respectively, may contain lead from the pesticide lead arsenate and the use of brass fittings in wine-dispensing equipment.

Screening

Screening can identify children with elevated blood lead levels and trigger appropriate interventions. Baltimore, the first place in the United States to do so, offered free blood lead testing of children beginning in 1935, mandated lead paint removal from housing in 1941, and assigned public health nurses to investigate cases and educate parents in the late 1940s. Under the 1971 Lead-Based Paint Poisoning Prevention Act, the CDC initiated the first mass screening nationwide with, about 400,000–500,000 children under age 6 years screened annually during the next several years. Follow-up of children with high blood lead levels showed that over 90% had received medical care, 75% of homes had been investigated, and 80% of residential lead paint hazards had been abated. In 1991 the CDC reduced the action level for childhood blood lead to 10 μg/dL and recommended universal blood lead screening of children aged 12–72 months unless it could be shown that their community did not have a childhood lead poisoning problem. By 1994, only half of the states had implemented the CDC guideline.

In 1997 the CDC recommended that states develop policies and actions for primary prevention of lead exposure, targeted screening programs, surveillance, and actions to manage children with elevated levels (Tables 4–9 and 4–10) (Centers for Disease Control and Prevention, 1997). The CDC specified that screening programs should be targeted at children up to age 6 years who have never been screened and have one or more risk factors. Among young children with elevated blood lead levels during NHANES III (1988–1994), only one-third had been previously screened (Kaufmann et al., 2000).

An analysis of the 1997 CDC guidelines suggested that it is most cost-effective to do universal screening in high-prevalence populations and targeted screening in low-prevalence populations. Targeted screening con-

TABLE 4–9. Model Childhood Lead Poisoning Prevention Policies and Actions

Policy	Action
Primary prevention	
Housing codes or statutes	Evaluate/control residential lead-based paint hazards
Lead education plan	Public lead education
Certified lead-abatement workers	Professional education/training
Medicaid policies requiring anticipatory guidance	Anticipatory guidance by child health-care providers
Plan to reduce exposures from industry and drinking water	Identify/control sources other than lead-based paint
Secondary prevention	
Screening plan; Medicaid screening policies; protocols for providers	Childhood blood lead screening
Policies and protocols for care, environmental management, follow-up	Follow-up care for children with elevated levels
Monitoring (surveillance)	
Policy requiring laboratories to report blood lead test results	Monitor children's blood lead levels
Certification/licensing procedures for safety of lead-hazard reduction activities; procedures for tracking lead-safe housing	Monitor older/deteriorated housing, hazard-reduction activities, lead-safe housing

Source: Centers for Disease Control and Prevention (1997).

sistent with the CDC guidelines would detect 90% of the cases at two-thirds the cost of universal screening. The CDC concluded that venous blood samples are more cost-effective than finger prick samples under either universal or targeted screening; finger prick samples yield higher false-positive rates because of contamination from lead on skin. The prevalence of elevated blood lead levels (≥ 10 $\mu g/dL$) among young children of lead-exposed workers was 52%, considerably above the U.S. population prevalence, indicating a need to reduce take-home lead exposures and to screen at-risk children for elevated blood lead levels (Roscoe et al., 1999).

The U.S. Preventive Services Task Force recommended that blood lead be measured at age 12 months for all children having identifiable risk factors or living in communities with a high or unknown prevalence of elevated blood lead levels (U.S. Preventive Services Task Force, 1996).

TABLE 4–10. Blood Lead Categories and Actions Recommended by the CDC

Level (μg/dL)	Recommended Action
<10	Reassess or rescreen in 1 year. No additional action necessary unless exposure sources change
10–14	Provide family lead education and follow-up testing; refer for social services if necessary
15–19	Provide family lead education and follow-up testing; refer for social services if necessary. If blood lead levels in this range persist (two venous blood lead levels in this range at least 3 months apart) or increase, proceed according to actions for blood lead levels of 20–44 μg/dL
20–44	Provide case management, clinical management, environmental investigation, and lead-hazard control
45–69	Within 48 hours, begin case management, clinical management, environmental investigation, and lead-hazard control
70+	Hospitalize child and begin medical treatment immediately. Begin case management, clinical management, environmental investigation, and lead-hazard control immediately

Source: Centers for Disease Control and Prevention (1997).

Although the Task Force recommended targeted screening, it noted that no randomized screening trials had been done and that most intervention studies on asymptomatic children had evaluated the impact on blood lead levels, not on health status. The health benefits of blood lead screening programs are limited by irreversible neurotoxic effects before screening and intervention, prolonged mobilization of lead from bone stores to blood postintervention, and continued contamination of house dust.

Surveillance

The CDC funded childhood blood lead surveillance systems and developed software to track those with elevated levels. Such systems were used to document the extent of the problem, justify preventive and screening programs, and reveal risks where none were expected including traditional medicines and ceramic ware. Large-scale population-based health examination surveys are also important for monitoring health outcome and health hazard exposure trends. Without NHANES, we would not have such clear evidence of the role of leaded gasoline as the major exposure source for the general population, including persons in all demographic subgroups, during the leaded gasoline era.

CONCLUSION

Proven Child Health Outcomes

- Moderate to high childhood exposure—central nervous system toxicity (ranging from headaches and agitation to somnolence, vomiting, coma, and convulsions), peripheral neuropathy, anemia, kidney damage.
- Low exposure—deficits on standardized tests of global intelligence, increased threshold for hearing.

Unresolved Issues and Knowledge Gaps

- Developmental effects—there is limited evidence that low-level prenatal lead exposure may cause fetal death, reduced birth weight, preterm delivery, birth defects (cardiac, neural tube, oral clefts), and reduced stature among preadolescent children.
- Neurotoxicity—there is limited evidence that low-level prenatal and/or early childhood lead exposure may cause learning and behavior problems during childhood and adolescence.
- Delayed effects—there is inadequate evidence to assess the influence of low-level childhood lead exposure on the risk of kidney cancer, other renal disease, hypertension, and neurologic disease during adulthood
- Knowledge gaps—the efficacy of blood lead screening programs in reducing adverse health effects has not been tested in a randomized trial.

Risk Management Issues

- Prevention
  - An estimated 900,000 American children aged 1–5 years in 1991–1994 had blood lead values above the CDC action level (10 μg/dL); recent research has shown cognitive and hearing deficits below this level.
  - Interventions to reduce soil, dust, or paint lead hazards have had limited success in reducing children's blood lead levels, probably because of recontamination from persistent lead sources and mobilization of bone lead.
  - Ingestion of soil, dust, food, and water contaminated from past and present lead sources continues to expose young children to varying degrees of lead contamination.
  - Only the virtual elimination of lead exposure during gestation and early childhood can protect children from adverse neurobehavioral effects of lead.

- Biomonitoring—the tracking of population blood lead levels in NHANES has enabled evaluation of preventive interventions and identification of continuing needs.

REFERENCES

Agency for Toxic Substances and Disease Registry. (1999). Toxicological profile for lead. Atlanta: Agency for Toxic Substances and Disease Registry.

Altmann L, Sveinsson K, Kramer U, Weishoff-Houben M, Turfeld M, Winneke G, Wiegand H. (1998). Visual functions in 6-year-old children in relation to lead and mercury levels. Neurotoxicol Teratol 20:9–17.

Andrews KW, Savitz DA, Hertz-Picciotto I. (1994). Prenatal lead exposure in relation to gestational age and birth weight: a review of epidemiologic studies. Am J Ind Med 26:13–32.

Annest JL, Pirkle JL, Makuc D, Neese JW, Bayse DD, Kovar MG. (1983). Chronological trend in blood lead levels between 1976 and 1980. N Engl J Med 308: 1373–7.

Aschengrau A, Zierler S, Cohen A. (1993). Quality of community drinking water and the occurrence of late adverse pregnancy outcomes. Arch Environ Health 48:105–13.

Baghurst PA, McMichael AJ, Wigg NR, Vimpani GV, Robertson EF, Roberts RJ, Tong SL. (1992). Environmental exposure to lead and children's intelligence at the age of seven years. The Port Pirie Cohort Study. N Engl J Med 327:1279–84.

Ballew C, Khan LK, Kaufmann R, Mokdad A, Miller DT , Gunter EW. (1999). Blood lead concentration and children's anthropometric dimensions in the Third National Health and Nutrition Examination Survey (NHANES III), 1988–1994. J Pediatr 134:623–30.

Banks EC, Ferretti LE, Shucard DW. (1997). Effects of low level lead exposure on cognitive function in children: a review of behavioral, neuropsychological and biological evidence. Neurotoxicology 18:237–81.

Bellinger DC, Stiles KM, Needleman HL. (1992). Low-level lead exposure, intelligence and academic achievement: a long-term follow-up study. Pediatrics 90:855–61.

Borja-Aburto VH, Hertz-Picciotto I, Rojas Lopez M, Farias P, Rios C, Blanco J. (1999). Blood lead levels measured prospectively and risk of spontaneous abortion. Am J Epidemiol 150:590–7.

Brody DJ, Pirkle JL, Kramer RA, Flegal KM, Matte TD, Gunter EW, Paschal DC. (1994). Blood lead levels in the U.S. population. Phase 1 of the Third National Health and Nutrition Examination Survey (NHANES III, 1988 to 1991). JAMA 272:277–83.

Burns JM, Baghurst PA, Sawyer MG, McMichael AJ, Tong SL. (1999). Lifetime low-level exposure to environmental lead and children's emotional and behavioral development at ages 11–13 years. The Port Pirie Cohort Study. Am J Epidemiol 149:740–9.

Byers RK, Lord EE. (1943). Late effects of lead poisoning on mental development. Am J Dis Child 66:471–94.

Centers for Disease Control and Prevention. (1991). Preventing lead poisoning in young children: a statement by the Centers for Disease Control. Atlanta: Centers for Disease Control and Prevention, Public Health Service, U.S. Department of Health and Human Services.

Centers for Disease Control and Prevention. (1997). Screening young children for lead poisoning: guidance for state and local public health officials. Atlanta: Centers for Disease Control and Prevention.

Centers for Disease Control and Prevention. (2000). Blood lead levels in young children—United States and selected states, 1996–1999. MMWR 49:1133–7.

Danish Environmental Protection Agency. (2001). Denmark's lead ban a world first. Located at http://www.mst.dk/news/02070000.htm.

Davey FD, Breen KC. (1998). Stimulation of sialyltransferase by subchronic low-level lead exposure in the developing nervous system. A potential mechanism of teratogen action. Toxicol Appl Pharmacol 151:16–21.

Dewailly E, Ayotte P, Bruneau S, Lebel G, Levallois P, Weber JP. (2001). Exposure of the Inuit population of Nunavik (Arctic Quebec) to lead and mercury. Arch Environ Health 56:350–7.

Dietrich KN, Ris MD, Succop PA, Berger OG, Bornschein RL. (2001). Early exposure to lead and juvenile delinquency. Neurotoxicol Teratol 23:511–8.

Fels LM, Wunsch M, Baranowski J, Norska-Borowka I, Price RG, Taylor SA, Patel S, De Broe M, Elsevier MM, Lauwerys R, and others. (1998). Adverse effects of chronic low level lead exposure on kidney function—a risk group study in children. Nephrol Dial Transplant 13:2248–56.

Fergusson JE, Schroeder RJ. (1985). Lead in house dust of Christchurch, New Zealand: sampling, levels and sources. Sci Total Environ 46:61–72.

Galke W, Clark S, Wilson J, Jacobs D, Succop P, Dixon S, Bornschein B, McLaine P, Chen M. (2001). Evaluation of the HUD lead hazard control grant program: early overall findings. Environ Res 86:149–56.

Gibson JL. (1892). Notes on lead-poisoning as observed among children in Brisbane. Proc Intercolonial Med Congr Aust 3:76–83.

Gonzalez-Cossio T, Peterson KE, Sanin LH, Fishbein E, Palazuelos E, Aro A, Hernandez-Avila M, Hu H. (1997). Decrease in birth weight in relation to maternal bone lead burden. Pediatrics 100:856–62.

Grosse SD, Matte TD, Schwartz J, Jackson RJ. (2002). Economic gains resulting from the reduction in children's exposure to lead in the United States. Environ Health Perspect 110:563–69.

Guilarte TR. (1997). Glutamatergic system and developmental lead neurotoxicity. Neurotoxicology 18:665–72.

Gulson BL, Mahaffey KR, Jameson CW, Mizon KJ, Korsch MJ, Cameron MA, Eisman JA. (1998). Mobilization of lead from the skeleton during the postnatal period is larger than during pregnancy. J Lab Clin Med 131:324–9.

Haynes E, Lanphear BP, Tohn E, Farr N, Rhoads GG. (2002). The effect of interior lead hazard controls on children's blood lead concentrations: a systematic evaluation. Environ Health Perspect 110:103–7.

Hertz-Picciotto I. (2000). The evidence that lead increases the risk for spontaneous abortion. Am J Ind Med 38:300–9.

Hertz-Picciotto I, Schramm M, Watt-Morse M, Chantala K, Anderson J, Osterloh J. (2000). Patterns and determinants of blood lead during pregnancy. Am J Epidemiol 152:829–37.

Hogan K, Marcus A, Smith R, White P. (1998). Integrated exposure uptake biokinetic model for lead in children: empirical comparisons with epidemiologic data. Environ Health Perspect 106(Suppl 6):1557–67.

Irgens A, Kruger K, Skorve AH, Irgens LM. (1998). Reproductive outcome in off-spring of parents occupationally exposed to lead in Norway. Am J Ind Med 34:431–7.

Johnston MV, Goldstein GW. (1998). Selective vulnerability of the developing brain to lead. Curr Opin Neurol 11:689–93.

Kaufmann RB, Clouse TL, Olson DR, Matte TD. (2000). Elevated blood lead levels and blood lead screening among U.S. children aged one to five years: 1988–1994. Pediatrics 106:E79.

Kim R, Hu H, Rotnitzky A, Bellinger D, Needleman H. (1995). A longitudinal study of chronic lead exposure and physical growth in Boston children. Environ Health Perspect 103:952–7.

Kristensen P, Irgens LM, Daltveit AK, Andersen A. (1993). Perinatal outcome among children of men exposed to lead and organic solvents in the printing industry. Am J Epidemiol 137:134–44.

Landrigan PJ, Gehlbach SH, Rosenblum BF, Shoults JM, Candelaria RM, Barthel WF, Liddle JA, Smrek AL, Staehling NW, Sanders JF. (1975a). Epidemic lead absorption near an ore smelter. The role of particulate lead. N Engl J Med 292: 123–9.

Landrigan PJ, Whitworth RH, Baloh RW, Staehling NW, Barthel WF, Rosenblum BF. (1975b). Neuropsychological dysfunction in children with chronic low-level lead absorption. Lancet 1:708–12.

Lanphear BP. (1998). The paradox of lead poisoning prevention. Science 281: 1617–8.

Lanphear BP, Dietrich K, Auinger P, Cox C. (2000). Cognitive deficits associated with blood lead concentrations <10 microg/dL in U.S. children and adolescents. Public Health Rep 115:521–9.

Lanphear BP, Matte TD, Rogers J, Clickner RP, Dietz B, Bornschein RL, Succop P, Mahaffey KR, Dixon S, Galke W, and others. (1998). The contribution of lead-contaminated house dust and residential soil to children's blood lead levels. A pooled analysis of 12 epidemiologic studies. Environ Res 79:51–68.

Lanphear BP, Roghmann KJ. (1997). Pathways of lead exposure in urban children. Environ Res 74:67–73.

Lin S, Hwang SA, Marshall EG, Marion D. (1998). Does paternal occupational lead exposure increase the risks of low birth weight or prematurity? Am J Epidemiol 148:173–81.

Loghman-Adham M. (1997). Renal effects of environmental and occupational lead exposure. Environ Health Perspect 105:928–39.

Mahaffey KR, Annest JL, Roberts J, Murphy RS. (1982). National estimates of blood lead levels: United States, 1976–1980: association with selected demographic and socioeconomic factors. N Engl J Med 307:573–9.

McElvaine MD, DeUngria EG, Matte TD, Copley CG, Binder S. (1992). Prevalence of radiographic evidence of paint chip ingestion among children with moderate to severe lead poisoning, St Louis, Missouri, 1989 through 1990. Pediatrics 89:740–2.

Needleman HL. (1997). Clamped in a straitjacket: the insertion of lead into gasoline. Environ Res 74:95–103.

Needleman HL, Gatsonis CA. (1990). Low-level lead exposure and the IQ of children. A meta-analysis of modern studies. JAMA 263:673–8.

Needleman HL, Gunnoe C, Leviton A, Reed R, Peresie H, Maher C, Barrett P. (1979). Deficits in psychologic and classroom performance of children with elevated dentine lead levels. N Engl J Med 300:689–95.

Needleman HL, Riess JA, Tobin MJ, Biesecker GE, Greenhouse JB. (1996). Bone lead levels and delinquent behavior. JAMA 275:363–9.

Osman K, Pawlas K, Schutz A, Gazdzik M, Sokal JA , Vahter M. (1999). Lead exposure and hearing effects in children in Katowice, Poland. Environ Res 80:1–8.

Pirkle JL, Brody DJ, Gunter EW, Kramer RA, Paschal DC, Flegal KM, Matte TD. (1994). The decline in blood lead levels in the United States. The National Health and Nutrition Examination Surveys (NHANES). JAMA 272:284–91.

Pirkle JL, Kaufmann RB, Brody DJ, Hickman T, Gunter EW, Paschal DC. (1998). Exposure of the U.S. population to lead, 1991–1994. Environ Health Perspect 106:745–50.

Pocock SJ, Smith M, Baghurst P. (1994). Environmental lead and children's intelligence: a systematic review of the epidemiological evidence. BMJ 309:1189–97.

President's Task Force on Environmental Health Risks and Safety Risks to Children. (2000). Eliminating childhood lead poisoning: a federal strategy targeting lead paint hazards. Washington, DC: U.S. Environmental Protection Agency.

Rabinowitz M, Needleman H, Burley M, Finch H, Rees J. (1984). Lead in umbilical blood, indoor air, tap water, and gasoline in Boston. Arch Environ Health 39:299–301.

Rice DC. (1992). Lead exposure during different developmental periods produces different effects on FI performance in monkeys tested as juveniles and adults. Neurotoxicology 13:757–70.

Roscoe RJ, Gittleman JL, Deddens JA, Petersen MR, Halperin WE. (1999). Blood lead levels among children of lead-exposed workers: a meta-analysis. Am J Ind Med 36:475–81.

Rothenberg SJ, Schnaas L, Perroni E, Hernandez RM, Martinez S, Hernandez C. (1999). Pre- and postnatal lead effect on head circumference: a case for critical periods. Neurotoxicol Teratol 21:1–11.

Schwartz BS, Lee BK, Lee GS, Stewart WF, Simon D, Kelsey K, Todd AC. (2000). Associations of blood lead, dimercaptosuccinic acid–chelatable lead, and tibia lead with polymorphisms in the vitamin D receptor and δ-aminolevulinic acid dehydratase genes. Environ Health Perspect 108:949–54.

Schwartz J. (1994). Low-level lead exposure and children's IQ: a meta-analysis and search for a threshold. Environ Res 65:42–55.

Schwartz J, Landrigan PJ, Feldman RG, Silbergeld EK, Baker EL Jr, von Lindern IH. (1988). Threshold effect in lead-induced peripheral neuropathy. J Pediatr 112:12–7.

Seifert B, Becker K, Helm D, Krause C, Schulz C, Seiwert M. (2000). The German environmental survey 1990/1992 (GerES II): reference concentrations of selected environmental pollutants in blood, urine, hair, house dust, drinking water and indoor air. J Expo Anal Environ Epidemiol 10:552–65.

Shen XM, Wu SH, Yan CH, Zhao W, Ao LM, Zhang YW, He JM, Ying JM, Li RQ, Wu SM, and others. (2001). Delta-aminolevulinate dehydratase polymorphism and blood lead levels in Chinese children. Environ Res 85:185–90.

Silbergeld EK. (1997). Preventing lead poisoning in children. Annu Rev Public Health 18:187–210.

Succop P, Bornschein R, Brown K, Tseng CY. (1998). An empirical comparison of lead exposure pathway models. Environ Health Perspect 106(Suppl 6):1577–83.

Thacker SB, Hoffman DA, Smith J, Steinberg K, Zack M. (1992). Effect of low-level body burdens of lead on the mental development of children: limitations of meta-analysis in a review of longitudinal data. Arch Environ Health 47:336–46.

Tong S. (1998). Lead exposure and cognitive development: persistence and a dynamic pattern. J Paediatr Child Health 34:114–8.

Turner AJ. (1897). Lead poisoning among Queensland children. Aust Med Gazette 16:475–9.

U.S. Department of Housing and Urban Development. (2001). National survey of lead and allergens in housing. Final report. Volume I: Analysis of lead hazards. Revision 6.0. Washington, DC: U.S. Department of Housing and Urban Development.

U.S. Environmental Protection Agency. (1998). Risk analysis to support standards for lead in paint, dust, and soil (EPA 747-R-97-006). Washington, DC: U.S. Environmental Protection Agency.

U.S. Environmental Protection Agency. (2000a). National air pollutant emission trends, 1900–1998. Research Triangle Park, NC: U.S. Environmental Protection Agency.

U.S. Environmental Protection Agency. (2000b). National primary drinking water regulations for lead and copper. Final rule. Fed Reg 65:1950–2015.

U.S. Environmental Protection Agency. (2001a). Lead. Identification of dangerous levels of lead. Final rule. Fed Reg 66:1206–40.

U.S. Environmental Protection Agency. (2001b). National ambient air quality standards (NAAQS). Washington, DC: U.S. Environmental Protection Agency.

U.S. Food and Drug Administration. (1993). Guidance document for lead in shellfish. Washington, DC: U.S. Food and Drug Administration.

U.S. Preventive Services Task Force. (1996). Guide to clinical preventive services. Washington, DC: U.S. Department of Health and Human Services.

Vinceti M, Rovesti S, Bergomi M, Calzolari E, Candela S, Campagna A, Milan M, Vivoli G. (2001). Risk of birth defects in a population exposed to environmental lead pollution. Sci Total Environ 278:23–30.

Watt GC, Britton A, Gilmour WH, Moore MR, Murray GD, Robertson SJ, Womersley J. (1996). Is lead in tap water still a public health problem? An observational study in Glasgow. BMJ 313:979–81.

Weiss B. (1990). Risk assessment: the insidious nature of neurotoxicity and the aging brain. Neurotoxicology 11:305–13.

World Health Organization. (2000a). Guidelines for air quality. Geneva: World Health Organization.

World Health Organization. (2000b). Guidelines for drinking water quality. Geneva: World Health Organization.

Yiin LM, Rhoads GG, Lioy PJ. (2000). Seasonal influences on childhood lead exposure. Environ Health Perspect 108:177–82.

5

Metals—Mercury, Arsenic, Cadmium, and Manganese

The previous chapter documents the child health threats posed by lead, the most intensely studied heavy metal. This chapter describes the known and potential health hazards of other metals and metalloids including mercury, arsenic, cadmium, and manganese. Except for mercury, it is the inorganic and organic derivatives of these elements that are potential child health hazards. In common with PCBs and certain other stable organochlorine compounds, cadmium and methylmercury tend to persist in environmental media and to bioaccumulate in certain foods eaten by humans. While lead, mercury, arsenic, and cadmium have no known essential role in human biology, inorganic manganese is an essential trace element required for the normal function of several important enzymes. Inhaled inorganic manganese, however, can cause neurotoxicity among occupationally exposed adults. Although high-level exposures to mercury (especially methylmercury) cause severe neurotoxicity among children and adults, there has been little epidemiologic research on the potential roles of dental amalgam (a widespread source of elemental mercury exposure), arsenic, cadmium, and manganese in adverse child health outcomes. This chapter summarizes current knowledge about these elements and points to the need for increased epidemiologic research and biomonitoring.

I. MERCURY

Mercury exists in the natural environment as methylmercury, mercuric sulfide (cinnabar ore), and mercuric chloride. Microbial biotransformation of inorganic mercury creates virtually all of the methylmercury found in environmental media. Synthetic organic mercurials have been used as antimicrobial preservatives in vaccines, other medicines, paints, and seed grain. Elemental mercury is a dense, shiny, silver-white metal that is liquid at room temperature and has a relatively high vapor pressure. Uses of elemental mercury have included mercury cathodes for electrolysis of sodium chloride to produce chlorine gas and caustic soda, extraction of gold from ore, dental amalgam for repairing carious teeth, thermometers, barometers, mercury vapor lamps, electrical switches, and religious remedies and rituals in Latin America and Asia. Environmental inorganic mercury is a minor source of mercury exposure but inorganic mercury products have been used as disinfectants in diaper washes and as analgesics in teething powders for infants. The major issues explored in Part I of this chapter are the uncertainties about potential health risks of low-level exposure to methylmercury from dietary sources and elemental mercury from dental amalgam and other sources.

METHYLMERCURY

Health Effects

Severe neurotoxicity of organic mercury was evident as early as 1866, when exposure in a chemistry laboratory killed two persons. Grave or fatal neurotoxic effects also occurred among syphilitics treated with diethylmercury (1887) and among workers engaged in organic mercury pesticide production during the early twentieth century. After acute adult methylmercury exposure, a latent period of several weeks or even a few months passes before symptoms appear. Methylmercury is extremely neurotoxic in the human fetus and the developing infant.

Molecular Mechanisms

About 95% of ingested methylmercury is absorbed and readily crosses placental and blood-brain barriers. After crossing the blood–brain and placental barriers, methylmercury enters tissues, where it is demethylated and oxidized to divalent mercury that readily reacts with sulfhydryl groups of proteins and thiols (e.g., tubulin, glutathione). Possible mechanisms for toxicity of methylmercury and divalent mercury include (Agency for Toxic Substances and Disease Registry, 1999b)

- Oxidative stress with generation of free radicals that attack protein and DNA
- Disruption of microtubule formation, impairing cell motility and control of chromosome movement during cell division
- Increased permeability of the blood–brain barrier
- Disruption of DNA replication and protein synthesis
- Interference with proteins involved in neuronal calcium metabolism

In experimental animals, prenatal low-level methylmercury exposure inhibits neuronal cell division and migration, key processes in the developing brain, causing widespread brain damage. Neonatal exposures cause focal cell loss, primarily in the cerebellum and occipital cortex.

Neurotoxicity: Epidemic Poisonings

Minamata. In 1953, a strange polio-like disease struck inhabitants of Minamata, Japan, most victims being coastal villagers who regularly ate fish from the adjacent bay. Onset of the epidemic coincided with the startup of acetaldehyde production at a coastal factory later shown to have used mercuric oxide as a catalyst. Investigators observed that stray cats developed neurotoxicity after eating local shellfish. A heat-stable compound present in shellfish and factory effluents caused neurotoxicity in experimental animals. The local government did not intervene at this stage, as requested by public health authorities, on the grounds that the causative agent was not identified with certainty. Researchers finally identified the neurotoxin as methylmercury in 1963, but it was not until 1968 that Japanese authorities officially recognized it as the causal agent and intervened.

Investigators identified over 2000 victims, including about 64 prenatally exposed infants (Harada, 1995). Affected infants generally appeared normal at birth but later developed signs and symptoms of severe neurotoxicity: mental retardation, abnormal reflexes, ataxia, dysarthria, involuntary movements, and cerebral palsy. None crawled, stood, or talked before age 3 years, and many could not walk at age 7 years. Some infants exhibited severe neurotoxic effects, while their mothers had mild or no symptoms. Autopsies of infants who died showed greatest brain damage among those exposed during the third trimester. Because they did not suspect mercury initially, investigators did not collect blood or hair samples but many families followed the Japanese custom of preserving a dried section of umbilical cord. Children born during 1950–1965, the peak period of acetaldehyde production, had the highest umbilical cord mercury levels. Fish mercury levels (10–30 $\mu g/g$) and average fish consumption (300 g/day) at Minamata were much higher than current levels in United States.

Iraq. Methylmercury and other synthetic organic mercurials were used for several decades during the early twentieth century to protect seeds from fungal damage and improve crop yields. Unwitting use of methylmercury-treated seed grain for food caused several recognized epidemics of severe neurotoxicity in Iraq during 1955–1972; the largest epidemic (1971–1972) involved over 6000 cases with several hundred deaths. Similar outbreaks occurred in other countries (Pakistan, Guatemala, Ghana), and these disastrous experiences finally led to worldwide bans of alkylmercurials for seed treatment.

As in Minamata, some prenatally exposed infants had substantial neurologic deficits even though their mothers reported no symptoms or only mild, transitory paresthesias (Amin-Zaki et al., 1979). Signs and symptoms among 32 prenatally exposed infants included microcephaly, irritability, exaggerated reactions to stimuli, and abnormal reflexes. Among eight infants with severe cerebral palsy, six were blind and two had minimal sight; among their mothers, peak hair mercury levels occurred during the third trimester (average, 444 $\mu g/g$). Among infants with milder signs, the lowest peak maternal hair mercury level during pregnancy was 32 $\mu g/g$. Up to age 4 months, blood methylmercury among infants exceeded maternal levels, consistent with continued exposure through breast milk. Follow-up of severe cases to age 5 years showed persistent neurologic abnormalities and delayed developmental milestones, such as, inability at age 2 years to walk two steps without support or respond to simple verbal communication.

Among 49 Iraqi children aged 2–16 years with high postnatal exposures, about half had severe effects including ataxia, dysarthria, visual deficits (blurred vision, constricted fields, blindness), hearing deficits, glove and stocking numbness and paresthesias, involuntary movements, and incontinence (Amin-zaki et al., 1978). The severity of neurologic abnormalities was associated with estimated blood mercury concentrations near the end of the exposure period (using a blood mercury half-life of 56 days and extrapolating back in time from current blood levels). The degree of recovery over a 2-year follow-up period was inversely related to the initial severity of signs and symptoms; all children had persistent hyperreflexia, even those with initially mild poisoning. About a third of the initially blind children had recovered partial sight, and about a third of the severely poisoned children remained physically and mentally incapacitated (Amin-zaki et al., 1978). A WHO expert group reviewed dose–response data from Iraq and estimated risks of fetal neurotoxicity of 5% and 30%, respectively, at maternal hair mercury levels of 10–20 $\mu g/g$ and 70+ $\mu g/g$ (World Health Organization, 1990).

Neurotoxicity: Environmental Exposures
Studies of several fish-eating populations exposed to methylmercury at levels considerably below those in Minamata and Iraq have not shown consistent evidence of neurotoxic effects (Myers and Davidson, 1998). Results from the two largest longitudinal studies, the Faroe Islands and Seychelles Islands birth cohort studies, are shown in Table 5–1. Faroe Islands residents eat diets rich in fish and marine mammals (pilot whales) containing relatively high concentrations of methylmercury, PCBs, and potentially protective antioxidants (selenium and vitamin E); the median maternal hair mercury level during pregnancy was 4.5 $\mu g/g$, much lower than at Minamata (41 $\mu g/g$) but higher than in the United States (<1 $\mu g/g$). Cord blood methylmercury levels were inversely related to scores on a standardized neurologic examination at age 2 weeks, independent of PCBs (Steuerwald et al., 2000). Breast-feeding was associated with higher infant hair mercury level at age 12 months and *early* developmental milestone attainment (sitting, creeping, and rising). Assessment at age 7 years, however, indicated that cord-blood mercury level was associated with deficits in language, attention, and visuospatial memory, independent of cord blood PCB level (Grandjean et al., 1999).

The Seychelles Islands study population is remote from polluting industry, consumes large amounts of fish but not whales, and has a low prevalence of tobacco and alcohol use among women. The median maternal prenatal hair mercury level during pregnancy was 5.9 $\mu g/g$, slightly higher than that of the Faroese women. Prenatal or postnatal mercury exposure indices were inconsistently related to developmental milestones or neurobehavioral scores up to age 5 years.

High-level prenatal methylmercury exposure causes similar behavioral and pathologic effects in young animals and humans, that is, mental retardation, cerebellar ataxia, primitive reflexes, dysarthria, and seizures. Relatively low prenatal exposures cause visual memory deficits, abnormal social behavior, and reduced growth at puberty in nonhuman primates, while low neonatal exposures produce visual spatial contrast sensitivity deficits. Monkeys exposed from birth to adulthood to low doses of methylmercury displayed visual recognition memory deficits during infancy, slower retrieval of treats, impaired fingertip vibration sense in middle age, and slight visual field deficits as adults (Rice and

TABLE 5–1. Major Birth Cohort Studies of Mercury and Neurobehavioral Effects

Main Author, Population	Population	Exposures and Associations
Faroe Islands		
Grandjean et al. (1992)	1023 mother–infant pairs; exposed to methylmercury, PCBs, and other contaminants mainly from eating pilot whales; marine fish minor source of exposure	Cord blood mercury—median, 24.2 μg/L; 75th percentile, 40 μg/L; maternal hair mercury—median, 4.5 μg/g; 13% exceeded 10 μg/g
Grandjean et al. (1995)	583 infants followed to age 12 months; recorded age first sat without support, crawled, and stood without support	Early milestone development associated with breast-feeding and increased infant hair mercury level at age 12 months but not with maternal hair (at delivery) or cord blood mercury level
Grandjean et al. (1997, 1999)	917 children tested at age 7 years; clinical examination and neurophysiologic and neuropsychologic tests	Inverse associations between cord blood and maternal hair mercury levels and scores on tests of language, attention, memory, and visuospatial and motor functions that persisted at maternal hair mercury levels below 10 μg/g; cord blood mercury most closely associated with language, attention, and memory deficits; concurrent child hair and blood mercury levels were less predictive but were inversely associated with visuospatial memory
Grandjean et al. (1998)	112 children whose maternal hair mercury level was 10–20 μg/g and 112 matched children whose maternal hair mercury level was <3 μg/g, age 7 years	High-exposure group had small deficits in motor function (especially fingertapping), language, and memory
Murata et al. (1999)	Reanalysis of data on brainstem auditory evoked potentials	Maternal hair and cord blood but not child's concurrent hair mercury level associated with brainstem auditory evoked potential abnormalities

Reference	Study description	Findings
Budtz-Jørgensen et al. (2000)	Estimated BMDs of cord blood mercury for deficits in attention, language, and verbal memory scores at age 7 years	95% confidence lower limit of estimated BMDs for cord blood mercury was about 5 μg/L (equivalent to a maternal hair mercury level of about 1 μg/g)
Grandjean et al. (2001)	435 children age 7 years; measured PCB levels in umbilical cord tissue	Association between cord tissue PCBs and deficits on 2 of 17 neuro-psychologic outcomes; possible interaction between PCBs and mercury in highest mercury tertile
Seychelles Islands		
Myers et al. (1995)	779 mother–infant pairs, methylmercury from marine fish; infants tested at age 6 months (visual recognition memory and developmental screening tests)	Maternal hair total mercury during pregnancy—median, 5.9 μg/g (range, 0.5–27 μg/g); no associations with neurodevelopmental scores at age 6.5 months
Davidson et al. (1995); Myers et al. (1997)	738 infants assessed at 19 months, 736 retested at 29 months (infant development and behavior)	No association between maternal hair mercury during pregnancy and psychomotor or mental development scores or age at first walking or talking
Axtell et al. (1998); Davidson et al. (1998); Myers et al. (2000); Palumbo et al. (2000)	711 children aged 5.5 years	No consistent associations between prenatal or postnatal mercury exposure indices and reduced neuropsychologic scores (including overall indices, subscales, and recombined subscales); positive association between postnatal mercury exposure and memory subscale scores
Crump et al. (2000)	Estimated maternal hair mercury BMDs for neurologic tests, neuropsychologic tests, and developmental milestone data at four follow-up examinations (age 6, 19, 29, and 66 months)	The average lower 95% confidence limit BMD for maternal hair mercury was about 25 μg/g (range, 19–30 μg/g)

Hayward, 1999). Animal studies have not yet replicated the usual pattern of human methylmercury exposure, that is, generally intermittent and related to fish consumption.

Other Effects

All three forms of mercury cumulate to higher levels in kidney than any other tissue and can cause toxicity ranging from increased urinary protein levels (indicative of renal tubular damage) to renal failure with nephrosis and necrosis of proximal tubules. For instance, infants dermally exposed to diapers washed with soap containing phenylmercury have increased urinary excretion of γ-glutamyl transpeptidase. After exposure to organic mercury, children are more susceptible than adults to skin changes (acrodynia or "pink disease") including rash followed by peeling skin on the palms of the hands and soles of the feet, itching, and joint pain. Acrodynia was more common in the past, when mercury-containing laxatives, worming medications, teething powders, and diaper rinses were widely used. There is limited animal and inadequate human evidence that methylmercury is carcinogenic, and the EPA concluded that it is unlikely to be a human carcinogen at exposure levels generally encountered from environmental sources.

Exposures

Given the high toxicity of mercury, it is surprising that only Germany and the United States appear to have collected nationally representative data on mercury levels in children and reproductive-age women (Table 5–2) (Centers for Disease Control and Prevention 2001b, 2001c; Seifert et al., 2000).

Exposure Biomarkers

Blood mercury, about 95% of which is bound to red blood cells, has a half-life of about 50 days and thus reflects recent exposure. The half-life of methylmercury in the blood of lactating women is about half that in non-lactating women due to excretion in breast milk. The cord blood mercury concentration is about 20%–30% higher than that of maternal blood and reflects fetal exposure during late gestation, the period of greatest susceptibility to neurotoxicity. Maternal blood and hair but not breast milk mercury levels are associated with methylmercury exposure from fish consumption. About 90% of methylmercury is excreted in bile/feces and the remainder in urine and breast milk. Incomplete development of biliary transport systems contributes to a longer half-life of methylmercury in infants compared to adults.

TABLE 5–2. Norms and Health-Based Limits for Selected Metals in Human Specimens

Sample	Norm or Limit
Mercury	
Blood (age 1–5 years)	1.4 μg/L (CI 0.7–4.8), 90th percentile[a]
Blood (age 6–14 years)	1.1 μg/L, 90th percentile[b]
Blood (women age 16–49 years)	6.2 μg/L (CI 4.7–7.9), 90th percentile[a]
Cord blood	5 μg/L (BMDL)[c]
Hair (age 1–5 years)	0.4 μg/g (CI 0.3–1.8), 90th percentile[d]
Hair (women age 16–49 years)	1.4 μg/g (CI 0.9–1.7), 90th percentile[d]
Maternal hair	1 μg/g (BMDL)[c]
	25 μg/g (BMDL)[e]
	10–20 μg/g (BMD)[f]
	12 μg/g (BMDL)[g]
Urine (age 6–14 years)	1.9 μg/g creatinine, 90th percentile[b]
Arsenic	
Urine (age 6–14 years)	14.1 μg/g creatinine, 90th percentile[b]
Cadmium	
Blood (age 1–19 years)	0.4 μg/L (CI 0.3–1.0), 90th percentile[a]
Blood (age 6–14 years)	0.3 μg/L, 90th percentile[b]
Urine (age 6–14 years)	0.15 μg/g creatinine, 90th percentile[b]

[a]Centers for Disease Control and Prevention (2001a).

[b]Seifert et al. (2000).

[c]Budtz-Jorgensen et al. (2000).

[d]Centers for Disease Control and Prevention (2001c).

[e]Crump et al. (2000).

[f]World Health Organization (1990).

[g]National Academy of Sciences (2000).

BMDL = benchmark dose limit (lower 95% confidence limit on BMD).

BMD = benchmark dose.

Hair grows at the rate of about 1 cm per month, and the mercury content in a given segment of hair is about 250-fold that in blood at the time the segment was formed. Maternal hair mercury levels correlate strongly with those in fetal brain, cord blood, and newborn hair; thus segmental hair mercury analysis is valuable for retrospective mercury exposure estimation. Published studies vary as to whether they measured total mercury or methylmercury, but over 80% of total mercury in hair from fish-eating populations is methylmercury. Women exposed during the major poisoning incidents had hair mercury levels of up to 700 μg/g in Minamata (median, 41 μg/g) and over 400 μg/g in Iraq. Mothers in longitudinal studies of fish-eating populations all had hair mercury levels below 40 μg/g.

United States and German biomonitoring surveys showed that mercury levels were generally low; in the United States, about 10% of women had hair mercury levels within one-tenth of potentially hazardous levels, indicating a relatively narrow margin of safety. Average hair mercury levels in local studies in the United States have usually been under 1 $\mu g/g$, that is, about the level expected for exposure at the EPA reference dose for methylmercury. A Canadian methylmercury screening program tested almost 40,000 aboriginal persons during 1972–1992 (Wheatley and Paradis, 1998). Inuit communities dependent on diets high in fish and sea mammals had the highest average cord blood and adult mercury levels; over 30% of reproductive-age Inuit women had hair methylmercury levels over 10 $\mu g/g$. Blood mercury levels varied substantially by season, corresponding to high consumption of fish and seafood in the early fall and early winter.

Risk Management

It was not until the late 1960s and 1970s that investigators discovered the ability of aquatic microbes to methylate mercury and the bioaccumulation of methylmercury from concentrations in water to 1 million-fold higher levels in predators such as tuna and marine mammals atop the aquatic food chain. By then, however, vast amounts of mercury from chlor-alkali, pulp and paper, mining, and other industries had been discharged into aquatic environments worldwide. The largest current users of mercury are chlor-alkali plants (production of chlorine and caustic soda) and electrical/electronic industries (electric lighting, wiring, switches, batteries).

Air

Analyses of mercury in peat and lake sediments in remote parts of North America indicate that mercury emissions into air have increased about fivefold since the beginning of the industrial period. The major sources of air emissions are coal-fired utility/industrial boilers (50%), municipal waste combustors (20%), and medical waste incinerators (10%). Future mercury emission levels will be heavily influenced by increasing use of coal to meet energy needs, especially since emissions from municipal and medical waste combustion declined 50%–75% during the 1990s in the United States.

Airborne mercury emissions from natural and anthropogenic sources disperse in the environment by long-range atmospheric transportation. Elemental mercury vapor tends to remain airborne, while inorganic mercury is rapidly cleared to soil and water compartments, deposition being enhanced by precipitation. Modeling indicates that the highest deposition rates of airborne mercury in the United States occur in the southern Great Lakes region, the Ohio River valley, the northeastern states, and other scattered areas. Because atmospheric mercury deposition accounts for much of the mercury in fish in the northeastern United States, even modest increases in atmospheric mercury loading could further elevate levels in fish. Air mercury levels over the Atlantic Ocean increased until about 1990 and have continued to increase in northern Canada and Alaska due to long-range transport of increasing global emissions.

Phenylmercuric acetate was used as a fungicide/bactericide to prolong the shelf life of interior latex paint up to 1990 in the United States and was the source for two reported cases of childhood mercury poisoning (acrodynia). At that time, the EPA permitted interior latex paint to contain up to 300 ppm mercury but did not require a label warning about the presence and concentration of mercury; paint used in the home of one patient actually contained about 950 ppm mercury, or three times the EPA limit. After application, phenylmercuric acetate apparently breaks down and releases elemental mercury. Air mercury levels were greatly elevated during application of latex paint and decreased rapidly thereafter but remained above background levels for at least several years, reflecting continued mercury release. Subsequent investigations showed that exposed children had higher urinary mercury levels than older persons. Even in homes where paint contained less than 200 ppm mercury, air mercury levels were up to 1.5 $\mu g/m^3$ (median, 0.3 $\mu g/m^3$), with some homes exceeding the ATSDR acceptable indoor concentration for continuous exposure of 0.5 $\mu g/m^3$ (Beusterien et al., 1991). By 1991, all registrations for mercury compounds in paints had been canceled by the EPA or voluntarily withdrawn by manufacturers. This occurrence shows the importance of regulatory measures to ensure that children are not exposed to toxicants in the indoor environment arising from the use of household products.

Reduced mercury emissions can be achieved through manufacturing controls (product substitution, process modification, and materials separation), coal cleaning, and flue gas treatment technologies. Specific examples of manufacturing controls include replacement of mercury cathodes in chlor-alkali plants, reduced use of mercury in household batteries and fluorescent lights, and removal of mercury-containing materials (e.g., batteries, fluorescent lights, thermostats) from wastes prior to incineration. Conventional cleaning methods reduce the coal mercury content by about half, and control devices on utility and industrial boilers can remove over 90% of mercury emissions.

Under the Clean Air Act, the EPA has set rules for municipal and medical waste incineration with the goal of reducing mercury emissions to 10% of 1995 levels. The EPA has also proposed mercury emission standards for hazardous waste incinerators and is evaluating reductions for industrial boilers, chlor-alkali plants, and Portland cement kilns. Other Clean Air Act regulations, including those for fine particulate matter ($PM_{2.5}$), will contribute to reduced mercury emissions. In 1998, the EPA required coal-fired power plants to monitor smokestack mercury emissions. Mercury consumption in the United States decreased by 75% between 1988 and 1996 due to federal bans on its use in latex paints, pesticides, and batteries, state regulation of emissions and products, and state-mandated recycling programs.

Water
The Castner Kellner method for the electrolytic production of sodium hydroxide and chlorine from brine was introduced in the late 1800s. Each plant required about 100 tons of elemental mercury for cathodes to start production and intermittent supplements to replace losses in cooling water. As shown through investigation at Minamata and other sites, effluents from such plants contaminated the aquatic environment and food chain with methylmercury. Mercury levels in aquatic environments remote from polluting industries and other forms of development correlate strongly with air levels. Hydroelectric dams create new or enlarged aquatic environments where mercury leaches from rocks and soil and enters the aquatic food chain. Average mercury concentrations in pike in northern Quebec increased fivefold after construction of the James Bay hydroelectric dams, thereby exposing aboriginal and other populations dependent on local fish to increased methylmercury levels. Massive amounts of liquid elemental mercury have been used to extract gold, silver, copper, and tin from ores. Between 1550 and 1880, an estimated 200,000 metric tons of elemental mercury were used in South American gold mining. This practice persists in the Amazon basin, exposing workers to elemental mercury and local populations to methylmercury-contaminated fish.

Food
Predatory fish, shellfish, and sea mammals comprise the main methylmercury exposure sources for the general population. Dietary exposures before and during pregnancy are important because the half-life of methylmercury in maternal tissues is 1–9 months. In fish-eating populations, children are exposed prenatally, during breast-feeding (methylmercury in breast milk), and by eating fish from an early age. All fish contain some mercury, mostly as methylmercury, and large carnivorous freshwater and marine fish and fish-eating mammals can have levels

above 1 $\mu g/g$, the current FDA action level; average levels of most commercially important marine fish are 0.1 $\mu g/g$ or lower. About 95% of methylmercury in ingested fish is absorbed. The EPA estimated that 7% of reproductive-age women and about 20% of all fish-eating children aged 3–6 years exceed the EPA methylmercury RfD (0.1 $\mu g/kg/day$) (Table 5–3) (U.S. Environmental Protection Agency, 1997).

The Minamata epidemic remains the only known occurrence of severe methylmercury poisoning due to fish consumption. The hazards of methylmercury in fish must be balanced against the nutritional benefits of fish, especially in indigenous populations dependent on fish as a major dietary component. Fish are excellent sources of selenium and omega-3 fatty acids, substances important in brain growth that may offset to some degree the neurotoxicity of low-level methylmercury contamination.

In general, the FDA and other regulatory agencies issue advisories for mercury in fish rather than promulgating limits. A Health Canada advisory states that (1) reproductive-age women and children should limit their consumption of swordfish, shark, and fresh or frozen tuna to one

TABLE 5–3. Guidelines and Standards for Chronic Exposure to Mercury

Exposure	Guideline or Limit	Agency
Air (elemental)[a]	0.2 $\mu g/m^3$	ATSDR[b]
	0.3 $\mu g/m^3$	EPA[c]
Air (inorganic)	1 $\mu g/m^3$ (annual average)	WHO[d]
Drinking water	1 $\mu g/L$ (total mercury)	WHO[e]
	2 $\mu g/L$ (inorganic mercury)	EPA[f]
Food (methylmercury)	0.1$\mu g/kg/day$	EPA[c]
	0.3 $\mu g/kg/day$	ATSDR[b]
	1.0 $\mu g/g$ (fish, edible portion)	FDA[g]
	Women who are pregnant or may become pregnant or are breast-feeding and children should not eat shark, swordfish, king mackerel, or tilefish	FDA[h]
Chronic oral intake (inorganic)	0.3 $\mu g/kg/day$	EPA[c]

[a]Inhalation, chronic exposure.
[b]Agency for Toxic Substances and Disease Registry (2002).
[c]U.S. Environmental Protection Agency (2001b).
[d]World Health Organization (2000a).
[e]World Health Organization (2000b).
[f]U.S. Environmental Protection Agency (2001a).
[g]U.S. Food and Drug Administration (2000).
[h]U.S. Food and Drug Administration (2001).

meal monthly, (2) mercury concentrations in these fish (0.5–1.5 μg/g) are above the Canadian guideline of 0.5 μg/g, but the nutritional value of fish justifies occasional consumption, and (3) mercury levels in canned tuna are usually well below 0.5 μg/g. The FDA analyses of canned tuna indicated that the average mercury level was 0.17 μg/g (range, <0.1–0.75 μg/g). The FDA recently advised pregnant women not to eat shark, swordfish, king mackerel, and tilefish because of their high methylmercury levels. Surveys of the Cree native Indian population in northern Quebec indicate that the prevalence of hair mercury levels greater than 15 μg/g declined from 14% to 3% during 1988–1994, a change attributed to education on avoidance of high-mercury fish species (Dumont et al., 1998). Mercury levels in meat, liver, and kidney from Swedish pigs declined during the 1980s, possibly due to reduced use of fish in pig feed.

Other Sources
Despite their extreme neurotoxicity, childhood exposure to organic mercury compounds continues. An estimated 7000–10,000 infants in Argentina were exposed to phenylmercury compounds used as disinfectants during commercial diaper washing; health outcomes included acrodynia and elevated urinary γ-glutamyl transferase levels (Gotelli et al., 1985). Until recently, sodium ethylmercurithiosalicylate (thimerosal) was used to prevent microbial contamination of vaccines and other biologics; three professional societies and the U.S. Public Health Service recommended rapid introduction of thimerosal-free vaccines (Centers for Disease Control and Prevention, 2000). As of late 2001, all routine pediatric vaccines were being produced in thimerosal-free or thimerosal-reduced (>95% reduction) formulations.

General Considerations
Given the extraordinary sensitivity of the developing fetus to methylmercury, reproductive-age women have the highest priority for preventive actions including

- Policies and actions to further reduce food-related exposure while preserving access to beneficial and traditional diets
- Surveillance to evaluate progress and identify residual problems
- Continued research on neurobehavioral and other potential health effects of low-level perinatal methylmercury exposure, including delayed effects in adulthood

Major uncertainties exist regarding a safe level for ingested methylmercury. The available data from Iraq and Minamata were inadequate for robust estimates of a NOAEL and an RfD. The EPA, however, set an RfD for methylmercury of 0.1 μg/kg/day in 1995 (Table 5–3) based on developmental delays and neurologic abnormalities among Iraqi children, incorporating an uncertainty factor of 10. The EPA plans to review its RfD for methylmercury using new data from the Faroe Islands, the Seychelles Islands, and the U.S. Great Lakes region.

The ATSDR based its MRL for methylmercury on data from the Seychelles Islands study, in which no adverse effects were evident; on the assumption that the average exposure among study participants (mean maternal hair mercury was 15.3 μg/g) was a NOAEL, the ATSDR set the MRL at 0.3 μg/kg/day. A benchmark analysis of the Seychelles Islands study assessed neurobehavioral and developmental milestone data at four follow-up examinations; the average lower 95% confidence limit on estimated BMDs for maternal hair mercury was about 25 μg/g (range, 19–30 μg/g) (Crump et al., 2000). Among the epidemiologic studies, only the Faroe Islands study has shown adverse effects (reduced performance on language, attention, and memory tests at age 7 years) at maternal hair mercury levels less than 10 μg/g (Grandjean et al., 1997). The National Academy of Sciences recently concluded that the RfD for methylmercury should be based on the BMD lower limit for abnormal scores on the Boston Naming Test in the Faroe Islands study (equivalent to a mercury level of 12 μg/g in maternal hair); because the Academy also recommended an uncertainty factor of at least 10, maternal hair mercury concentrations should be no higher than 1.2 μg/g (National Academy of Sciences, 2000).

ELEMENTAL AND INORGANIC MERCURY

Health Effects

Dental amalgam is the major source of elemental mercury and (after oxidation in tissues) inorganic mercury exposure in the general population. Elemental mercury is highly lipophilic, and about 70%–80% of inhaled material is absorbed and disseminated in blood; it readily crosses the blood-brain and placental barriers and enters tissues, where it is rapidly oxidized to divalent mercury. The longest half-life of mercury in tissues occurs in brain, while kidneys accumulate mercury to levels about ten times those in other tissues (Agency for Toxic Substances and Disease Registry, 1999b).

Most evidence of the health effects of elemental mercury comes from adult studies. Acute exposure to very high levels of elemental mercury vapor can cause pulmonary edema, respiratory distress, and death; the nervous system and the kidneys are the most sensitive targets at lower exposure levels. Neurotoxic effects in children accidentally exposed to moderately high levels include dizziness, insomnia, peripheral neuropathy (numbness and tingling in the hands and feet), tremors, and irritability. Although major debates about the safety of dental amalgam have occurred since its introduction in the 1800s, the potential child health effects of prenatal and childhood exposure to this source remain virtually unresearched and unknown.

Mercurous chloride, also known as *calomel*, was used to treat many ailments beginning in the eighteenth century and in teething powders during the 1940s, causing many childhood poisonings. Even in recent years, there have been mercury poisoning cases caused by Mexican products containing calomel for treatment of acne and other skin conditions (Centers for Disease Control and Prevention, 1996a). Renal toxicity of divalent mercury appears to be related mainly to actions on enzymes and transport proteins that take up mercury in proximal tubular cells. A small fraction of persons, possibly due to genetic susceptibility, produce anti-glomerular basement membrane and anti-DNA antibodies in response to inorganic mercury exposure, and some develop autoimmune glomerulonephritis. Inorganic mercury triggers an autoimmune syndrome in susceptible rodents including autoreactive T cells, high IgE, anticollagen types I and II IgGs, glomerulonephropathy, and gastrointestinal necrotizing vasculitis.

Exposures

The estimated percentage of total mercury uptake attributable to dental amalgam is about 30% for children and 50% for adults, making it the single largest source for the general population (Richardson, 1995). Amalgam dental fillings continually release elemental mercury vapor that is inhaled and readily absorbed through the lungs. The average number of carious permanent teeth per person among children aged 2–10 years decreased from 2.3 in NHANES I to 1.4 in NHANES III; corresponding values for persons aged 6–18 years were, respectively, 4.4 and 1.9 (Brown et al., 2000). Release of mercury vapor from amalgam increases about five-fold when chewing, brushing, or consuming hot beverages; mouth breathing, common in children, increases exposure.

The number of dental amalgam fillings in children and adults is associated with blood, breast milk, and urinary mercury levels. Inhaled elemental mercury is transported in blood to tissues and oxidized to inorganic mercury, which is transported mainly in plasma and excreted in urine; plasma and urinary mercury levels appear to be the best indices of mercury uptake from dental amalgam fillings. Placental mercury levels are strongly correlated with maternal blood levels and with the number of amalgam fillings (Ask et al., 2002).

Estimated infant mercury exposure from breast-feeding was up to

0.3 μg/kg/day (approximately half as inorganic mercury and half as methylmercury) (Oskarsson et al., 1996). The number of amalgam fillings estimated to cause exposure at the tolerable daily intake level for mercury vapor (0.014 μg/kg/day) was one for toddlers and children, three for teenagers, and four for adults (Richardson, 1995). A survey of urban homes showed that the average mercury concentration in house dust samples (1.7 μg/g) was 30 times that in soil samples, suggesting the existence of important indoor sources (Rasmussen et al., 2001). Drinking water is a minor source of mercury exposure.

Risk Management

Child health issues related to elemental mercury include its widespread use in dental amalgam and the difficulty of recognizing sporadic cases caused by exposures such as accidental indoor spillage or religious practices. Although Egyptians used a mercury amalgam in dentistry over 1500 years ago, widespread use has occurred only during the past 150 years. Dental amalgam causes continuous exposure to mercury; on precautionary grounds alone, this argues for not using amalgam among children and reproductive-age women. Removal of amalgam causes an exponential decline of blood, plasma, and urinary mercury levels, with values at 2 months being about 60% of preremoval levels. The importance of dental amalgam should decrease as prevalence rates of dental caries decline (fluoridation and fluoride supplements) and as the use of substitute materials increases.

Potential indoor sources of elemental mercury exposure include broken switches, thermostats, and thermometers and religious practices. Mercury can easily be obtained for religious or cultural purposes including sprinkling on the floor of a home or car, burning in a candle, and mixing with perfume. Many users are not aware of its toxicity and may be exposed to indoor air mercury levels far above occupational exposure limits. If mercury is spilled on floors, it tends to remain in cracks and carpets and emit dense mercury vapor; sporadic childhood poisoning cases from such sources continue to be reported (Centers for Disease Control and Prevention, 1996b).

CONCLUSIONS

Proven Child Health Outcomes

- Moderate to high prenatal exposure to methylmercury can cause severe neurotoxic effects ranging from abnormal reflexes, irritability, delayed milestones, and visual disturbances to cerebral palsy, micro-cephaly, blindness, and major cognitive deficits.

- Postnatal exposure to high methylmercury levels can cause ataxia, dysarthria, visual deficits (including blindness), hearing deficits, pe-ripheral neuropathy, and involuntary movements.
- Neurotoxic effects in children accidentally exposed to moderately high levels of elemental mercury include dizziness, insomnia, peripheral neuropathy, tremors, and irritability.
- Inorganic mercury (mercurous chloride) used in teething powders dur-ing the early twentieth century caused many childhood poisonings (acrodynia) characterized by irritability, stomatitis, insomnia, and erythema of the hands, feet, and other areas.
- All three forms of mercury can cause increased urinary protein excre-tion indicative of renal tubular damage.

Unresolved Issues and Knowledge Gaps

- Neurotoxic effects of low-level prenatal or childhood exposure to methylmercury from diet. The two major birth cohort studies of pre-natal maternal exposure to fish or marine mammals contaminated by methylmercury at levels well below those in Minamata, but higher than those in the general population, have produced conflicting results:
  - The Faroes Islands study showed that cord blood mercury levels were associated with significant deficits in language, attention, and visuo-spatial memory at age 7 years, independent of cord blood PCB levels.
  - The Seychelles Islands study showed no consistent associations be-tween prenatal or postnatal mercury exposure indices and develop-mental milestones or neurobehavioral scores up to age 5 years.
- The health effects of exposure to elemental mercury from dental amal-gam during fetal development and childhood, if any, remain unknown.
- Knowledge gaps exist concerning neurobehavioral and other potential health effects of low-level perinatal methylmercury exposure.

Risk Management Issues

- Prevention—policies and actions are required to further reduce mercury emissions and education to reduce consumption of highly contaminated aquatic foods.
- Biomonitoring—biomonitoring of children and reproductive-age women is needed to measure progress in reducing perinatal mercury exposure (only the United States and Germany have implemented national track-ing of mercury levels in children).

II. OTHER METALS AND METALLOIDS

In contrast to the relatively well-known effects of mercury on children, most epidemiologic research on arsenic, cadmium, and manganese has involved occupationally and environmentally exposed adults. Arsenic and cadmium can affect a vast array of biochemical and nutritional processes by binding to sulfhydryl groups, generating free radicals, inhibiting antioxidative enzymes, and depleting intracellular glutathione. Countering such effects are metallothioneins (MTs), small cysteine-rich proteins that bind metals and scavenge free radicals. Tissues vary in their MT content and their susceptibility to metals; for example, testes have very low levels of MT, and cadmium exposure triggers Leydig cell death and decreased testosterone production. Cadmium and arsenic compounds inhibit DNA repair systems and are well-known carcinogens in experimental animals and humans.

Arsenic

Arsenic, a metalloid with both metallic and nonmetallic physicochemical properties, occurs naturally in rocks, soil, water, air, plants, and animals and has four valency states (0, -3, $+3$, and $+5$). Inorganic arsenates (pentavalent arsenic) dominate in aerobic surface waters and arsenites (trivalent arsenic) in anaerobic groundwaters (U.S. Environmental Protection Agency, 2000). Although organic arsenic has been considered to be relatively nontoxic, recent evidence suggests otherwise.

Health Effects

Molecular Mechanisms
About 50%–70% of absorbed inorganic arsenate is rapidly reduced in vivo to arsenite; the latter reacts readily with tissue components and inhibits many enzymes. In humans, arsenite is methylated to metabolites (monomethylarsonic acid, dimethylarsinic acid, and trimethylarsine oxide) that are excreted more rapidly. Arsenic may contribute to carcinogenicity in humans by inhibiting DNA repair, causing DNA methylation and oxidative stress, and inhibiting transcription of the hTERT gene (which encodes the reverse transcriptase subunit of human telomerase), causing chromosome end-to-end fusions and other abnormalities. Reduction of pentavalent to trivalent arsenic in vivo may be viewed as an activation pathway, as the trivalent form is more reactive with sulfhydryl groups of tissue components. Although methylation of inorganic arsenic

is still commonly viewed as a detoxification pathway, methylated and di-methylated trivalent arsenicals are more potent cytotoxins, genotoxins, and enzyme inhibitors (Thomas et al., 2001). Dimethylarsinic acid (DMA) is genotoxic and a complete carcinogen in rodents.

Developmental Effects
Inorganic arsenic crosses the human placenta, but there has been little re-search on adverse developmental outcomes. Ecologic and case-control studies have shown elevated risks of spontaneous abortion, birth defects, and/or stillbirths in areas with elevated drinking water or airborne ar-senic levels (Ahmad et al., 2001; Aschengrau et al., 1989; Hopenhayn-Rich et al., 2000; Ihrig et al., 1998; Zierler et al., 1988). Prenatal exposure to high-dose inorganic arsenic caused neural tube birth defects, growth re-tardation, and fetal death in hamsters, mice, rats, and rabbits. The Na-tional Research Council and the ATSDR concluded that there is insuffi-cient evidence to judge if inorganic arsenic can affect reproduction or development in humans (Agency for Toxic Substances and Disease Reg-istry, 2000a; National Academy of Sciences, 1994).

Cancer and Other Chronic Diseases
Several major agencies concluded that arsenic compounds cause skin, lung, bladder, and kidney cancers in humans (International Agency for Research on Cancer, 1980; National Academy of Sciences, 1999; U.S. Environmental Protection Agency, 1994). These conclusions were based mainly on epi-demiologic studies of adults occupationally exposed to airborne arsenic and populations exposed to drinking water containing high arsenic lev-els. The National Academy of Sciences recently concluded that chronic ex-posure to drinking water with arsenic levels less than 50 μg/L is associ-ated with increased risks of bladder and lung cancers (National Academy of Sciences, 2001). An estimated 4–7 excess lifetime cancer cases per 10,000 persons would occur at chronic exposure levels as low as 3 μg/L.

There have been very few epidemiologic studies of the potential role of arsenic in childhood cancer. Exposure to airborne arsenic and other metals (lead, cadmium) from smelters was associated with a doubling of the childhood cancer risk in an ecologic study (Wulff et al., 1996). Chil-dren in northern Chile exposed to drinking water containing 750–800 μg/L arsenic developed skin pigmentation and keratoses (Smith et al., 2000). Lymphocytes from children and women exposed to inorganic ar-senic in drinking water at levels of about 200 μg/L displayed an increased frequency of micronuclei and trisomy compared to less exposed controls (Dulout et al., 1996). Epidemiologic studies of adults exposed to relatively high levels of inorganic arsenic from drinking water or arsenical drugs have shown increased risks of several types of cancer, skin hyperpigmentation/keratoses in areas not exposed to the sun, peripheral neuropathy, cardiovascular disease, anemia, and diabetes.

Exposures

Ingested trivalent and pentavalent soluble inorganic arsenic compounds are readily absorbed and transported in blood and are excreted mainly in urine. The National Academy of Sciences noted that urinary total inorganic arsenic measurement avoids interference from organic arsenic in seafood and better reflects recent and ongoing exposure than blood, hair, or nail levels. Among persons exposed to arsenic in drinking water, children had higher urinary arsenic levels than adults, reflecting their higher daily intake of water per unit body weight. The German Environmental Survey showed that the 90th percentile urinary arsenic level among children was 14.1 μg/g creatinine (Table 5–2). Geometric mean urinary levels among children who consumed fish less than or more than once weekly, respectively, were 5.9 and 10.5 μg/L (Seifert et al., 2000). The half-life of arsenic in blood is only 1 hour and is strongly influenced by recent exposure; hair and nails are subject to contamination. Breast milk arsenic levels are quite low even in areas with high levels in drinking water.

Risk Management

Food, drinking water, and soil are the main potential arsenic exposure sources for children. Children living near point sources of arsenic are at risk of increased exposure, particularly from soil and drinking water. An estimated 13% of the general U.S. population exceed the EPA RfD for inorganic arsenic (0.3 μg/kg/day).

Air
Combustion of fossil fuels and wastes, mining, smelting, pulp and paper production, glass manufacturing, and cement manufacturing are the main industrial sources of airborne arsenic. Although air is a minor exposure source for the general population, young children in zinc and copper smelter communities may have elevated blood and urinary arsenic levels.

Water
Millions of persons in Bangladesh are exposed to high drinking water arsenic levels from deep wells installed to reduce gastrointestinal infections related to contaminated surface water; more localized problems exist in other regions including India, China, Taiwan, Chile, and Argentina. The

EPA estimated that 5.4% of groundwater and only 0.7% of surface water sources in the United States have average arsenic levels above 10 μg/L. High groundwater arsenic levels occur in some western states with sulfide mineral deposits high in arsenic. The National Academy of Sciences assessed epidemiologic data on drinking water arsenic levels and adult cancer and concluded that cancer risks are significant even at the former EPA arsenic drinking water standard (50 μg/L). In 2001 the EPA reduced its arsenic drinking water standard from 50 to 10 μg/L, to be effective 3–5 years after approval (Table 5–4).

Food

Marine fish (e.g., tuna) and shellfish have the highest mean arsenic levels in Canadian and American total diet studies. Current evidence indicates that organic arsenic compounds in fish and shellfish (arsenobetaine and arsenocholine) are excreted rapidly in urine and do not pose a significant risk to humans.

Other Sources

Arsenic, cadmium, and mercury were the metals in indoor and outdoor dust samples in Louisiana that most frequently exceeded EPA risk-based concentrations (Lemus et al., 1996). The last agricultural application involving inorganic arsenic pesticides was voluntarily canceled in 1993, but young children continue to be at risk of unintentional arsenic poisoning from arsenic-based rodenticides. The EPA recently began a review of the potential for child exposure to chromated copper arsenate (CCA), widely used in pressure-treated wood. Leaching from CCA-treated wood used in playground structures and decks can raise arsenic and chromium lev-

TABLE 5–4. Guidelines and Standards for Chronic Exposure to Inorganic Arsenic

Exposure	Guideline or Limit	Agency
Air	1.5×10^{-3} per μg/m^3 (unit risk)	WHO[a]
Drinking water	10 μg/L	WHO[b]
	10 μg/L	EPA[c]
Total oral exposure	0.3 μg/kg/day	ATSDR[d]
	0.3 μg/kg/day	EPA[e]

[a] World Health Organization (2000a); because arsenic is a human carcinogen, the WHO specifies a unit risk (excess lifetime cancer risk of inorganic arsenic).

[b] World Health Organization (2000b).

[c] U.S. Environmental Protection Agency (2001a).

[d] Agency for Toxic Substances and Disease Registry (2002).

[e] U.S. Environmental Protection Agency (2001b).

els in underlying sand or soil, including both trivalent and the more toxic hexavalent chromium. There have been no measurements of arsenic levels in children exposed to CCA-treated wood but adult workers handling arsenic-treated wood have elevated urinary arsenic levels (Jensen et al., 1991).

CADMIUM

Elemental cadmium is a relatively rare, soft, extremely toxic metal used in many products including batteries, pigments, metal coatings, plastics, and metal alloys. Cadmium is ubiquitous in natural environments, usually as inorganic salts. Adults exposed to high levels of inorganic cadmium may develop kidney dysfunction, lung diseases, disturbed calcium metabolism, and osteomalacia.

Health Effects

Endemic itai-itai ("ouch-ouch") disease occurred in the downstream basin of the Jinzu River in Japan beginning about 1912, the name coming from the cries of victims suffering from severe bone pain. Although chronic cadmium poisoning was suspected as a possible cause during the late 1950s, it was not until 1968 that the Japanese government completed research and concluded that the source was rice grown in water contaminated with cadmium from a mine. Health outcomes included irreversible, progressive kidney damage, calcium loss, and osteomalacia (Iwata et al., 1993). The delayed onset and progression of kidney damage reflect the cumulation and persistence of cadmium in tissues. There appear to have been no epidemiologic studies of the potential health effects of prenatal and childhood cadmium exposure.

Molecular Mechanisms

Cadmium enters cells through calcium channels, cumulates intracellularly, and interferes with the uptake and functions of several essential metals (including calcium, zinc, selenium, chromium, and iron). At noncytotoxic doses, cadmium interferes with *p53* and other transcription factors, enhancing the genotoxicity of direct mutagens. Tumor suppressor *p53* is a zinc-dependent DNA transcription factor that controls DNA repair, survival, proliferation, and differentiation in cells with DNA damage; inactivation of this gene by mutation is a key event in many human cancers. Cadmium also interferes with chromosome spindle formation and appears to cause chromosome aberrations among occupationally exposed men. Most cadmium in vivo is bound to MT, but this low molecular weight complex can enter plasma, be excreted into the renal glomerular filtrate, and be reabsorbed in renal tubular cells that split the complex and are exposed to the toxic effects of free cadmium. In liver, cadmium binds to mitochondrial protein sulfhydryl groups and triggers oxidative stress and liver cell injury. Although inhaled cadmium is taken up by olfactory axonal projections, it appears that it is not transported into other parts of the brain.

Reproductive and Developmental Effects
Human evidence is insufficient to assess the potential role of cadmium in prenatal and childhood development. Animals experienced fetal growth deficits and skeletal malformations after prenatal exposure and testicular atrophy from high postnatal exposure.

Kidney
Urinary excretion of small proteins (α1-microglobulin, β2-microglobulin, retinol-binding protein, and N-acetyl-β-D-glucosaminidase) is a sensitive indicator of renal tubular cell injury caused by cadmium and certain other nephrotoxins. A cross-sectional study showed a borderline association between urinary cadmium and small proteins in children (Noonan et al., 2002).

Cancer
The IARC classifies cadmium as a known human carcinogen, while the EPA deems it a probable human carcinogen (International Agency for Research on Cancer, 1994; U.S. Environmental Protection Agency, 1994). Men occupationally exposed to inhaled cadmium dust and fumes had elevated lung cancer risks. In experimental animals, inhaled cadmium caused lung cancer, while ingested cadmium caused leukemia, testicular tumors, and proliferative prostatic lesions; there appear to have been no epidemiologic studies of the potential role of cadmium in childhood cancer.

Other Effects
The few epidemiologic studies of cadmium and cognitive function in children have yielded inconclusive findings because of inadequate exposure assessment and lack of control for potential confounders. Prenatal exposure of rodents to relatively low cadmium levels caused adverse neurobehavioral effects (Agency for Toxic Substances and Disease Registry, 1999a). Other potential effects, based on very limited epidemiologic evi-

dence, include reduced serum free thyroxine (T4) levels and suppressed immediate hypersensitivity and IgG levels.

Exposures

Blood and urine cadmium levels in humans are both good indicators of dietary cadmium intake, the main exposure source among nonsmokers in the general population. Iron deficiency, relatively prevalent among reproductive-age women, increases gastrointestinal cadmium absorption. Blood and hair cadmium levels in children are related to residential proximity to zinc and copper smelters. Cord blood cadmium levels are associated with maternal blood levels but are about tenfold lower; pregnant smokers have higher blood and placental cadmium levels than nonsmokers. At low exposure levels, blood cadmium reflects exposure during the past 2–3 months, while urine cadmium indicates the body burden, particularly that in kidney. Hair is not an ideal indicator, as it is prone to external contamination by airborne cadmium.

The German Environmental Survey and NHANES III appear to provide the only nationally representative cadmium exposure data (Table 5–2) (Centers for Disease Control and Prevention 2001b; Paschal et al., 2000; Seifert et al., 2000). The 90th percentile blood cadmium levels for children in the German Environmental Survey and NHANES III (1999), respectively, were 0.3 and 0.4 $\mu g/L$. During 1988–1994, about 0.2%–0.5% of U.S. children aged 6–19 years had urine cadmium concentrations above 5 $\mu g/g$ creatinine, the current WHO health-based exposure limit (Paschal et al., 2000). Results from NHANES III, however, indicate that the likelihood of renal tubular damage (indicated by urine microalbumin levels above 30 $\mu g/mL$) increased by 1% for each 10% increase in urinary cadmium above the median 0.23 $\mu g/g$ creatinine (Paschal et al., 2000).

Cadmium levels in diet, blood, and urine in Japan and in cadaver kidneys in Sweden decreased by about 40% over the past 10–20 years, possibly due to changed dietary habits or reduced food contamination. A considerable fraction of the adult cadmium body burden may arise from exposures during childhood, when gastrointestinal absorption rates are higher.

Risk Management

Sources

The main industrial sources of airborne cadmium include metal production, waste incineration, battery production, fossil fuel combustion, and cement production. Airborne cadmium, mainly in respirable particulate matter, ranges from 5 ng/m^3 in rural areas to 15 ng/m^3 in urban areas, 60 ng/m^3 in industrial areas, and 300 ng/m^3 near metal smelters. Drinking water usually contains less than 1 μg/L but can reach 10 μg/L in areas influenced by anthropogenic activities. Agricultural soil cadmium levels increase with use of phosphate or sewage sludge fertilizers; food crops readily take up soil cadmium.

Food is the main source of cadmium intake by children and non-smoking adults, with amounts averaging 10–50 μg/day but up to tenfold higher in polluted areas. Compared to breast-fed children, dietary cadmium intake may be up to 12 times higher in infants fed soy-based or cereal-based formula; the estimated weekly intake at age 6 months is 3.1 μg/kg, below the WHO provisional tolerable weekly intake based on kidney effects in adults (7 μg/kg) (Eklund and Oskarsson, 1999). Cadmium intake may be higher if the water used to make the formula also contains cadmium. Only 5%–10% of ingested cadmium is absorbed, but this increases if diets are deficient in zinc, iron, or calcium. The main dietary sources of cadmium in the U.S. adult population are liver, potatoes, spinach, iceberg lettuce, and pasta; this is consistent with evidence that leafy vegetables and grain crops readily take up cadmium from soil contaminated by the use of phosphate or sewage sludge fertilizers. Cereals and shellfish are the main sources of cadmium exposure among non-smoking Swedes.

Uptake of cadmium by rice varies with soil cadmium levels; concentrations in rice varied from less than 10 ng/g (geometric mean) in Australia, Finland, Spain, and the United States to 30 ng/g or more in China, Japan, Italy, and Colombia. Most food crops other than rice contain sufficient zinc to inhibit absorption of ingested cadmium. Surveys of non-smoking women aged 20–50 years in Asia showed that most cadmium was from the diet, with rice alone accounting for about 40%. Northern indigenous populations who regularly consume organ meat, particularly the liver and kidney of caribou, moose, and seal liver, may have cadmium intakes above the EPA RfD for food (Table 5–5). Drinking water usually contains very low cadmium levels (<1 μg/L), with important exceptions such as water contaminated by leaching from waste disposal sites or certain plumbing materials (Agency for Toxic Substances and Disease Registry, 1999a).

Intervention

The EPA RfDs for cadmium are based on the observation that a renal cortex cadmium concentration of 200 μg/g is the highest level not associated with significant proteinuria in adults. Given the toxicity of cadmium

TABLE 5–5. Guidelines and Standards for Chronic Exposure to Cadmium

Exposure	Guideline or Limit	Agency
Air	5 ng/m^3 (average annual)	WHO[a]
Drinking water	3 μg/L	WHO[b]
	5 μg/L	EPA[c]
Oral (food)	1 μg/kg/day	EPA[d]
Total oral	0.2 μg/kg/day	ATSDR[e]

[a]World Health Organization (2000a).

[b]World Health Organization (2000b).

[c]U.S. Environmental Protection Agency (2001a).

[d]U.S. Environmental Protection Agency (2001b).

[e]Agency for Toxic Substances and Disease Registry (2002).

in adults and its accumulation in tissues, especially kidney, it would be prudent to minimize exposures during pregnancy and childhood.

MANGANESE

Manganese is a transition element closely related to iron, an essential nutrient, and an integral part of several enzymes. Although manganese has 11 possible valence states, the main forms found in mammalian tissues are di-, tri-, and tetravalent cations. Metallic manganese is employed primarily in steel production, while inorganic manganese compounds are components of dry-cell batteries, matches, fireworks, glazes, varnishes, ceramics, and nutritional supplements. Synthetic organic manganese compounds include the fuel additive methylcyclopentadienyl manganese tricarbonyl (MMT) and the fungicides maneb and mancozeb. Given the neurotoxicity of inhaled manganese among occupationally exposed adults and the susceptibility of the developing nervous system to neurotoxins, some jurisdictions have banned MMT use on precautionary grounds.

Health Effects

Ingested manganese is relatively nontoxic because of low absorption rates and homeostatic mechanisms. Inhaled manganese can cause adverse developmental and respiratory effects and neurotoxicity similar to Parkinson's disease in occupationally exposed persons and experimental animals.

Molecular Mechanisms

The brain has a high energy requirement, making it susceptible to defects in mitochondrial function, a feature common to Parkinson's disease, Huntington's disease, and Friedreich's ataxia. Manganese disrupts mitochondrial functions by (1) competing with iron, notably in certain iron-dependent mitochondrial enzymes, (2) catalyzing dopamine oxidation to a reactive quinone that generates reactive oxygen species that damage mitochondrial DNA, and (3) inhibiting aconitase, an enzyme essential for mitochondrial energy production. Trivalent manganese appears to be a much more potent generator of reactive oxygen species than divalent manganese. Manganese accumulates in astrocytes and is only slowly eliminated from the brain; its persistence in mitochondria may explain progressive loss of function after exposure ends (Aschner et al., 1999).

Rodent models indicate that inhaled manganese may enter the brain via projections of olfactory neurons. Gastrointestinally absorbed manganese is transported in blood bound to plasma proteins including transferrin; transferrin bound manganese enters the brain by binding to transferrin-receptors in cerebral capillaries and migrates to basal ganglia via axonal transport. Because they compete for the same receptors, iron deficiency promotes brain uptake of manganese; given the high prevalence of iron deficiency globally, this could be an important determinant of manganese toxicity.

Neurotoxicity

Children on parenteral nutrition containing relatively high manganese levels have developed signs of neurotoxicity including tremors and seizures. There have been no adequate studies of children exposed to environmental manganese. A case report, however, noted marked verbal and visual memory deficits but normal cognitive function in a child aged 10 years exposed for 5 years to drinking water high in manganese (1.2 mg/L; compare this to the EPA MCL of 0.05 mg/L) (Woolf et al., 2002). Compared to unexposed children, those exposed to manganese in drinking water contaminated by sewage irrigation had increased hair manganese levels and reduced scores on short-term memory, manual dexterity, and visuoperceptual speed tests (He et al., 1994). An epidemiologic study in Greece revealed an association between drinking water manganese levels and neurotoxicity scores among adults (Kondakis et al., 1989). Endemic motor neuron disease and other chronic neurologic disorders among certain island populations in the western Pacific have been linked to diets low in calcium and iron and high in manganese, about half the cases developing during early childhood (Cawte et al., 1989).

Neurotoxic effects among men occupationally exposed to inhaled manganese for many years include tremor, reduced response speed, possible memory and intellectual deficits, and mood changes (Agency for Toxic Substances and Disease Registry, 2000b; Mergler and Baldwin, 1997). Among Quebec adults exposed to ambient airborne manganese, those with higher blood manganese levels had reduced ability to perform regular, rapid, and precise pointing movements, lower maximum rotation speeds in rapid alternating movements, and increased tremor (Beuter et al., 1999).

Manganese is a cumulative neurotoxin in experimental animals, causing adverse effects at relatively low levels when inhaled. Neurotoxic effects of manganese are linked to its accumulation in basal ganglia, especially the globus pallidus. Although the animal evidence of neurotoxicity is extensive, a NOAEL has not been established. Among rats exposed to ingested manganese, neonates but not adults had an increased acoustic startle response.

Other Effects

Studies of animals perinatally exposed to manganese by various routes have shown adverse effects including transient ataxia, decreased hypothalamic dopamine levels, reduced birth weight, skeletal abnormalities (club foot), and reduced size of testes and seminal vesicles (Agency for Toxic Substances and Disease Registry, 2000b). No studies have assessed the potential carcinogenicity of inhaled manganese in humans or animals; one animal study of ingested manganese revealed an increased incidence of pancreatic tumors, but several other studies were negative. The EPA designated manganese as not classifiable for carcinogenicity in humans.

Exposures

The EPA estimated that if MMT were used in all unleaded gasoline, about 5%–10% of people would be exposed to airborne manganese levels exceeding $0.1 \ \mu g/m^3$, a potential inhalation RfC. Canada appears to be the only country that has adopted MMT as the major replacement for tetraethyl lead. Tailpipe emissions of manganese from combustion of fuel containing MMT occur mainly as fine particulate ($PM_{2.5}$). Mean ambient manganese levels in Canadian cities ($12 \ ng/m^3$) are higher than those in California ($3 \ ng/m^3$), where MMT use has been restricted (Wallace and Slonecker, 1997). Airborne $PM_{2.5}$ manganese levels generally declined during recent years in the United States but not in Canada. Blood and urine manganese levels, respectively, appear to reflect the body burden and recent exposures (Agency for Toxic Substances and Disease Registry, 2000b).

Risk Management

Sources

Food is the main source of manganese for the general population, with air and water contributing about 1% of the daily intake. Combustion of MMT produces manganese oxides. Average airborne manganese levels in high and low traffic density areas of Montreal, respectively, were 24 ng/m³ and 15 ng/m³ (Loranger and Zayed, 1997). Manganese levels over time at both sites were significantly correlated with changes in traffic density. About 40% of inhaled manganese is absorbed.

Intervention

The EPA set the RfC for airborne manganese at 0.4 μg/m³ in 1990 and reduced it to 0.05 μg/m³ in 1993 based on neurobehavioral deficits in workers exposed to airborne manganese (Table 5–6). Unresolved risk assessment issues included the need to extrapolate from subchronic to chronic exposures, lack of reproductive and developmental toxicity data, and unknown differences in the toxicity of different forms of manganese. The EPA RfD for ingested manganese is 140 μg/kg/day for adults; an RfD for children has not been developed.

In 1976, MMT was introduced into the U.S. fuel supply, to raise octane ratings and reduce engine knock, but its use was restricted to leaded gasoline in 1977. The Ethyl Corporation subsequently applied to the EPA several times for permission to use MMT in unleaded gasoline. The EPA initially denied these applications on the grounds of concern about the impact on exhaust hydrocarbon emissions; later, the EPA based its denial on public health concerns related to inhaled particu-

TABLE 5–6. Guidelines and Standards for Chronic Exposure to Manganese

Exposure	Guideline or Limit	Agency
Air	0.15 μg/m³ (annual average)	WHO[a]
	0.05 μg/m³	EPA[b]
	0.04 μg/m³	ATSDR[c]
Drinking water	500 μg/L	WHO[d]
	50 μg/L	EPA[a]
Oral RfD	140 μg/kg/day	EPA[b]

[a] World Health Organization (2000a).
[b] U.S. Environmental Protection Agency (2001b).
[c] Agency for Toxic Substances and Disease Registry (2002).
[d] World Health Organization (2000b).

late manganese emissions (Davis, 1999). The Ethyl Corporations's subsequent challenge succeeded because the Clean Air Act allows the EPA to ban a fuel additive only if it interferes with any emission control device or system.

Canada legislated a ban on importation of MMT in 1997. A consortium of 21 automotive manufacturers supported this decision on the grounds that MMT interferes with antipollution devices and can harm human health by increasing toxic contaminant emissions. The ban was overturned in 1998 after a challenge by the Ethyl Corporation under the North American Free Trade Act, again giving precedence to economic concerns over public health and the precautionary principle. The Council on Scientific Affairs of the American Medical Association concluded that it.would be prudent to call for more research and testing before MMT is introduced widely into the U.S. gasoline supply (Lyznicki et al., 1999).

CONCLUSIONS

Proven Health Outcomes

- Arsenic
  - Large doses of inorganic arsenic can cause severe acute toxicity and death.
  - Chronic occupational exposure, mainly by inhalation, can cause lung cancer in adults.
  - Chronic environmental exposure, mainly by ingestion of contaminated drinking water, can cause skin, lung, bladder, and kidney cancers, peripheral vascular disease, and skin pigmentation and keratoses in adults.
- Cadmium
  - Chronic high-level exposure to ingested cadmium can cause severe kidney disease and osteomalacia in adults.
  - Men occupationally exposed to inhaled cadmium dust and fumes have an elevated lung cancer risk.

Unresolved Issues and Knowledge Gaps

- Arsenic—there is inadequate evidence to assess the role of chronic environmental exposure in developmental effects (fetal deaths, birth defects, low birth weight), childhood cancer, and delayed effects (hypertension, diabetes).

- Cadmium—there is inadequate evidence to assess the role of environmental cadmium in childhood renal disease; cadmium can cause reduced fetal growth, skeletal malformations, leukemia, and testicular cancer in animals, but its role in these conditions in humans is unknown.
- Manganese—although inhaled manganese can cause neurotoxic and other adverse health effects in occupationally exposed men and experimental animals, there has been almost no research on its potential effects on human prenatal development and child health.
- Knowledge gaps—the potential role of arsenic, cadmium, and manganese in fetal and child health is still to be investigated.

Risk Management Issues

- Prevention
  - Arsenic—drinking water standards for arsenic should be reduced to 10 μg/L as soon as possible; the potential for childhood exposure to arsenic from CCA-treated wood requires early assessment.
  - Cadmium—use of cadmium-contaminated sewage sludge on land for food crops should be avoided.
  - Manganese—use of the fuel additive MMT in countries such as Canada requires assessment for its potential neurotoxic effects on the human fetus and the developing child.
- Biomonitoring—Germany and the United States appear to be the only countries with population-based biomonitoring systems for measuring exposures to metals and other environmental toxicants among children.

REFERENCES

Agency for Toxic Substances and Disease Registry. (1999a). Toxicological profile for cadmium. Atlanta: Agency for Toxic Substances and Disease Registry.

Agency for Toxic Substances and Disease Registry. (1999b). Toxicological profile for mercury (update). Atlanta: Agency for Toxic Substances and Disease Registry.

Agency for Toxic Substances and Disease Registry. (2000a). Toxicological profile for arsenic. Atlanta: Agency for Toxic Substances and Disease Registry.

Agency for Toxic Substances and Disease Registry. (2000b). Toxicological profile for manganese. Atlanta: Agency for Toxic Substances and Disease Registry.

Agency for Toxic Substances and Disease Registry. (2002). Minimal risk levels (MRLs) for hazardous substances. Located at http://www.atsdr.cdc.gov/mrls.html.

Ahmad SA, Sayed MH, Barua S, Khan MH, Faruquee MH, Jalil A, Hadi SA, Talukder HK. (2001). Arsenic in drinking water and pregnancy outcomes. Environ Health Perspect 109:629–31.

Amin-Zaki L, Majeed MA, Clarkson TW, Greenwood MR. (1978). Methylmercury poisoning in Iraqi children: clinical observations over two years. BMJ 1:613–6.

Amin-Zaki L, Majeed MA, Elhassani SB, Clarkson TW, Greenwood MR, Doherty RA. (1979). Prenatal methylmercury poisoning. Clinical observations over five years. Am J Dis Child 133:172–7.

Aschengrau A, Zierler S, Cohen A. (1989). Quality of community drinking water and the occurrence of spontaneous abortion. Arch Environ Health 44:283–90.

Aschner M, Vrana KE, Zheng W. (1999). Manganese uptake and distribution in the central nervous system (CNS). Neurotoxicology 20:173–80.

Ask K, Akesson A, Berglund M, Vahter M. (2002). Inorganic mercury and methylmercury in placentas of Swedish women. Environ Health Perspect 110:523–6.

Axtell CD, Myers GJ, Davidson PW, Choi AL, Cernichiari E, Sloane-Reeves J, Cox C, Shamlaye C, Clarkson TW. (1998). Semiparametric modeling of age at achieving developmental milestones after prenatal exposure to methylmercury in the Seychelles child development study. Environ Health Perspect 106: 559–63.

Beusterien KM, Etzel RA, Agocs MM, Egeland GM, Socie EM, Rouse MA, Mortensen BK. (1991). Indoor air mercury concentrations following application of interior latex paint. Arch Environ Contam Toxicol 21:62–4.

Beuter A, Edwards R, deGeoffroy A, Mergler D, Hundnell K. (1999). Quantification of neuromotor function for detection of the effects of manganese. Neurotoxicology 20:355–66.

Brown LJ, Wall TP, Lazar V. (2000). Trends in total caries experience: permanent and primary teeth. J Am Dent Assoc 131:223–31.

Budtz-Jorgensen E, Grandjean P, Keiding N, White RF, Weihe P. (2000). Benchmark dose calculations of methylmercury-associated neurobehavioural deficits. Toxicol Lett 112–13:193–9.

Cawte J, Kilburn C, Florence M. (1989). Motor neurone disease of the western Pacific: do the foci extend to Australia? Neurotoxicology 10:263–70.

Centers for Disease Control and Prevention. (1996a). Update: mercury poisoning associated with beauty cream—Arizona, California, New Mexico, and Texas, 1996. MMWR 45:633–5.

Centers for Disease Control and Prevention. (1996b). Mercury exposure among residents of a building formerly used for industrial purposes—New Jersey, 1995. MMWR 45:422–4.

Centers for Disease Control and Prevention. (2000). Summary of the joint statement on thimerosal in vaccines. American Academy of Family Physicians, American Academy of Pediatrics, Advisory Committee on Immunization Practices, Public Health Service . MMWR 49:622, 631.

Centers for Disease Control and Prevention. (2001a). National report on human exposure to environmental chemicals. Located at http://www.cdc.gov/nceh/dls/report/PDF/CompleteReport.pdf.

Centers for Disease Control and Prevention. (2001b). National report on human exposure to environmental chemicals. Selection of chemicals for the report. Located at http://www.cdc.gov/nceh/dls/report/totalreport/substance.htm

Centers for Disease Control and Prevention. (2001c). Blood and hair mercury levels in young children and women of childbearing age—United States, 1999. MMWR 50:140–3.

Crump KS, Van Landingham C, Shamlaye C, Cox C, Davidson PW, Myers GJ, Clarkson TW. (2000). Benchmark concentrations for methylmercury obtained from the Seychelles Child Development Study. Environ Health Perspect 108: 257–63.

Davidson PW, Myers GJ, Cox C, Axtell C, Shamlaye C, Sloane-Reeves J, Cernichiari E, Needham L, Choi A, Wang Y, and others. (1998). Effects of prenatal and postnatal methylmercury exposure from fish consumption on neurodevelopment: outcomes at 66 months of age in the Seychelles Child Development Study. JAMA 280:701–7.

Davidson PW, Myers GJ, Cox C, Shamlaye CF, Marsh DO, Tanner MA, Berlin M, SloaneReeves J, Cernichiari E, Choisy O, and others. (1995). Longitudinal neurodevelopmental study of Seychellois children following in utero exposure to methylmercury from maternal fish ingestion: outcomes at 19 and 29 months. Neurotoxicology 16:677–88.

Davis JM. (1999). Inhalation health risks of manganese: an EPA perspective. Neurotoxicology 20:511–8.

Dulout FN, Grillo CA, Seoane AI, Maderna CR, Nilsson R, Vahter M, Darroudi F, Natarajan AT. (1996). Chromosomal aberrations in peripheral blood lymphocytes from Native Andean women and children from northwestern Argentina exposed to arsenic in drinking water. Mutat Res 370:151–8.

Dumont C, Girard M, Bellavance F, Noel F. (1998). Mercury levels in the Cree population of James Bay, Quebec, from 1988 to 1993/94. CMAJ 158:1439–45.

Eklund G, Oskarsson A. (1999). Exposure of cadmium from infant formulas and weaning foods. Food Addit Contam 16:509–19.

Gotelli CA, Astolfi E, Cox C, Cernichiari E, Clarkson TW. (1985). Early biochemical effects of an organic mercury fungicide on infants: "dose makes the poison." Science 227:638–40.

Grandjean P, Budtz-Jorgensen E, White RF, Jorgensen PJ, Weihe P, Debes F, Keiding N. (1999). Methylmercury exposure biomarkers as indicators of neurotoxicity in children aged 7 years. Am J Epidemiol 150:301–5.

Grandjean P, Weihe P, Burse VW, Needham LL, Storr-Hansen E, Heinzow B, Debes F, Murata K, Simonsen H, Ellefsen P, and others. (2001). Neurobehavioral deficits associated with PCB in 7-year-old children prenatally exposed to seafood neurotoxicants. Neurotoxicol Teratol 23:305–17.

Grandjean P, Weihe P, Jorgensen PJ, Clarkson T, Cernichiari E, Videro T. (1992). Impact of maternal seafood diet on fetal exposure to mercury, selenium, and lead. Arch Environ Health 47:185–95.

Grandjean P, Weihe P, White RF. (1995). Milestone development in infants exposed to methylmercury from human milk. Neurotoxicology 16:27–33.

Grandjean P, Weihe P, White RF, Debes F. (1998). Cognitive performance of children prenatally exposed to "safe" levels of methylmercury. Environ Res 77: 165–72.

Grandjean P, Weihe P, White RF, Debes F, Araki S, Yokoyama K, Murata K, Sorensen N, Dahl R, Jorgensen PJ. (1997). Cognitive deficit in 7-year-old children with prenatal exposure to methylmercury. Neurotoxicol Teratol 19:417–28.

Harada M. (1995). Minamata disease: methylmercury poisoning in Japan caused by environmental pollution. Crit Rev Toxicol 25:1–24.

He P, Liu DH, Zhang GQ. (1994). Effects of high-level-manganese sewage irrigation on children's neurobehavior. Chung Hua Yu Fang I Hsueh Tsa Chih 28:216–8.

Hopenhayn-Rich C, Browning SR, Hertz-Picciotto I, Ferreccio C, Peralta C, Gibb H. (2000). Chronic arsenic exposure and risk of infant mortality in two areas of Chile. Environ Health Perspect 108:667–73.

Ihrig MM, Shalat SL, Baynes C. (1998). A hospital-based case-control study of still-births and environmental exposure to arsenic using an atmospheric dispersion model linked to a geographical information system. Epidemiology 9:290–4.

International Agency for Research on Cancer. (1980). IARC monographs on the evaluation of carcinogenic risks to humans. Vol. 23. Arsenic and arsenic compounds. Lyon, France: International Agency for Research on Cancer.

International Agency for Research on Cancer. (1994). Beryllium, cadmium, mercury, and exposures in the glass manufacturing industry. Lyon, France: International Agency for Research on Cancer.

Iwata K, Saito H, Moriyama M, Nakano A. (1993). Renal tubular function after reduction of environmental cadmium exposure: a ten-year follow-up. Arch Environ Health 48:157–63.

Jensen GE, Christensen JM, Poulsen OM. (1991). Occupational and environmental exposure to arsenic—increased urinary arsenic level in children. Sci Total Environ 107:169–77.

Kondakis XG, Makris N, Leotsinidis M, Prinou M, Papapetropoulos T. (1989). Possible health effects of high manganese concentration in drinking water. Arch Environ Health 44:175–8.

Lemus R, Abdelghani AA, Akers TG, Horner WE. (1996). Health risks from exposure to metals in household dusts. Rev Environ Health 11:179–89.

Loranger S, Zayed J. (1997). Environmental contamination and human exposure assessment to manganese in the St. Lawrence River ecozone (Quebec, Canada) using an environmental fate/exposure model: GEOTOX. SAR QSAR Environ Res 6:105–19.

Lyznicki JM, Karlan MS, Khan MK. (1999). Manganese in gasoline. Council on Scientific Affairs, American Medical Association. J Occup Environ Med 41:140–3.

Mergler D, Baldwin M. (1997). Early manifestations of manganese neurotoxicity in humans: an update. Environ Res 73:92–100.

Murata K, Weihe P, Araki S, Budtz-Jorgensen E, Grandjean P. (1999). Evoked potentials in Faroese children prenatally exposed to methylmercury. Neurotoxicol Teratol 21:471–2.

Myers GJ, Davidson PW. (1998). Prenatal methylmercury exposure and children: neurologic, developmental, and behavioral research. Environ Health Perspect 106(Suppl 3):841–7.

Myers GJ, Davidson PW, Palumbo D, Shamlaye C, Cox C, Cernichiari E, Clarkson TW. (2000). Secondary analysis from the Seychelles Child Development Study: the child behavior checklist. Environ Res 84:12–9.

Myers GJ, Davidson PW, Shamlaye CF, Axtell CD, Cernichiari E, Choisy O, Choi A, Cox C, Clarkson TW. (1997). Effects of prenatal methylmercury exposure from a high fish diet on developmental milestones in the Seychelles Child Development Study. Neurotoxicology 18:819–29.

Myers GJ, Marsh DO, Davidson PW, Cox C, Shamlaye CF, Tanner M, Choi A, Cernichiari E, Choisy O, Clarkson TW. (1995). Main neurodevelopmental study of Seychellois children following in utero exposure to methylmercury from a maternal fish diet: outcome at six months. Neurotoxicology 16:653–64.

National Academy of Sciences. (1994). Science and judgment in risk assessment. Washington, DC: National Academy Press.

National Academy of Sciences. (1999). Arsenic in drinking water. Washington, DC: National Academy Press.

National Academy of Sciences. (2000). Toxicological effects of methylmercury. Washington, DC: National Academy Press.

National Academy of Sciences. (2001). Arsenic in drinking water. 2001 update. Washington, DC: National Academy Press.

Noonan CW, Sarasua SM, Campagna D, Kathman SJ, Lybarger JA, Mueller PW. (2002). Effects of exposure to low levels of environmental cadmium on renal biomarkers. Environ Health Perspect 110:151–5.

Oskarsson A, Schultz A, Skerfving S, Hallen IP, Ohlin B, Lagerkvist BJ. (1996). Total and inorganic mercury in breast milk in relation to fish consumption and amalgam in lactating women. Arch Environ Health 51:234–41.

Palumbo DR, Cox C, Davidson PW, Myers GJ, Choi A, Shamlaye C, Sloane-Reeves J, Cernichiari E, Clarkson TW. (2000). Association between prenatal exposure to methylmercury and cognitive functioning in Seychellois children: a reanalysis of the McCarthy Scales of Children's Ability from the main cohort study. Environ Res 84:81–8.

Paschal DC, Burt V, Caudill SP, Gunter EW, Pirkle JL, Sampson EJ, Miller DT, Jackson RJ. (2000). Exposure of the U.S. population aged 6 years and older to cadmium: 1988–1994. Arch Environ Contam Toxicol 38:377–83.

Rasmussen PE, Subramanian KS, Jessiman BJ. (2001). A multi-element profile of housedust in relation to exterior dust and soils in the city of Ottawa, Canada. Sci Total Environ 267:125–40.

Rice DC, Hayward S. (1999). Comparison of visual function at adulthood and during aging in monkeys exposed to lead or methylmercury. Neurotoxicology 20:767–84.

Richardson GM. (1995). Assessment of mercury exposure and risks from dental amalgam. Ottawa: Health Canada.

Seifert B, Becker K, Helm D, Krause C, Schulz C, Seiwert M. (2000). The German environmental survey 1990/1992 (GerES II): reference concentrations of selected environmental pollutants in blood, urine, hair, house dust, drinking water and indoor air. J Expo Anal Environ Epidemiol 10:552–65.

Smith AH, Arroyo AP, Mazumder DN, Kosnett MJ, Hernandez AL, Beeris M, Smith MM, Moore LE. (2000). Arsenic-induced skin lesions among Atacameno people in northern Chile despite good nutrition and centuries of exposure. Environ Health Perspect 108:617–20.

Steuerwald U, Weihe P, Jorgensen PJ, Bjerve K, Brock J, Heinzow B, Budtz-Jorgensen E, Grandjean P. (2000). Maternal seafood diet, methylmercury exposure, and neonatal neurologic function. J Pediatr 136:599–605.

Thomas DJ, Styblo M, Lin S. (2001). The cellular metabolism and systemic toxicity of arsenic. Toxicol Appl Pharmacol 176:127–44.

U.S. Environmental Protection Agency. (1994). Cadmium. Located at http://www.epa.gov/iris/subst/0141.htm.

U.S. Environmental Protection Agency. (1997). Mercury study report to Congress. Research Triangle Park, NC: U.S. Environmental Protection Agency.

U.S. Environmental Protection Agency. (2000). 40 CFR Parts 141 and 142. National drinking water regulations; arsenic and clarifications to compliance and new source contaminants monitoring; proposed rule. Fed Reg 65:38888–983.

U.S. Environmental Protection Agency. (2001a). Current drinking water standards. Washington, DC: U.S. Environmental Protection Agency.

U.S. Environmental Protection Agency. (2001b). IRIS substance list. Located at http://www.epa.gov/iris/subst/index.html

U.S. Food and Drug Administration. (2000). Action levels for poisonous or deleterious substances in human food and animal feed. Located at http:// www.cfsan.fda.gov/~lrd/fdaact.html.

U.S. Food and Drug Administration. (2001). An important message for pregnant women and women of childbearing age who may become pregnant about the risks of mercury in fish. Located at http://vm.cfsan.fda.gov/~dms/admehg. html

Wallace L, Slonecker T. (1997). Ambient air concentrations of fine (PM2.5) manganese in U.S. national parks and in California and Canadian cities: the possible impact of adding MMT to unleaded gasoline. J Air Waste Manag Assoc 47:642–52.

Wheatley B, Paradis S. (1998). Northern exposure: further analysis of the results of the Canadian aboriginal methylmercury program. Int J Circumpolar Health 57(Suppl 1):586–90.

Woolf A, Wright R, Amarasiriwardena C, Bellinger D. (2002). A child with chronic manganese exposure from drinking water. Environ Health Perspect 110:613–16.

World Health Organization. (1990). Environmental health criteria 101. Methylmercury. Geneva: International Programme on Chemical Safety.

World Health Organization. (2000a). Guidelines for air quality. Geneva: World Health Organization.

World Health Organization. (2000b). Guidelines for drinking water quality. Geneva: World Health Organization.

Wulff M, Hogberg U, Sandstrom A. (1996). Cancer incidence for children born in a smelting community. Acta Oncol 35:179–83.

Zierler S, Theodore M, Cohen A, Rothman KJ. (1988). Chemical quality of maternal drinking water and congenital heart disease. Int J Epidemiol 17:589–94.

6

PCBs, Dioxins, and Related Compounds

Polyhalogenated aromatic hydrocarbons (PHAHs) comprise a large group of semi-volatile chemicals that are stable at high temperatures, highly soluble in lipids, and resistant to biodegradation. Unfortunately, these properties enable PHAHs to disperse and persist in the environment, to bioaccumulate in terrestrial and aquatic food chains, and to cause unforeseen adverse health effects among wildlife and humans. All of us probably have detectable PHAHs in our bodies, the concentrations of PCBs generally being much higher than those of other PHAHs.

Chlorinated, brominated, and mixed halogenated PHAHs have similar structures and toxicity but widely variable potencies; major subgroups include biphenyls, dibenzo-p-dioxins, and dibenzofurans (Table 6–1). Monsanto, the sole manufacturer of PCBs in the United States, produced about 700,000 tons during the period 1929–1979, annual output peaking in 1970 at 43,000 tons. Given their high heat capacity and stability, PCBs were ideal for uses in heat-resistant solvents, sealants, and lubricants; and as dielectric fluids in electrical transformers, fluorescent light ballasts, and other electrical equipment. The most intensely studied PHAH is 2,3,7,8-tetrachloro-p-dibenzodioxin (TCDD), one of the most potent known toxicants (Schiestl et al., 1997).

This chapter describes the health threats to children of the widespread use and dispersion of these highly toxic chemicals. The PCBs illustrate a

TABLE 6–1. PHAHs: Types and Acronyms

	Polychlorinated	*Polybrominated*
Dibenzo-*p*-dioxins	PCDDs	PBDDs
Biphenyls	PCBs	PBBs
Dibenzofurans	PCDFs	PBDFs
Diphenylethers	PCDEs	PBDEs
Naphthalenes	PCNs	PBNs

recurrent theme: the banning of a toxicant after recognition of severe human health impacts but continued use of chemically similar substances with ill-defined human health risks. The key role of the aryl hydrocarbon receptor in the toxicity of coplanar dioxin-like PHAHs and current knowledge of adverse health effects in humans and experimental animals are discussed. The identified exposure sources and pathways point to the interventions needed to further reduce environmental contamination and human exposures. See also Chapter 7 (Pesticides) and Chapter 8 (Hormonally Active Agents) for further discussion of the potential effects of PHAHs and related compounds on reproductive system development and function.

HEALTH EFFECTS

Several events led to the discovery of the toxicity of PCBs, dioxins, and related compounds:

- A major outbreak of chloracne (a severe acne-like skin eruption) occurred at a trichlorophenol plant in West Virginia after a reactor explosion in 1949. Only later was it realized that combustion of trichlorophenol can generate large amounts of TCDD and dioxin-like compounds, now known to cause chloracne.
- The deaths of millions of chickens from chick edema in the United States during the late 1950s and 1960s were linked to poultry feeds contaminated by fat-soluble chlorinated aromatic compounds, including polychlorinated dibenzo-*p*-dioxins (PCDDs); the contamination was traced to pentachlorophenol used in hide-stripping operations followed by removal of fat and alkaline hydrolysis to produce fatty acids for animal feeds. Pentachlorophenol is soluble in fat and yields PCDDs during alkaline hydrolysis.

- Investigation of unexpected gas chromatographic peaks during analyses of tissues from fish and marine mammals revealed the bioaccumulation of PCBs and DDT/DDE in the aquatic food chain.
- Outbreaks of an apparently new illness occurred in Japan (1968) and Taiwan (1979) characterized by severe acne-like skin eruptions and other signs and symptoms in children and adults and by low birth weight, pigmentation, developmental delays, and cognitive deficits in prenatally exposed infants. Both outbreaks were traced to leakage of PCBs and other PHAHs from heat-exchange coils.

Epidemiologic studies have focused on populations exposed to PHAHs through diet (consumption of highly contaminated cooking oils or moderately tainted fish), occupation, and industrial accidents. In general, PHAH exposures of these populations involved mixtures, precluding definitive assignment of toxic effects to specific congeners. Some health effects attributed to PCBs, for example, may have been caused by other PHAHs.

Molecular Mechanisms

The three major PHAH families each have two aromatic rings but differ in how the rings are joined (Fig. 6–1). The major families comprise over 400 members (congeners) that vary by the number and placement of chlorine or bromine atoms. Among PCBs, those with zero or one chlorine in the ortho position (positions 2, 2', 6, or 6' on biphenyl (see Fig. 6–1) are

TABLE 6–2. Equitoxic Levels of Selected PHAHs in the Diet of Rhesus Macaque Monkeys

Compound	Level (ng/g)
Aroclor 1242	100,000
Arcola 1248	25,000
Firemaster FF-1	25,000
3,4,3',4'-Tetrachlorobiphenyl	1,000
3,4,5,3',4',5'-Hexachlorodibenzofuran	1,000
2,3,7,8-Tetrachlorodibenzofuran	50
2,3,4,6,7,8-Hexachlorodibenzo-p-dioxin	5
2,3,6,7-Tetrachlorodibenzo-p-dioxin	0.5–2
2,3,7,8-Tetrachlorodibenzo-p-dioxin	1.0

Source: McNulty (1985).

Equitoxicity based on red, swollen eyelids and elevated fingernails after 1 month and severe morbidity or death after 2 months.

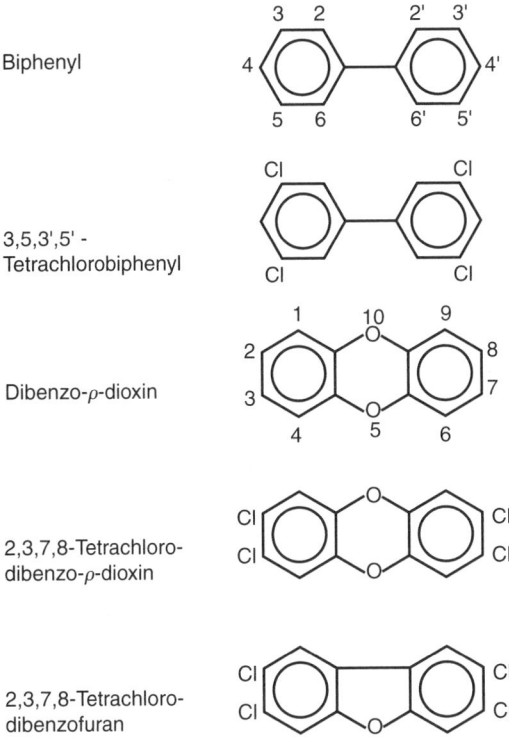

Biphenyl

3,5,3',5' - Tetrachlorobiphenyl

Dibenzo-*p*-dioxin

2,3,7,8-Tetrachloro-dibenzo-*p*-dioxin

2,3,7,8-Tetrachloro-dibenzofuran

FIGURE 6–1. Structure of biphenyls, dioxins, and selected chlorinated congeners.

often called *coplanar* because they have a flat configuration. Less than 10% of PHAH congeners, those with chlorine and/or bromine in at least the 2, 3, 7, and 8 positions, have dioxin-like toxicity; certain halogenated benzenes and naphthalenes have similar toxicity (U.S. Environmental Protection Agency, 2000b). Congeners with zero, one, or two or more chlorine atoms in the ortho position, respectively, have high, intermediate, or low AhR affinities and dioxin-like toxicities. The toxicity of PHAHs varies widely, with PCDDs and polychlorinated dibenzofurans (PCDFs) generally being much more potent than PCBs (Table 6–2). Among the 209 PCB congeners, the 13 coplanar members with four or more chlorines have dioxin-like toxicity. Some evidence, however, suggests that noncoplanar PCB congeners are more neurotoxic than coplanar compounds and may act through AhR-independent mechanisms.

AhR-Mediated Toxicity
TCDD and dioxin-like compounds appear to have three main biochemical effects: enzyme induction and modulation of multiple growth factors

and hormones (Birnbaum, 1995). The reproductive, developmental, immunologic, and carcinogenic effects of dioxin-like PHAHs occur at extremely low body-burden levels in experimental animals and are mediated by AhR, a ligand-dependent transcription factor. The AhR occurs in human tissues and functions similarly to that in rodents but generally has lower affinity for PHAHs, possibly explaining the higher susceptibility of rodents to PHAH toxicity. When activated by TCDD or other ligands, AhR dimerizes with AhR nuclear translocator (Arnt) and binds with high affinity to enhancer elements in the upstream region of several oncogenes and genes that encode growth factors, hormones, hormone receptors, cytochrome P450 enzymes (*CYP1A1, CYP1A2, CYP1B1*), and electrophile response element (*EPRE*) genes (Safe, 2001). Upregulation of these genes can enhance or mitigate the effects of toxicants and hormones; for instance, *CYP1A1* and *CYP1A2* increase the metabolism of endogenous and exogenous substances to reactive oxygenated metabolites and cause oxidative stress, a major signal for triggering apoptosis. The most potent known inducer of the *CYP1A1* gene is TCDD.

The ability of dioxin-like PHAHs to cause wasting, immunosuppression, birth defects, chloracne, and cancer in experimental animals and/or humans may arise from persistent AhR activation due to their strong binding affinity and long biologic half-life. Knockout mice missing the AhR gene are not susceptible to TCDD and are resistant to benzo[a]pyrene-induced tumors, demonstrating the key role of AhR in carcinogenesis. The duration of health effects depends on the half-lives of congeners in body fat; for example, recovery is rapid from certain PHAH congeners with short half-lives but protracted for persistent congeners.

Toxic Equivalency
A PHAH congener is dioxin-like if it binds to AhR, causes dioxin-like effects, and bioaccumulates. Toxic equivalency factors (TEFs) for PHAHs are the ratios of the toxicity of specific congeners relative to that of TCDD. There is no universally accepted set of TEFs, and congener-specific TEFs may vary among species; TEFs developed by the U.S. EPA and the WHO are widely used. The toxic equivalent (TEQ) of each congener in a mixture is the product of its TEF and its molar concentration; the sum of TEQs in a mixture is the amount of TCDD estimated to equal the toxicity of the mixture. Although use of TEQs entails uncertainties, they address the need to assess health risks of the mixed PHAH exposures among humans. For instance, the affinity of TCDD for AhR is about 10,000 times that of hexachlorobenzene, but the latter occurs at much higher concentrations, comprising up to 60% of total TEQ in breast milk in some countries.

AhR-Independent Mechanisms
Ortho-substituted (noncoplanar) PCB congeners appear to cause neurotoxic effects through AhR-independent mechanisms in experimental
animals. Reduced dopamine levels in the caudate nucleus, putamen, and
hypothalamus of adult monkeys exposed to commercial PCB mixtures
are associated with brain tissue PCB residues composed almost entirely
of di-ortho-substituted congeners. Noncoplanar PCB congeners are the
most potent in reducing dopamine levels and disrupting calcium transport in human pheochromocytoma cells in vitro. Finally, the ability of ortho-substituted PCBs to bind with high affinity to the thyroid hormone
transport protein transthyretin may contribute to the neurotoxicity of prenatal PCB exposure.

Reproduction

See Chapter 8 (Hormonally Active Agents) for discussion of the potentially adverse effects of dioxins, PCBs, and related compounds on reproductive health.

Development

In 1968, a 3-year-old girl with severe acne-like skin lesions visited a der-
matology clinic in Japan and became the first recognized case of a new
disease called *Yusho* (oil disease). About 1800 persons were eventually
recognized to have Yusho, characterized in older children and adults by
chloracne, eye discharge, hyperpigmentation, fatigue, nausea, elevated
serum triglyceride levels, and reduced sensory nerve conduction velocity (Urabe and Asahi, 1985). Prenatally exposed infants experienced increased perinatal mortality, intrauterine growth retardation, small head
circumference, eye discharges, hyperpigmentation (skin, nails, buccal cav-
ity), gingival hyperplasia, precocious dentition, and abnormal skull cal-
cification (Yamashita and Hayashi, 1985). Lengthy investigations identified the cause to be cooking oil contaminated by PCBs leaking through a
heating coil during rice oil production. Subsequent studies revealed other
highly toxic contaminants, including PCDFs, polychlorinated triphenyls,
and polychlorinated quaterphenyls in the contaminated oil and blood and
adipose tissue samples from exposed persons.

In 1979, acne-like skin lesions occurred among the students and staff
of a school for blind children in Taiwan; over 2000 *Yucheng* (oil disease)
cases were eventually recognized. Some children developed severe, scarring chloracne (Fig. 6–2). Follow-up at ages of up to 6 years showed that

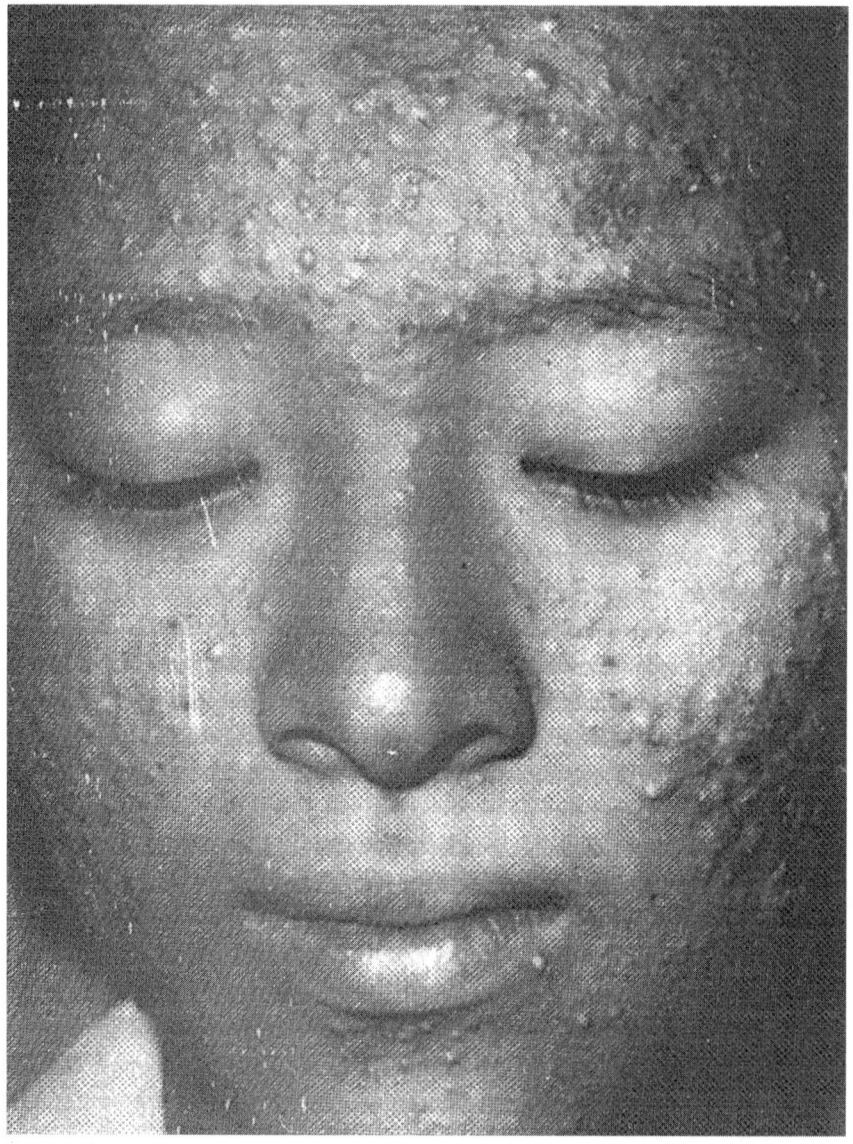

FIGURE 6–2. Chloracne on the face of a Yusho case (Urabe and Asahi, 1985).

prenatally exposed Yucheng children had delayed developmental mile-stones, abnormal behaviors, lower stature and weight, gingival hyper-trophy, tooth chipping, acne or acne scars, hyperpigmentation, lymphad-enopathy, hirsutism, hypertelorism (eyes abnormally far apart), and short metacarpal bones (Rogan et al., 1988). Despite the close clinical resem-blance to Yusho and epidemiologic evidence showing an association with a specific brand of rice oil, several months passed before Taiwanese authorities formally recognized the cause and prohibited further distribution of the oil. PCDFs, PCBs, and PCDDs, respectively, contributed 53%, 35%, and 12% of the dioxin-TEQ in the contaminated cooking oil.

The Yusho and Yucheng incidents showed that high prenatal exposures to PCBs and other dioxin-like PHAHs can cause low birth weight and structural and functional abnormalities. A review concluded that there is inconsistent evidence in populations exposed to relatively low-level PCBs (from background sources such as fish) of inverse associations between maternal PCB levels and birth weight or gestation length (Longnecker et al., 1997); recent European studies, however, have shown fairly consistent associations between maternal PCB or dioxin-TEQ exposure indices and low birth weight (Patandin et al., 1998; Rylander et al., 1998; Vartiainen et al., 1998). Prenatal PCB exposures were associated with growth deficits during early childhood in three cohort studies (Blanck et al., 2002; Gladen et al., 2000; Jacobson et al., 1990). Follow-up of daughters of women prenatally exposed to polybrominated biphenyls (PBBs) showed a strong inverse association between maternal serum PCBs, but not PBBs, and weight adjusted for height at ages 5–24 years (average difference of 11 pounds for maternal serum PCB levels above the median versus below the median) (Blanck et al., 2002). Stature at age 10 years was not associated with blood PCB levels measured at age 8 years (Karmaus et al., 2002).

An explosion at a trichlorophenol plant in Seveso, Italy, in 1976 exposed the surrounding population to relatively pure TCDD. The ratio of male:female births was reduced among the highest exposure group at Seveso (Mocarelli et al., 2000) but not among Yusho infants (Yoshimura et al., 2001). Among the 26 births in the most contaminated part of Seveso, 2 had minor structural defects and none had major malformations. An early case-control study showed an increased risk of some birth defects related to likely paternal exposure to Agent Orange in Vietnam, but later studies found no consistent associations between paternal serum TCDD levels and risks of fetal death, birth defects, preterm birth, intrauterine growth retardation, infant death, or altered sex ratio.

Developmental effects of TCDD in experimental animals include fetal death, cleft palate, hydronephrosis (caused by ureteral epithelial hyperplasia), hypomineralization of teeth, ovarian atrophy, cleft phallus (female), reduced size of testes and male accessory sex glands (especially the ventral prostate), delayed testicular descent, reduced anogenital distance (males), reduced growth, thymic atrophy, and immunosuppression (Agency for Toxic Substances and Disease Registry, 1998) (see also Chapter 8, Hormonally Active Agents).

Neurotoxicity

Epidemiologic Studies

Although some Yusho infants had reduced head circumference, there appear to have been no follow-up studies to assess neurobehavioral function. Yucheng children had global IQ deficits of about 5 points at ages 4–7 years; those born up to 6 years after their mothers' exposure were just as affected as those born within 2 years of exposure (Chen et al., 1992). These findings are consistent with the long half-lives of many PHAH congeners in vivo; serum PCB and PCDF levels in Yucheng women 14 years after exposure were still 10–100 times higher than those of controls. A birth cohort study of children whose mothers were exposed to PCBs from eating contaminated Lake Michigan fish showed that prenatal PCB exposure was associated with weak reflexes and an increased startle response at birth, visual recognition memory deficits during infancy, verbal and numerical memory deficits at age 4 years, and full-scale and verbal IQ deficits at age 11 years (Jacobson and Jacobson, 1996). Children with the highest prenatal PCB exposure had an average full-scale IQ deficit of 6 points, independent of potential confounders, and were two to three times more likely to score poorly on verbal comprehension, freedom from distractibility, and written word comprehension. Benchmark dose analyses of the Lake Michigan cohort were conducted for four PCB-related cognitive outcomes: full-scale IQ, word comprehension, and average reaction time at age 11 years and the McCarthy Memory Scale at age 4 years (Jacobson et al., 2002); the estimated benchmark dose for a 5% increased incidence of full-scale IQ deficits was 0.36–0.63 μg/g (average lipid-adjusted PCB level in cord and maternal serum and breast milk).

A systematic review of seven cohort studies of prenatal PCB exposure and neurologic development noted associations with abnormal reflexes among newborn infants, reduced motor skills among infants, and cognitive deficits at about age 4 years; importantly, lactational PCB exposure was not clearly associated with any adverse neurologic effect (Ribas-Fito et al., 2001). A recent German study, however, reported independent effects of prenatal and postnatal PCB exposures on cognitive deficits at age 42 months (Walkowiak et al., 2001). Although divergent from most other studies, this finding is consistent with evidence that postnatal exposure of monkeys to a relatively low dose of PCBs can cause learning deficits (Rice, 1997).

Cognitive deficits observed in Michigan but not in North Carolina might be attributable to differences in exposure levels. For example, a later study showed that persons who averaged one meal of Great Lakes fish per week had mean serum dioxin-TEQ and PCB-TEQ levels, respectively, about twofold and tenfold those of nonconsumers (Anderson et al., 1998).

Other possible differences include "spiking" of serum PCB levels among fish eaters (serum PCB levels increase two- to fivefold after a PCB-contaminated fish meal and require a week to return to baseline levels) and the presence of toxic contaminants other than PCBs in Lake Michigan fish.

Toxicologic Studies
Perinatal exposure of rodents and nonhuman primates to PCBs causes neurotoxic effects involving motor activity (increased open field activity during early life, hypoactivity as adults), cognitive function (decreased active avoidance learning, increased errors in radial arm maze, decreased performance on spatial and nonspatial discrimination reversal tasks), and altered dopamine levels in several brain regions (Agency for Toxic Substances and Disease Registry, 2000). Prenatal PCB exposure also causes markedly low serum thyroxine (T4) levels in experimental animals; perinatal hypothyroidism is a known cause of cognitive deficits in animals and humans and may contribute to the neurotoxicity of PCBs. Although neurotoxicity of PCBs may relate mainly to noncoplanar congeners, coplanar PCBs may also be important; for instance, rats perinatally exposed to 3,3',4,4',5-pentachlorobiphenyl developed low-frequency hearing deficits at doses as low as 1 μg/kg/day (Crofton and Rice, 1999). There has been little research on neurotoxicity of TCDD in animals.

Cancer

Dioxins
The IARC concluded that TCDD is a human carcinogen based on limited human evidence from occupationally exposed persons, strong evidence of carcinogenicity in experimental animals, and a shared mechanism (AhR) in animals and humans. The IARC concluded that the human carcinogenicity of other dioxins and furans could not be determined. The EPA independently concluded that TCDD is a human carcinogen, other dioxins are probable human carcinogens, and general population exposure levels to TCDD may increase the lifetime (up to age 70 years) absolute cancer risk by as much as 0.1–1.0% (U.S. Environmental Protection Agency, 2000b).

Few studies of TCDD and childhood cancer have been conducted. People exposed as children to TCDD at Seveso had statistically insignificant excesses of ovarian cancer, Hodgkin's disease, myeloid leukemia, and thyroid cancer (Pesatori et al., 1993). Given the limited exposure assessment, the small number of highly exposed children, and the usual long latency of human cancers, longer follow-up is needed to assess potential cancer risks. Children living near municipal or hospital incinerators, potential sources of TCDD exposure, had a twofold increased risk of leukemia and other cancers (Knox, 2000). The EPA concluded that existing epidemiologic data are insufficient to assess the risk of childhood cancer from TCDD exposure. However, TCDD is a potent animal carcinogen, causing cancer (usually at multiple sites) in all species tested at doses as low as 1 ng/kg/day. Rats exposed prenatally to a single low dose of TCDD develop more mammary gland terminal end buds, the breast structures most susceptible to carcinogenesis; such animals are more susceptible as adults to chemically induced breast cancer.

PCBs and Related Compounds

The IARC concluded that several PCB mixtures are reasonably anticipated to be human carcinogens based on sufficient evidence in animal studies and inadequate human evidence (International Agency for Research on Cancer, 1987). Cohort studies of occupationally exposed adults showed slightly increased risks of skin melanoma and liver, biliary tract, gallbladder, colorectal, and hematopoietic cancers. In experimental animals, PCBs caused liver cancer and hyperplasia of the bile duct, gallbladder, and urinary tract, with the higher chlorinated PCBs being most potent. The EPA estimated that lifetime ingestion of PCBs at a rate of 1 μg/kg/day would cause an extra 77 cancer cases per 10,000 persons.

Population-based epidemiologic studies have shown associations between PCBs and adult cancers, including non-Hodgkin's lymphoma (Rothman et al., 1997) and breast cancer. Although a review concluded that the epidemiologic evidence concerning PCBs and breast cancer was mixed and inconclusive, two subsequent well-conducted studies showed associations with breast adipose tissue levels of specific PCB congeners (Aronson et al., 2000; Holford et al., 2000). Breast adipose tissue PCB levels reflect cumulative exposure in the target organ of interest and likely provide a better indicator of the breast cancer risk. Studies that assessed total blood PCB levels may be misleading because breast tissue levels of specific PCB congeners are only weakly correlated with blood levels and specific PCB congeners vary widely with respect to estrogenic activity, affinity for AhR, cytochrome P450 response, and half-lives in vivo. Apart from a small case-control study of childhood leukemia in Germany showing no associations with PCB, DDE, hexachlorocyclohexane, or dieldrin levels in bone marrow fat (Scheele et al., 1992), the role of PCBs in childhood cancer remains virtually unexplored.

Immune System

Yucheng children reexamined at ages 8–16 years were much more likely than matched controls to have experienced recent middle ear infections but had normal immunologic markers (Chao et al., 1997; Yu et al., 1998). Among Dutch children, current plasma PCB levels were associated with recurrent middle ear infections, chicken pox, and allergies but not with antibody levels, leukocyte counts, or T-cell markers (Weisglas-Kuperus et al., 2000). Among Inuit infants, the risk of otitis media before age 1 year was associated with prenatal exposure to DDE, hexachlorobenzene, and dieldrin but not PCBs (Dewailly et al., 2000).

The EPA and the ATSDR assessed the immunologic effects of dioxins, PCBs, and related PHAHs in humans and experimental animals and concluded that (Agency for Toxic Substances and Disease Registry, 1998, 2000; U.S. Environmental Protection Agency, 2000a)

- No consistent exposure-related immunologic effects have been observed in adult humans exposed to PCDDs at levels several orders of magnitude above background levels.
- Yucheng infants and infants whose mothers ate fish or marine mammals contaminated by PCBs and other organochlorine compounds had increased infections (middle ear infections, bronchitis) during early infancy.
- The immune system is one of the most sensitive targets for dioxins in experimental animals. Perinatal exposure to low TCDD doses causes thymic gland atrophy, and much lower doses disrupt specific immune receptor functions, with a reduced antibody response and decreased host resistance to infections.
- TCDD and related PHAHs should be considered nonspecific immunosuppressants, at least until better data are available.

Endocrine System

See Chapter 8 (Hormonally Active Agents) for discussion of potential effects of dioxins and related compounds on the endocrine system.

Chloracne

Chloracne is the earliest clinically recognizable and most consistent health effect of exposure to dioxin-like PHAHs in several species, including humans and monkeys. Based on TCDD levels in soil and a limited number of blood samples, chloracne was the only dose-related health effect among the local population at Seveso; 88% of the 187 cases diagnosed by an expert panel were children. Chloracne developed in children over a period of 3 days to 2 weeks after the explosion; lipid-adjusted serum TCDD levels were highest among those most severely affected and were several orders of magnitude higher than adipose tissue levels among U.S. children

TABLE 6-3. TCDD Levels among Seveso Children
Aged 3-14 Years with Chloracne and U.S. Populations

	pg/g Fat
Grade 4 (severe chloracne)	12,100–56,000[a]
Grade 3	828–7,420[a]
U.S. children	2[b]
U.S. general population	5.4[c]

[a]Serum. Mocarelli et al. (1991).
[b]Adipose tissue (Orban et al., 1994).
[c]Whole blood (Needham et al., 1996).

(Table 6-3). Children but not adults with serum TCDD levels below 10,000 pg/g fat developed chloracne, suggesting that children were more susceptible. The Seveso incident caused the greatest documented human TCDD exposures, the highest blood TCDD levels occurring among six children with grade 4 chloracne (12,100–56,000 ng/L) (Pocchiari et al., 1979). All children with chloracne soon after exposure were clear of lesions by 6 years after the incident.

Based on levels in blood samples and contaminated cooking oil, persons (mainly children) who developed chloracne in the Yusho and Yucheng incidents had average exposures to PCDFs of 4–6 μg/kg, measured as 2,3,4,7,8-pentachlorodibenzofuran equivalents (PEQ) (Ryan et al., 1990). These exposures are toxicologically equivalent to TCDD levels known to cause chloracne in monkeys and are about 200 times higher than current body burden levels in North American populations. It is possible that TCDD causes chloracne by interfering with the regulatory role of retinol (vitamin A) and retinoic acid in skin epithelial cell proliferation and differentiation.

Other Effects

Some of the children exposed to PCBs and other PHAHs during the Yusho and Yucheng incidents had natal teeth, discoloration of teeth during infancy, and tooth chipping during later childhood. Combined prenatal and postnatal PCB exposure has been linked to enamel defects in permanent teeth. Lactational exposure to dioxin-TEQs in Finland was associated with the frequency and severity of mineralization defects in permanent first molars at relatively low exposure levels; such changes may provide a lifelong visible indicator of exposure to TCDD and dioxin-like compounds

(Alaluusua et al., 1999). After a single postnatal dose of TCDD, young adult male rats experienced defective dentin and enamel formation, possibly due to interference with vitamin A by TCDD.

EXPOSURES

Internal Dose Indices

The body PHAH burden is stored mainly in adipose tissue and the liver. Until the late 1980s, the gold standard for TCDD body burden assessment required a biopsy of adipose tissue, a highly invasive procedure. After the discovery that lipid-based TCDD concentrations are similar in adipose tissue, liver, and serum, and with the the development of sensitive analytic methods, blood analysis became the most common method for estimating human exposure to TCDD and other PHAHS. But the correlation between serum and adipose tissue levels of individual PCB congeners varies substantially; also, the relative amounts of coplanar PCBs in adipose tissue vary more among individuals than do PCDD and PCDF levels. The persistence of individual PCB congeners in blood varies widely; after cessation of chronic exposure, the half-lives of nine PCB congeners in monkeys ranged from a few months to about 8 years.

Internal Dose Estimates

After 13 years of follow-up, serum PCB and PCDF levels among Yucheng women were still one to two orders of magnitude higher than those in controls and were inversely associated with the total duration of breast-feeding, consistent with the importance of lactation as a PHAH excretory mechanism. Dioxin-TEQ levels in placental samples from Yucheng women were up to 1000 times those observed in American women. Compared to unexposed persons, frequent consumers of Great Lakes fish had twofold higher mean serum TEQs for dioxins and furans and tenfold higher TEQs for coplanar PCBs (Anderson et al., 1998). Monitoring data for PHAH levels in the general population are virtually nonexistent; a small German study of neonates showed relatively low cord blood levels of individual PCB congeners and hexachlorobenzene, consistent with a substantial decline during 1994–1998 (Lackmann, 2002). The CDC plans to include dioxins, furans, and PCBs in NHANES in future years (Centers for Disease Control and Prevention 2001).

Breast milk PHAH levels reflect the body burden of reproductive-age women and the potential for prenatal and lactational infant exposure. Although limited by small sample sizes and methodologic differences, existing data suggest that breast milk dioxin-TEQ levels declined by about 50% in several countries during the period 1970–1998 (LaKind et al., 2001). To the extent that there has been a real decrease, this would be consistent with reduced PHAH emissions.

Breast milk PCB levels in Canada have decreased since 1982 (Craan and Haines, 1998). However, PCB levels in breast milk from Inuit women in the Canadian Arctic were up to ten times those in southern Canada, reflecting high consumption of contaminated traditional foods (Dewailly et al., 1993). In Sweden, total breast milk dioxin-TEQ decreased by about two-thirds during recent decades, but polybrominated diphenyl ethers (PBDEs) increased sharply (see Fig. 6–3) (Noren and Meironyte, 2000). If the latter trend continues, PBDEs will displace PCBs and DDT as the leading breast milk organochlorines during the next 15–30 years.

RISK MANAGEMENT

The PHAHs from manufacturing or combustion processes and waste disposal disperse widely through evaporation, long-range airborne transport, and deposition into soil and water, persisting in and cycling between

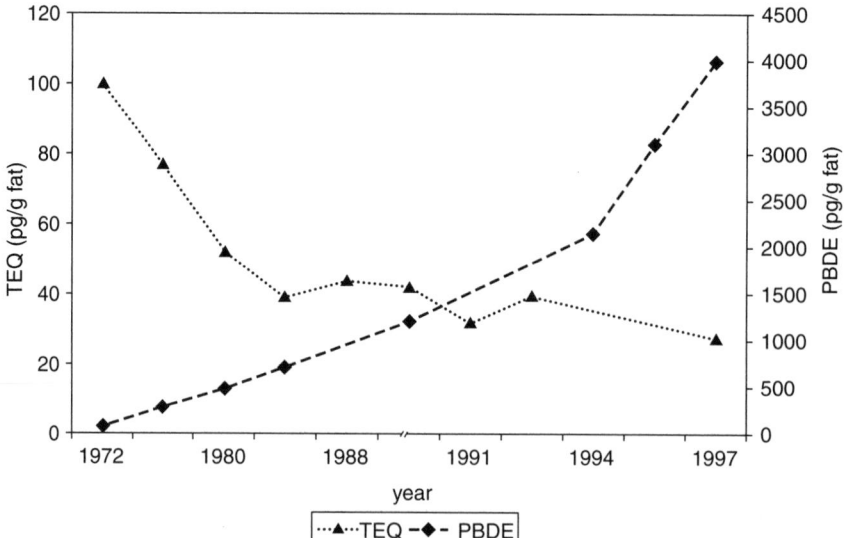

FIGURE 6–3. Breast milk contaminant levels, Sweden, 1972–1997 (chart is based on data in Noren and Meironyte, 2000). PBDE = polybrominated diphenyl ethers; TEQ = TCDD toxic equivalents.

environmental compartments and biota. Widely used during the mid-twentieth century, PCBs are now tightly controlled chemicals but substantial amounts remain in use, mainly in electrical equipment manufactured before the 1979 ban. Large amounts of PCBs from electrical equipment removed from service and other sources remain in storage and waste disposal sites, subject to fires that generate extremely toxic PCDFs and PCDDs. The EPA estimates that up to 200 chemical processes, including production of chlorinated solvents, paints, printing inks, plastics, and detergent bars, may inadvertently generate PCBs.

In general, PCDDs and PCDFs arise unintentionally through four main processes: (1) combustion of wastes and fossil fuels, (2) metal smelting, refining, and processing (including the reprocessing of scrap metal from cars and other products containing plastics), (3) production, use, and disposal of chlorinated organic compounds, and (4) production of chlorine-bleached wood pulp. Other sources include photolysis of highly chlorinated phenols and reservoir sources, that is, contaminated soils, sediments, biota, and water.

Airborne concentrations of PCDDs, PCDFs, and PCBs in Europe and the United States were low before the 1930s, increased until about 1970, and then declined. Total PCBs in Great Lakes sediments and biota decreased during the 1970s and 1980s, but this trend slowed during the 1990s. Industrial production of chlorinated organic chemicals and chlorine use by pulp and paper mills increased during 1930–1970, followed by a period of increasing pollution abatement activities. The latter included elimination of most open burning, particulate controls on combustors, the phase-out of leaded gas, bans on PCBs, 2,4,5-trichlorophenoxyacetic acid (2,4,5-T), and hexachlorophene and restrictions on the use of pentachlorophenol. Emissions of PCDD and PCDF in the United States declined about 80% during 1987–1995, mainly due to reduced municipal and medical waste incinerator emissions.

Food

Sources
The vast majority of dioxin-TEQ intake is from dietary sources, especially meat and dairy products (Table 6–4). The primary pathways for PCDDs in the human diet are air-plant-animal and air-water-fish, with bioaccumulation factors generally higher for congeners with a higher chlorine content. Dairy products from cows grazed on pasture contaminated by the application of sewage sludge (as fertilizer) can raise the daily dietary intake of PCDDs and PCDFs by up to 40%. Among pregnant Dutch women, dairy products and oils of animal origin contributed, respectively,

TABLE 6–4. Estimated Average Daily Intake
of Dioxin-TEQ by the U.S. Population

Source/Pathway	Intake (pg/day)
Air	0.4
Water	0.004
Soil (ingestion)	0.02
Food sources (total)	34.4
Fruits and vegetables	1.2
Dairy products	8.0
Beef	18.0
Fish	6.7
Eggs	0.5
Total intake	34.8

Source: Travis (1991).

about 50% and 25% of dietary intake of PCDDs and coplanar PCBs. In the United Kingdom, the estimated daily dietary intake of PCDD/PCDF and PCB TEQs each declined by about 70% during 1982–1992. Similarly, estimated adult daily PHAH intakes in the United States peaked about 1970 and then declined.

Breast milk is the major exposure source during infancy, far exceeding prenatal exposures. Infants absorb 90%–100% of tetra and higher chlorinated PCB congeners from breast milk. A U.S. national survey showed that average total dioxin-TEQ intakes in breast-fed infants (42 pg/kg/day) were 10–20 times those in adolescents or adults (Schecter et al., 2001); in all age groups, average daily intakes exceeded the ATSDR MRL for chronic exposure (1 pg/kg/day) (Table 6–5). Infant blood PCB levels increase with the duration of breast-feeding and may be up to fivefold higher than those of formula-fed children. The total daily TEQ intake among breast-fed infants in Holland is about 110–120 pg/kg, substantially higher than the tolerable daily intake for the general population set by the WHO (1–4 pg/kg). Breast milk PHAH levels decline by over 50% after prolonged breast-feeding, reflecting the importance of lactation as an excretory mechanism.

Children consume more food per unit body weight than adults and substantially more for specific foods such as milk. Analysis of hamburgers, pizza, deep-fried chicken, and ice cream showed that daily total dioxin-TEQ exposure (per unit body weight) from consumption of these foods would be almost fourfold higher for children than adults (Schecter and Li, 1997). Dairy products, meat, and processed foods, respectively, contributed 43%–50%, 14%–19%, and 15%–23% of PCB/dioxin-TEQ in-

TABLE 6–5. Standards and Guidelines for TCDD or Dioxin TEQs

Medium	Standard	Agency
Air	Emission limits	EPA[a]
Drinking water	3×10^{-8} mg/L	EPA[b]
Foods of animal origin		
Milk and dairy products	5 pg/g fat	France[c]
Pork and derived products	3 pg/g fat	Belgium[d]
Soil[e]		
Action level	≥1 ng/g	ATSDR
Evaluation level	>0.05 and <1 ng/g	ATSDR
Screening level	≤0.05 ng/g	ATSDR
Total daily intake		
MRL (chronic exposure)	1 pg/kg/day	ATSDR[f]
TCDD and dioxin-like compounds	1–4 pg/kg/day	WHO[g]

[a]The EPA has regulations for release of dioxin-like compounds from air sources and from pulp and paper mills into water bodies.

[b]U.S. Environmental Protection Agency (2001).

[c]France (World Health Organization, 2001).

[d]Belgium (World Health Organization, 2001).

[e]Dioxin-TEQ (De Rosa et al., 1997).

[f]Agency for Toxic Substances and Disease Registry (2002).

[g]Van Leeuwen et al. (2000).

take among toddlers (Patandin et al., 1999). In the United States, average dioxin-TEQ levels were highest in farm-grown freshwater fish fillets (1.7 pg/g), intermediate in ocean fish, beef, chicken, pork, sandwich meat, eggs, cheese, ice cream, and human milk (0.33–0.51 pg/g), and lowest in a simulated vegan diet (0.09 pg/g) (Schecter et al., 2001). Intake of dietary dioxins in some European countries has declined by about 50% since the late 1980s.

Intervention
Dietary intervention during pregnancy would make little difference in fetal exposure; effective intervention will require lifelong reduced PHAH dietary intake, especially from foods of animal origin. In its three risk assessments of PHAHs since 1987, the WHO each time has concluded that there are known benefits of breast-feeding, that evidence of harm from PHAHs is insufficient to limit breast-feeding or to eliminate specific foods from the diet, that reducing the release of PHAHs to the environment is the best way to minimize human exposures, and that it should continue to endorse breast-feeding (Brouwer et al., 1998).

Since the 1970s, fish advisories have been used to reduce consumption of contaminated sport fish, especially by women. Although almost 10% of Great Lakes States residents consume regional sport fish, less than half of exposed women are aware of the advisories. During 1986–1989, Mohawk women at Akwasasne in New York had breast milk PCB levels almost double those of nonaboriginal women and associated with fish consumption; after issuance of fish advisories and decreased local fish consumption, breast milk PCB levels declined to general population levels by 1990–1992. See Table 6–6 for reference doses and standards for PCBs.

Air and Water

Sources

The EPA estimates that PCDD/PCDF releases totaled about 3.3 kg TEQ in the United States during 1995 compared to about 14 kg in 1987. Reduced municipal and medical waste incinerator releases accounted for most of the improvement, but these sources plus burning of refuse in barrels still comprise about 70% of quantifiable emissions. Outdoor air has generally been a minor direct source of human TCDD exposure, with important exceptions including the Seveso incident. Low levels of PCBs are widely found in surface waters but rarely occur at high levels in groundwater because of their low solubility; exceptions include groundwater contaminated by leachates from hazardous waste sites. Chlorine bleached pulp and paper production has been a major source of dioxins in water.

Intervention

The Clean Air Act and the Clean Water Act require the EPA to set emissions limits and ambient water quality criteria for TCDD (Table 6–5). The

TABLE 6–6. Standards and Guidelines for PCBs

Medium	Standard
Drinking water	0.5 μg/L[a]
Food[b,c]	
Eggs	0.3 μg/g fat
Milk	1.5 μg/g fat
Poultry	3 μg/g fat
Fish (edible portion)	2 μg/g
Red meat	3 μg/g fat

[a]U.S. Environmental Protection Agency (2001).

[b]U.S. Food and Drug Administration (2000b).

[c]U.S. Food and Drug Administration (2000a).

1998 pulp and paper effluent guidelines should eliminate 96% of TCDD discharges from this industry, once the largest industrial source of TCDD in water. The EPA maximum contaminant level for TCDD in public drinking water is 3×10^{-8} mg/L. Virtual elimination of PHAH air emissions is essential to reduce population exposures to these toxicants over the long term, including prenatal and lactational exposures at critical stages of growth and development. The May 2001 Stockholm Convention legally binds the United States, the European countries, and several other countries to (1) regulate 16 persistent organochlorine compounds, ban production and use of 8 organochlorine pesticides, and ban production and limit uses of PCBs, (2) require the use of the best available technology to limit air emissions from major stationary sources of PCDDs, PCDFs, and certain other toxicants, (3) limit PCDD/PCDF emissions from waste incinerators, (4) reduce total national air emissions below the levels for a reference year, and (5) manage stockpiles of waste persistent organochlorine pollutants (POPs) in an environmentally sound manner.

Other Sources

Urban levels of the higher chlorinated PCDD congeners generally exceed those in rural areas and are associated with local combustion sources including incinerators. Sludges contaminated with PHAH from pulp and paper mills and sewage treatment plants have been widely used as agricultural soil enhancers. Although food crops take up only small amounts of PHAHs from soil, continuation of this practice could cause higher uptakes in the future as PHAHs accumulate in soil.

There has been no systematic survey of dioxins in commercial products. Pentachlorophenol (PCP) and the herbicide 2,4,5-T were banned because of concern about their content of dioxins and other PHAHs. The EPA reported that 14% of 2,4-D samples contained 1,2,3,7,8-pentachlorodibenzo-p-dioxin, a congener that is as potent as TCDD. Manufacturers have cooperated with the EPA to prevent the manufacturing of new products significantly contaminated with TCDD. The FDA and the Consumer Product Safety Commission concluded that dioxins in paper and paper products including coffee filters, food packaging, tampons, surgical dressings, and diapers do not pose a significant health risk. Pentachlorophenol is ubiquitous in the environment because of past uses in wood preservation.

The PHAHs are chemicals of concern in many of the Superfund hazardous waste sites, the best known being Love Canal (New York) and Times Beach (Missouri). In 1999, the EPA proposed regulations to limit dioxins in cement kiln dust and sludges from pulp and paper and sewage treatment plants used as soil additives. The recent EPA TCDD assessment concluded that the human cancer risk related to current background levels of dioxins is 0.1 to 1.0% (U.S. Environmental Protection Agency, 2000b). The EPA did not recommend an RfD because, under its traditional approach, it would have been two to three orders of magnitude lower than current background exposure levels. The WHO used noncarcinogenic animal toxicity data and human body burden data to set a tolerable daily intake of dioxin-TEQ at 1–4 pg/kg (World Health Organization, 2000).

CONCLUSIONS

Proven Health Effects

- Prenatal exposure to relatively high amounts of PCBs (contaminated by other PHAHs) can cause intrauterine growth retardation, eye discharges, increased pigmentation, developmental delays, and cognitive deficits.
- Relatively high exposure to TCDD can cause chloracne, with children possibly being more susceptible than adults.
- The IARC and the EPA concluded that TCDD can cause cancer in humans; the excess lifetime cancer risk of current population TCDD exposure levels may be as high as 1.0%.

Unresolved Issues and Knowledge Gaps

- Developmental effects—there is limited evidence that low-level preconceptual and gestational exposure to PCBs and related PHAHs may cause fetal deaths, intrauterine growth retardation, and preterm delivery and that high-level prenatal exposure may cause developmental abnormalities (hypertelorism, natal teeth).
- Neurotoxicity
  - There is limited epidemiologic evidence that preconceptual and prenatal maternal exposure to PCBs and related PHAHs from dietary and/or other background environmental sources can cause abnormal reflexes among newborn infants, reduced motor skills among infants, and cognitive deficits in children
  - There is inadequate evidence to assess the possible independent roles of lactational PCB exposure, coplanar versus noncoplanar PCB congeners, and prenatal PHAH-induced thyroid suppression in causing neurotoxicity
- Cancer
  - Occupational PCB exposure is a probable cause of cancer in adults.
  - There is limited evidence that cumulative exposure to PCBs and related PHAHs may cause adult cancers including breast cancer and

non-Hodgkin's lymphoma; the relative importance of PHAH exposure during childhood and adulthood is unknown.
  - The potential role of PHAHs in childhood cancers is unknown.
- Other toxicity
  - There is inadequate evidence to assess the role of perinatal PHAH exposure in the development of the endocrine, reproductive, and immune systems; TCDD and related PHAHs should be considered nonspecific immunosuppressants at least until better data are available.
  - There is limited evidence that perinatal PHAH exposure may affect preadolescent growth (reduced stature).

Risk Management Issues

- Prevention
  - Although PCB production ceased in 1979 and emissions of other PHAHs have generally decreased, PHAHs persist throughout the global environment and bioaccumulate in aquatic and terrestrial food chains.
  - Foods, particularly breast milk, dairy products, fish, meat, and poultry, continue to be the major sources of PHAH uptake for the general population.
  - The benefits of breast-feeding appear to outweigh the potential neurobehavioral effects of lactational PHAH exposure.
  - It is necessary to reduce PHAH emissions and human exposures through various strategies including
    Replacement of chlorine and chlorine-containing products with safer alternatives
    Reduced incineration of chlorine-containing products and emission controls to further reduce PHAH emissions from incinerators
    Continued modification of industrial processes to reduce inadvertent production of PHAH contaminants
    Reduced use of PHAH-contaminated sludge on croplands
- Biomonitoring
  - Breast milk dioxin-TEQ levels have decreased by about 50% in several countries during recent decades, with the notable exception of dioxin-like PCDEs; relatively high levels persist in populations dependent on contaminated fish and sea mammals.

REFERENCES

Agency for Toxic Substances and Disease Registry. (1998). Toxicological profile for chlorinated dibenzo-*p*-dioxins (update). Atlanta: Agency for Toxic Substances and Disease Registry.

Agency for Toxic Substances and Disease Registry. (2000). Toxicological profile for polychlorinated biphenyls (update). Atlanta: Agency for Toxic Substances and Disease Registry.
Agency for Toxic Substances and Disease Registry. (2002). Minimal risk levels (MRLs) for hazardous substances. Located at http://www.atsdr.cdc.gov/mrls.html.
Alaluusua S, Lukinmaa PL, Torppa J, Tuomisto J, Vartiainen T. (1999). Developing teeth as biomarker of dioxin exposure. Lancet 353:206.
Anderson HA, Falk C, Hanrahan L, Olson J, Burse VW, Needham L, Paschal D, Patterson D Jr, Hill RH Jr. (1998). Profiles of Great Lakes critical pollutants: a sentinel analysis of human blood and urine. The Great Lakes Consortium. Environ Health Perspect 106:279–89.
Aronson KJ, Miller AB, Woolcott CG, Sterns EE, McCready DR, Lickley LA, Fish EB, Hiraki GY, Holloway C, Ross T, and others. (2000). Breast adipose tissue concentrations of polychlorinated biphenyls and other organochlorines and breast cancer risk. Cancer Epidemiol Biomarkers Prev 9:55–63.
Birnbaum LS. (1995). Developmental effects of dioxins. Environ Health Perspect 103(Suppl 7):89–94.
Blanck HM, Marcus M, Rubin C, Tolbert PE, Hertzberg VS, Henderson AK, Zhang RH. (2002). Growth in girls exposed in utero and postnatally to polybrominated biphenyls and polychlorinated biphenyls. Epidemiology 13:205–10.
Brouwer A, Ahlborg UG, van Leeuwen FX, Feeley MM. (1998). Report of the WHO working group on the assessment of health risks for human infants from exposure to PCDDs, PCDFs and PCBs. Chemosphere 37:1627–43.
Centers for Disease Control and Prevention. (2001). National report on human exposure to environmental chemicals. Selection of chemicals for the report. Located at http://www.cdc.gov/nceh/dls/report/totalreport/substance.htm.
Chao WY, Hsu CC, Guo YL. (1997). Middle-ear disease in children exposed prenatally to polychlorinated biphenyls and polychlorinated dibenzofurans. Arch Environ Health 52:257–62.
Chen YC, Guo YL, Hsu CC, Rogan WJ. (1992). Cognitive development of Yu-Cheng ("oil disease") children prenatally exposed to heat-degraded PCBs. JAMA 268:3213–8.
Craan AG, Haines DA. (1998). Twenty-five years of surveillance for contaminants in human breast milk. Arch Environ Contam Toxicol 35:702–10.
Crofton KM, Rice DC. (1999). Low-frequency hearing loss following perinatal exposure to 3,3',4,4',5-pentachlorobiphenyl (PCB 126) in rats. Neurotoxicol Teratol 21:299–301.
De Rosa CT, Brown D, Dhara R, Garrett W, Hansen H , Holler J, Jones D, Jordan-Izaguirre D, O'Connor R, Pohl H, and others. (1997). Dioxin and dioxin-like compounds in soil, Part I: ATSDR interim policy guideline. Agency for Toxic Substances and Disease Registry. Toxicol Ind Health 13:759–68.
Dewailly E, Ayotte P, Bruneau S, Gingras S, Belles-Isles M, Roy R. (2000). Susceptibility to infections and immune status in Inuit infants exposed to organochlorines. Environ Health Perspect 108:205–11.
Dewailly E, Ayotte P, Bruneau S, Laliberte C, Muir DC, Norstrom RJ. (1993). Inuit exposure to organochlorines through the aquatic food chain in Arctic Quebec. Environ Health Perspect 101:618–20.
Gladen BC, Ragan NB, Rogan WJ. (2000). Pubertal growth and development

and prenatal and lactational exposure to polychlorinated biphenyls and dichlorodiphenyl dichloroethene. J Pediatr 136:490–6.

Holford TR, Zheng T, Mayne ST, Zahm SH, Tessari JD, Boyle P. (2000). Joint effects of nine polychlorinated biphenyl (PCB) congeners on breast cancer risk. Int J Epidemiol 29:975–82.

International Agency for Research on Cancer. (1987). Overall evaluations of carcinogenicity: an updating of IARC Monographs Volumes 1 to 42 (Supplement 7). Lyon, France: International Agency for Research on Cancer.

Jacobson JL, Jacobson SW. (1996). Intellectual impairment in children exposed to polychlorinated biphenyls in utero. N Engl J Med 335:783–9.

Jacobson JL, Jacobson SW, Humphrey HE. (1990). Effects of exposure to PCBs and related compounds on growth and activity in children. Neurotoxicol Teratol 12:319–26.

Jacobson JL, Janisse J, Banerjee M, Jester J, Jacobson SW, Ager JW. (2002). A benchmark dose analysis of prenatal exposure to polychlorinated biphenyls. Environ Health Perspect 110:393–8.

Karmaus W, Asakevich S, Indurkhya A, Witten J, Kruse H. (2002). Childhood growth and exposure to dichlorodiphenyl dichloroethene and polychlorinated biphenyls. J Pediatr 140:33–9.

Knox E. (2000). Childhood cancers, birthplaces, incinerators and landfill sites. Int J Epidemiol 29:391–7.

Lackmann GM. (2002). Polychlorinated biphenyls and hexachlorobenzene in full-term neonates. Reference values updated. Biol Neonate 81:82–5.

LaKind JS, Berlin CM, Naiman DQ. (2001). Infant exposure to chemicals in breast milk in the United States: what we need to learn from a breast milk monitoring program. Environ Health Perspect 109:75–88.

Longnecker MP, Rogan WJ, Lucier G. (1997). The human health effects of DDT (dichlorodiphenyltrichloroethane) and PCBs (polychlorinated biphenyls) and an overview of organochlorines in public health. Annu Rev Public Health 18:211–44.

McNulty WP. (1985). Toxicity and fetotoxicity of TCDD, TCDF and PCB isomers in rhesus macaques (*Macaca mulatta*). Environ Health Perspect 60:77–88.

Mocarelli P, Needham LL, Marocchi A, Patterson DG Jr, Brambilla P, Gerthoux PM, Meazza L, Carreri V. (1991). Serum concentrations of 2,3,7,8-tetrachlorodibenzo-p-dioxin and test results from seleced residents of Seveso, Italy. J Toxicol Environ Health 32:357–66.

Mocarelli P, Gerthoux PM, Ferrari E, Patterson DG Jr, Kieszak SM, Brambilla P, Vincoli N, Signorini S, Tramacere P, Carreri V, and others. (2000). Paternal concentrations of dioxin and sex ratio of offspring. Lancet 3555:1858–63.

Needham LL, Patterson DG Jr, Burse VW, Paschal DC, Turner WE, Hill RH Jr. (1996). Reference range data for assessing exposure to selected environmental toxicants. Toxicol Ind Health 12:507–13.

Noren K, Meironyte D. (2000). Certain organochlorine and organobromine contaminants in Swedish human milk in perspective of past 20–30 years. Chemosphere 40:1111–23.

Orban JE, Stanley JS, Schwemberger JG, Remmers JC. (1994). Dioxins and dibenzofurans in adipose tissue of the general U.S. population and selected subpopulations. Am J Public Health 84:439–45.

Patandin S, Dagnelie PC, Mulder PG, Op de Coul E, van der Veen JE, Weisglas-Kuperus N, Sauer PJ. (1999). Dietary exposure to polychlorinated biphenyls and dioxins from infancy until adulthood: a comparison between breast-feeding, toddler, and long-term exposure. Environ Health Perspect 107:45–51.

Patandin S, Koopman-Esseboom C, de Ridder MA, Weisglas-Kuperus N, Sauer PJ. (1998). Effects of environmental exposure to polychlorinated biphenyls and dioxins on birth size and growth in Dutch children. Pediatr Res 44:538–45.

Pesatori AC, Consonni D, Tironi A, Zocchetti C, Fini A, Bertazzi PA. (1993). Cancer in a young population in a dioxin-contaminated area. Int J Epidemiol 22: 1010–3.

Pocchiari F, Silano V, Zampieri A. (1979). Human health effects from accidental release of tetrachlorodibenzo-p-dioxin (TCDD) at Seveso, Italy. Ann NY Acad Sci 320:311–20.

Ribas-Fito N, Sala M, Kogevinas M, Sunyer J. (2001). Polychlorinated biphenyls (PCBs) and neurological development in children: a systematic review. J Epidemiol Commun Health 55:537–46.

Rice DC. (1997). Effect of postnatal exposure to a PCB mixture in monkeys on multiple fixed interval-fixed ratio performance. Neurotoxicol Teratol 19:429–34.

Rogan WJ, Gladen BC, Hung KL, Koong SL, Shih LY, Taylor JS, Wu YC, Yang D, Ragan NB, Hsu CC. (1988). Congenital poisoning by polychlorinated biphenyls and their contaminants in Taiwan. Science 241:334–6.

Rothman N, Cantor KP, Blair A, Bush D, Brock JW, Helzlsouer K, Zahm SH, Needham LL, Pearson GR, Hoover RN, and others. (1997). A nested case-control study of non-Hodgkin lymphoma and serum organochlorine residues. Lancet 350:240–4.

Ryan JJ, Gasiewicz TA, Brown JF Jr. (1990). Human body burden of polychlorinated dibenzofurans associated with toxicity based on the Yusho and Yucheng incidents. Fundam Appl Toxicol 15:722–31.

Rylander L, Stromberg U, Dyremark E, Ostman C, Nilsson-Ehle P, Hagmar L. (1998). Polychlorinated biphenyls in blood plasma among Swedish female fish consumers in relation to low birth weight. Am J Epidemiol 147:493–502.

Safe S. (2001). Molecular biology of the Ah receptor and its role in carcinogenesis. Toxicol Lett 120:1–7.

Schecter A, Cramer P, Boggess K, Stanley J, Papke O, Olson J, Silver A, Schmitz M. (2001). Intake of dioxins and related compounds from food in the U.S. population. J Toxicol Environ Health A 63:1–18.

Schecter A, Li L. (1997). Dioxins, dibenzofurans, dioxin-like PCBs, and DDE in U.S. fast food, 1995. Chemosphere 34:1449–57.

Scheele J, Teufel M, Niessen KH. (1992). Chlorinated hydrocarbons in the bone marrow of children: studies on their association with leukaemia. Eur J Pediatr 151:802–5.

Schiestl RH, Aubrecht J, Yap WY, Kandikonda S, Sidhom S. (1997). Polychlorinated biphenyls and 2,3,7,8-tetrachlorodibenzopdioxin induce intrachromosomal recombination in vitro and in vivo. Cancer Res 57:4378–83.

Travis CC, Hattemer-Frey HA. (1991). Human exposure to dioxin. Sci Total Environ 104:97–127.

U.S. Environmental Protection Agency. (2000a). Exposure and human health reassessment of 2,3,7,8-tetrachlorodibenzo-p-dioxin (TCDD) and related compounds, part III: integrated summary and risk characterization for 2,3,7,8-tetrachloro-p-dioxin (TCDD) and related compounds. Washington, DC: U.S. Environmental Protection Agency.

U.S. Environmental Protection Agency. (2000b). Exposure and human health reassessment of 2,3,7,8-tetrachlorodibenzo-*p*-dioxin (TCDD) and related compounds. Washington, DC: U.S. Environmental Protection Agency.

U.S. Environmental Protection Agency. (2001). Current drinking water standards. Washington, D.C: U.S. Environmental Protection Agency.

U.S. Food and Drug Administration. (2000a). Action levels for poisonous or deleterious substances in human food and animal feed. Washington, DC: U.S. Food and Drug Administration.

U.S. Food and Drug Administration. (2000b). Food and drugs chapter 1: Unavoidable contaminants in food for human consumption and food-packaging material. Washington, DC: U.S. Government Printing Office.

Urabe H, Asahi M. (1985). Past and current dermatological status of Yusho patients. Environ Health Perspect 59:11–5.

van Leeuwen FX, Feeley M, Schrenk D, Larsen JC, Farland W, Younes M. (2000). Dioxins: WHO's tolerable daily intake (TDI) revisited. Chemosphere 40:1095–101.

Vartiainen T, Jaakkola JJ, Saarikoski S, Tuomisto J. (1998). Birth weight and sex of children and the correlation to the body burden of PCDDs/PCDFs and PCBs of the mother. Environ Health Perspect 106:61–6.

Walkowiak J, Wiener JA, Fastabend A, Heinzow B, Kramer U, Schmidt E, Steingruber HJ, Wundram S, Winneke G. (2001). Environmental exposure to polychlorinated biphenyls and quality of the home environment: effects on psychodevelopment in early childhood. Lancet 358:1602–7.

Weisglas-Kuperus N, Patandin S, Berbers GA, Sas TC, Mulder PG, Sauer PJ, Hooijkaas H. (2000). Immunologic effects of background exposure to polychlorinated biphenyls and dioxins in Dutch preschool children. Environ Health Perspect 108:1203–7.

World Health Organization. (2000). Consultation on assessment of the health risk of dioxins; re-evaluation of the tolerable daily intake (TDI): executive summary. Food Addit Contam 17:223–40.

World Health Organization. (2001). Joint FAO/WHO food standards programme. Codex committee on food additives and contaminants. Thirty-third Session, The Hague, The Netherlands, 12–16 March 2001. Position paper on dioxins and dioxin-like PCBs. Located at http://www.who.int/fsf/Chemicalcontaminants/fa01_29e.pdf.

Yamashita F, Hayashi M. (1985). Fetal PCB syndrome: clinical features, intrauterine growth retardation and possible alteration in calcium metabolism. Environ Health Perspect 59:41–5.

Yoshimura T, Kaneko S, Hayabuchi H. (2001). Sex ratio in offspring of those affected by dioxin and dioxin-like compounds: the Yusho, Seveso, and Yucheng incidents. Occup Environ Med 58:540–1.

Yu ML, Hsin JW, Hsu CC, Chan WC, Guo YL. (1998). The immunologic evaluation of the Yucheng children. Chemosphere 37:1855–65.

7
Pesticides

Conventional pesticides comprise a diverse group of substances intended to destroy, repel, or control organisms identified as pests. Some are broad-spectrum biocides and others are relatively selective, targeting specific organisms such as insects, fungi, or plants. By 1999, the EPA had registered almost 900 active ingredients in pesticides, including 350 approved for use on food crops. The discovery during the 1960s of toxic effects in wildlife linked to bioaccumulation of organochlorines in food chains contributed to public concern and decisions of the U.S. government to form the Environmental Protection Agency (EPA) in 1970 and to ban the use of DDT on food crops in 1972. *Pesticides in the Diets of Infants and Children* was a landmark report documenting the vulnerability of children to pesticides and the potential for disrupting growth and development processes (National Academy of Sciences, 1993). This report noted that tests conducted by manufacturers usually involved sexually mature animals and did not assess neurobehavioral, immunologic, and endocrine effects of prenatal and early-life pesticide exposures.

Milestones in the history of pesticide development include:

- Use of elemental sulfur and oil mixtures as insecticides by the Greeks and Romans

- Fungicidal and insecticidal applications of inorganic sulfur and arsenic compounds during the nineteenth century
- Development of synthetic organic pesticides during the 1930s and the early post–World War II era; for example, DDT was registered for use on 334 crops by 1961
- Introduction during the 1960s and 1970s of organophosphate (OP) insecticides, highly toxic but less persistent compounds that generally do not bioaccumulate
- Use during the 1980s and 1990s of natural plant pyrethrins and synthetic pyrethroids, nonpersistent insecticides effective at low doses with relatively low toxicity
- Introduction during the 1990s of genetically modified plants, pesticide-resistant crops, and relatively nontoxic biopesticides (microbials, plant pesticides, pheromones)

This chapter explores pesticides with respect to acute poisonings, developmental toxicity, developmental neurotoxicity, carcinogenicity, and exposure issues. Other topics include the new measures under the 1996 Food Quality Protection Act (FQPA) that address the unique exposure patterns and susceptibility of children.

HEALTH EFFECTS

Major classes and examples of active ingredients in conventional pesticides are shown in Table 7–1. Herbicides comprise about half of the 5 billion pounds of active ingredients used globally each year. Almost 80% of these active ingredients are used in agriculture and forestry, the remainder being used by industry and homeowners. Pesticide formulations incorporate so-called inert substances, that is, ingredients not claimed to be pesticidally active (e.g., surfactants, dyes, suspending agents, preservatives, and emulsifiers). The EPA has registered about 1600 inert ingredients including 56 substances for which it has significant concern about carcinogenicity, reproductive and developmental toxicity, and neurotoxicity (U.S. Environmental Protection Agency, 1999a, 2001b).

Susceptibility

The developing fetus and child are at risk of adverse effects from pesticides because of their unique characteristics and their potential for higher exposures than adults.

TABLE 7–1. Classes and Examples of Conventional Pesticides

Class	Subclasses	Examples
Antimicrobials—substances used to destroy or suppress the growth of harmful bacteria, viruses, fungi, algae, protozoa	Fungicides	Vinclozolin, procymidone, iprodione, ziram, ferbam, thiram, maneb, mancozeb, zineb, benomyl, captan, methylmercury, pentachlorophenol, hexachlorobenzene
	Algicides	Copper sulfate, lithium hypochlorite, pentachlorophenol, various herbicides
	Nonselective biocides	Methyl bromide, phosphine gas
Biopesticides—pesticides derived from natural materials including animals, plants, bacteria, and certain minerals	Microbials	Bacillus thuringiensis (used as an insecticide)
	Plant pesticides	Pyrethrins (insecticides)
	Pheromones	11-Hexadecenal, many other compounds
Herbicides—agents used to destroy unwanted plants	Selective	Chlorophenoxy herbicides—2,4-D, 2,4,5-T; other—atrazine, cyanazine, alachlor, metolachlor, acetochlor
	Nonselective	Paraquat, diquat, glyphosate
Insecticides—any substance used to destroy insects	OPs	Chlorpyrifos, malathion
	N-methyl carbamates	Aldicarb, aminocarb, carbaryl, carbofuran
	Organochlorines	DDT, hexachlorocyclohexanes, aldrin, dieldrin, endrin, endosulfan, heptachlor, chlordane, toxaphene, chlordecone
	Other	Pyrethroids—allethrin, permethrin
Rodenticides—pesticides specially designed to kill rodents	Anticoagulants	Hydroxycoumarins, indandiones
	Other	Vitamin D_3, bromethalin, zinc phosphide, strychnine

Immature Detoxification Systems

Liver metabolism of xenobiotics increases dramatically during early infancy with some enzymes not maturing until age 5 years or later. Several OP insecticides, for instance, are activated by cytochrome P450 systems to oxons, and the latter are inactivated by plasma and liver paraoxonases, enzymes that do not reach adult levels until at least age 6 months.

Developmental Molecular Targets

Normal development of the nervous system requires a complex array of precisely timed events including neuronal proliferation, migration, differentiation, synapse formation, gliogenesis, myelination, and programmed cell death (apoptosis) that appear to depend in part on early-life neurotransmitter systems. Transient bursts of anticholinesterase (AChE) expression coincide with periods of axonal outgrowth in neonatal primate brains, and some selective AChE inhibitors suppress neurite outgrowth in neuroblastoma cells in vitro. Anticholinesterase exists as intracellular monomers and dimers before synapse formation and as cell surface tetramers afterward, paralleling a functional change from generating and stabilizing synapses to enabling neurotransmission. In humans, nicotinic cholinergic receptors are maximally expressed in the brainstem at mid-gestation and may mediate adverse effects of maternal smoking on brain development (Eskenazi and Castorina, 1999).

Prenatal exposure of experimental animals to nicotine or chlorpyrifos inhibits DNA synthesis, triggers apoptosis, and causes reduction of neuron populations in brain regions enriched in cholinergic innervation. Repeated exposure to OPs during gestation or the early postnatal period causes persistent reduced brain AChE activity and deficits in learning, locomotion, and balance. In neonatally exposed rats, chloropyrifos also causes reduced expression of the adenyl cyclase cascade signaling system that serves global functions in the coordination of cell differentiation during development. Development of serotonergic and noradrenergic neurons depends on GABA. Prenatal exposure of rats to dieldrin reduces the expression of developing GABA receptor subunits.

Exposure

Young children may have higher pesticide exposures than adults because they have (1) a higher intake of air, water, and food per unit body weight per day, (2) a larger skin surface area per unit body weight (dermal absorption is an important exposure route for many pesticides), (3) markedly higher intake per unit body weight per day of certain foods (e.g., apple juice), and (4) behaviors that favor pesticide uptake, such as hand–mouth behavior and frequent contact with potentially contaminated surfaces (floors, carpets, lawns).

Poisonings

There appear to be no accurate estimates of the global burden of pesticide poisoning among children. The Toxic Exposure Surveillance System (TESS) of the American Association of Poison Control Centers covers 96% of the U.S. population. During 2000, TESS received reports of 54,544 childhood pesticide exposures attributed to insecticides (41%), rodenticides (36%), insect repellents (16%), and herbicides (6%); about 25% of all exposures were treated in a health care facility, mostly on a precautionary basis (Litovitz et al., 2001). The main causes of moderate or severe poisonings were OPs (alone or in combination), pyrethins, piperonyl butoxide/pyrethin mixtures, herbicides, and carbamate insecticides.

Because they are used in and around homes, bait and tracking rodenticides are one of the leading causes of poisoning among young children; fortunately, most cases are mild and do not require medical intervention. Severe neurotoxicity, including coma, seizures, and death, has occurred after ingestion or excessive dermal exposure to N,N-diethyl-m-toluamide (DEET) (Briassoulis et al., 2001). Some type II pyrethroids have acute oral toxicities comparable to those of OPs (salivation, hyperexcitability, choreoathetosis, seizures, sympathetic activation). In contrast to adults, the major clinical signs in children with severe carbamate and OP poisoning involve central nervous system (CNS) depression and hypotonia rather than the cholinergic symptoms seen in adults.

During the late 1950s, about 4000 persons in Turkey (mainly children) developed porphyria cutanea tarda. This condition includes fragile skin, blisters, sores, and small cysts on sun-exposed skin areas caused by increased liver porphyrin production and photosensitization; at least several hundred infants died, apparently from exposure through breast milk (Gocmen et al., 1989). Investigation linked the illness to consumption of foods prepared from wheat seed grain treated with the fungicide hexachlorobenzene (HCB). Many breast-fed children of exposed mothers died from pembe yara ("pink sore"), a condition including weakness, convulsions, and skin lesions from photosensitization. The most frequent clinical symptoms observed during a follow-up study of victims 20 years later were severe scarring from skin lesions, hyperpigmentation, arthritis, small hands, hypertrichosis, short stature, weakness, paresthesias, and cogwheeling. Release of methyl isocyanate from an insecticide production plant in Bhopal, India, during 1984 was the worst pesticide-related poisoning incident to date, exposing at least 200,000 persons and causing over 3000 deaths.

Development

Among the relatively few epidemiologic studies of pesticides and fetal development reported to date, most have had limited statistical power and crude exposure assessment.

Fetal Death

A review of pre-1998 epidemiologic studies concluded that parental pesticide exposure may increase the risk of early and late fetal deaths; although fetal deaths could not be attributed to specific pesticides, there were associations with broad pesticide categories such as organochlorines and carbamates (Arbuckle and Sever, 1998). Fetal deaths before 12 weeks were associated with both paternal and maternal preconceptual pesticide exposure (especially to herbicides and thiocarbamates), while later fetal deaths were associated with postconception exposure (Arbuckle et al., 1999, 2001). There is also limited evidence of associations between early fetal deaths and serum HCB or DDE levels (Jarrell et al., 1998; Korrick et al., 2001) and between late fetal deaths and maternal residential proximity to agricultural use of restricted pesticides (Bell et al., 2001b).

Fetal Growth and Gestational Length

The few epidemiologic studies of pesticide exposure and fetal growth and gestational length have produced mixed results. There were exposure–risk relationships between third trimester maternal serum DDE levels and intrauterine growth retardation and preterm birth in a recent study that took advantage of stored serum samples collected during 1959–1966, when DDT exposures were much higher than today (Longnecker et al., 2001). Two analytic studies of paternal occupational exposure to herbicides showed no relation to intrauterine growth retardation (IUGR) and inconsistent evidence of a link to preterm delivery (Michalek et al., 1998; Savitz et al., 1997). Maternal but not paternal occupational exposure to PCP was associated with IUGR (Dimich-Ward et al., 1996; Karmaus and Wolf, 1995). There was no relation between birth weight and community exposure to malathion or parental occupation as farmers (Kristensen et al., 1997; Thomas et al., 1992). In one of the few studies to examine postnatal growth, stature at intervals up to age 8 years was inversely associated with blood DDE in girls but not boys (Karmaus et al., 2002).

Birth Defects

Two reviews of epidemiologic studies of pesticide exposure and birth defects concluded that the evidence is suggestive but inconclusive (Garcia, 1998; Nurminen, 1995). In these studies, the main indicator of pesticide exposure was parental occupational exposure in agriculture and the most frequent associations were with limb reduction defects and orofacial clefts. Epidemiologic studies published since these reviews have shown:

- Orofacial clefts—associated with paternal occupational pesticide exposure (Shaw et al., 1999).
- Limb reduction defects—associated with maternal occupational and residential pesticide exposure (Engel et al., 2000; Shaw et al., 1999).
- Genital defects—cryptorchidism was associated with adipose tissue heptachlor levels (Hosie et al., 2000) and maternal but not paternal occupational pesticide exposure (Weidner et al., 1998); neither cryptorchidism nor hypospadias was associated with maternal serum DDT/DDE levels (Longnecker et al., 2002).
- Neural tube defects—associated with residential pesticide use and maternal residence within 0.25 mile of agricultural crops (Shaw et al., 1999) and paternal occupational exposure to phenoxy herbicides (National Academy of Sciences, 2001).
- Cardiac defects—associated with maternal first trimester pesticide exposure, with some evidence of higher risks with herbicide and rodenticide exposure (Loffredo et al., 2001).
- Late fetal deaths from birth defects—associated with maternal residential proximity to agricultural pesticide use during gestational weeks 3–8 (especially pyrethroid and organochlorine pesticides) (Bell et al., 2001a, 2001c).

Reproductive Toxicity

Men occupationally exposed during production of the organochlorine insecticide chlordecone and the nematocide 1,2-dibromo-3-chloropropane (DBCP) developed greatly reduced sperm counts and infertility; DBCP was also linked to Y chromosome nondisjunction in the sperm of exposed men. Animal studies showed that DBCP caused testicular atrophy at the lowest dose tested and several types of cancer in rodents. In addition, DBCP covalent binds to DNA and causes single-strand DNA breaks in round spermatids at low doses. Chlordecone binds to the estrogen receptor and has estrogenic activity in vivo, but the mechanism by which it causes oligospermia remains uncertain. Occupational exposure during application of pesticides has been associated with reduced semen quality in men and reduced fertility in women. See also Chapter 8 (Hormonally Active Agents) for a discussion of hormonally active pesticides.

Neurotoxicity

Compared to studies of lead, mercury, and PCBs, few epidemiologic studies have assessed the developmental neurotoxicity of pesticides. Also, most pesticides and other commercial chemicals have not been tested in animals for developmental neurotoxicity. Hypothesized effects of perinatal pesticide exposure in humans include social and emotional development deficits, autism, cerebral palsy, and mental retardation (Goldman and Koduru, 2000). Most insecticides are designed to target a variety of neuroreceptors and ion channels causing effects such as hyperexcitation and paralysis in target species, but they are also neurotoxic in human and animal bystanders. In one of the few epidemiologic studies of neurobehavioral development and perinatal pesticide exposure, there was no association between cord blood DDE levels and scores on the Fagan Test of Infant Intelligence at ages 6 or 12 months (Darvill et al., 2000). Occupational exposure of older children (and adults) to OPs, carbamates, and some other pesticides may cause prolonged suppression of AChE, visual disturbances, and peripheral neuropathy.

Cancer

Children may be exposed to pesticides used in and around homes and schools, residues in food and water, airborne drift from agricultural use, and carry-home residues by occupationally exposed parents. Recent reviews of childhood cancers and pesticide exposure concluded that (1) reported associations were modest but stronger when exposure was assessed in more detail, (2) most childhood cancers associated with pesticide exposure are the same types linked to pesticide exposure in adults, but the associations among children tend to be stronger, and (3) methodologic limitations preclude strong conclusions (Daniels et al., 1997; Zahm and Ward, 1998). Pesticide exposures linked to specific childhood cancers included

- Brain cancer—in-home, pet, and garden use of pesticides and parental occupational pesticide exposure (including exposure–risk relationships)
- Leukemia—parental occupational pesticide exposure and in-home and garden use of pesticides during pregnancy or childhood (exposure–risk relationships in two studies that assessed children's direct exposure to pesticides)
- Non-Hodgkin's lymphoma, Wilms' tumor, Ewing's sarcoma—postnatal exposure indices

Recent studies have increased the evidence of associations between residential or parental pesticide exposure indices and childhood brain cancer, acute lymphatic leukemia, non-Hodgkin's lymphoma, and kidney cancer (mainly Wilms' tumor) (see, e.g., Cordier et al., 2001; Daniels et al., 2001; Feychting et al., 2001; Krajinovic et al., 2002). Insecticide exposure during year 2 of infancy appeared to confer a higher risk of childhood leukemia than later exposures (Ma et al., 2002). Children with certain poly-morphisms of phase I and phase II enzymes involved in the metabolism of xenobiotics had substantially increased risks of acute lymphoblastic leukemia, and there was evidence of positive interactions between *CYP1A1* polymorphisms and pesticide exposure (Infante-Rivard et al., 1999; Krajinovic et al., 2002; Sinnett et al., 2000).

Because of the relative rarity of childhood cancer, most etiologic stud-ies of childhood cancer have used a case-control design and may be sub-ject to recall bias. Some have argued that many natural biocides in foods are rodent carcinogens at high doses and that carcinogenic risks of syn-thetic pesticides at levels found in foods are likely minimal. The limited epidemiologic evidence of a role for pesticides in childhood cancer, how-ever, is consistent with the following evidence:

- Epidemiologic studies of adult cancers
  - Although one reviewer concluded that evidence of associations be-tween herbicide exposure and soft tissue sarcomas, non-Hodgkin's lymphoma, leukemia, and ovarian cancer was limited (Dich et al., 1997), the National Academy of Sciences concluded that there was sufficient evidence of an association between herbicide and/or TCDD exposure and soft tissue sarcomas, non-Hodgkin's lym-phoma, and Hodgkin's disease (National Academy of Sciences, 2001).
  - There were interactions between serum anti-Epstein-Barr virus anti-body and p,p'-DDE, HCB, or chlordane levels as risk factors for hairy cell leukemia (Nordstrom et al., 2000).
- Genotoxicity—cytogenetic studies of fumigant and herbicide applica-tors have shown sister chromatid breaks and exchanges in peripheral lymphocytes at bands that contain oncogenes and genes involved in tumor suppression and apoptosis including bands 14q32 and 18q21, the most common sites of chromosomal rearrangements in non-Hodgkin's lymphoma.
- Carcinogenicity risk assessments—the EPA concluded that pesticide ac-tive ingredients include 5 known, 71 probable, and 82 possible human carcinogens, many of which are still registered for use on foods.

Immunotoxicity

In one of the few epidemiologic studies of immunologic abnormalities and pesticide exposure among children, combined blood DDE plus PCB or DDE plus HCB levels were associated with otitis media; blood DDE was also associated with a history of asthma and elevated IgE levels (Karmaus et al., 2001).

EXPOSURES

Potential indicators of pesticide exposures among children and reproductive-age adults include environmental levels (air, water, soil, house dust, food) and internal dose. Epidemiologic studies and environmental surveys revealed that the pesticides most frequently used in homes or yards include chlorpyrifos, diazinon, DEET, dichlorvos, malathion, piperonyl butoxide, pyrethrins, 2-methyl-4-chlorophenoxyacetic acid (MCPA), 2,4-D, cygon, propoxur, chlordane, carbaryl, and heptachlor. In agricultural areas, children may be exposed to pesticides through various media including substantially higher house dust concentrations of OPs compared to nonagricultural families (Lu et al., 2000). Among California children living in agricultural areas with intense pesticide use, the highest-ranked pesticides (weighted by amount used and carcinogenic potential in experimental animals) were propargite, methyl bromide, trifluralin, simazine, molinate, and metam sodium (Gunier et al., 2001).

Environmental pesticide monitoring and human activity survey data enable exposure estimates, but actual uptake can be measured only through biomonitoring of human tissues and fluids (Fenske et al., 2000). Breast milk, adipose tissue, and blood samples contain measurable amounts of many fat-soluble, persistent contaminants including organochlorine pesticides, while urine analyses may detect evidence of recent exposure to nonpersistent pesticides and some organochlorines. Some biochemical effects of pesticides reflect the internal dose (e.g., cholinesterase depression reflects recent exposure to AChE insecticides), while others are nonspecific (e.g., chromosome aberrations).

Blood and Adipose Tissue

Dichlorodiphenyldichloroethylene, the major long-lived metabolite of DDT, was detected in 99% of blood serum and adipose tissue samples from U.S. national surveys in the late 1970s (median maternal serum DDE level was 25 μg/L during the early 1960s), but average concentrations have decreased severalfold since then. Over 90% of adipose tissue samples contained multiple organochlorine pesticide metabolites indicative of past and continuing exposure to these persistent, bioaccumulative compounds.

Plasma butyrylcholinesterase (BChE) and red blood cell AChE levels are the most sensitive indicators of OP and carbamate insecticide uptake;

for example, red blood cell AChE is 12–14 times more sensitive to chlorpyrifos than brain or retinal AChE (Chen et al., 1999). The plasma BChE level is normally depressed during the first two trimesters of pregnancy among younger women but is still strongly correlated with self-reported pesticide exposure status. Hemoglobin adducts of pesticides or their metabolites are detectable after exposure to several urea and carbamate insecticides. The frequency of chromosome damage, as indicated by micronuclei in peripheral lymphocytes, has been associated with occupational exposure to pesticides, especially among persons with certain phase II enzyme polymorphisms.

Urine

About 75% of registered OPs are metabolized in vivo to dimethyl and other dialkyl phosphate metabolites excreted in urine. Population-based surveys have shown high prevalence rates among children of urinary metabolites of several pesticides including chlorpyrifos (80%–90%), PCP (100%), p-dichlorobenzene (a widely used toilet deodorant and moth repellent) (96%), lindane (54%), and 2,4-D (20%). During recent decades, the prevalence of the main urinary chlorpyrifos metabolite increased substantially, while that of PCP decreased markedly. Organophosphate metabolites were detected in 95%–100% of meconium samples from neonates in New York City, indicating fetal exposure (Whyatt and Barr, 2001). Concentrations of chlorpyrifos and other OPs in house dust and of their metabolites in children's urine samples were associated with parental occupational exposure and residential proximity to treated farmland (Fenske et al., 2000, 2002). Based on urinary metabolite levels, children living near orchards are more likely than unexposed children to exceed EPA acute and chronic RfDs for azinphosmethyl and phosmet.

Among the U.S. population aged 6–59 years, the 90th percentile urinary dimethyl phosphate level was 10.1 μg/g (Centers for Disease Control and Prevention, 2001). As in children, the most frequently detected urinary pesticide metabolite among adults during NHANES III was 2,5-dichlorophenol (98%), indicative of ubiquitous exposure to p-dichlorobenzene (Table 7–2). Compared to NHANES II (1976–1980), the prevalence of detectable chlorpyrifos (metabolite) in urine increased fivefold (from 6% to 31%) during NHANES III (1988–1994), while that of PCP decreased by about half (from 72% to 39%). Biomonitoring of urinary metabolites and red blood cell cholinesterase levels in agricultural workers has been used to assess pesticide exposure.

TABLE 7–2. Prevalence of Pesticide Urinary Metabolites, NHANES III (1988–1994)

Metabolite	Parent Pesticide	Prevalence (%)	95th Percentile Concentration ($\mu g/g$ creatinine)
2,5-Dichlorophenol	*p*-Dichlorobenzene	98	670
1-Naphthol	Naphthalene, carbaryl	86	36
3,5,6-Trichloro-2-pyridinol	Chlorpyrifos	82	8
2-Naphthol	Naphthalene	81	18
Pentachlorophenol	Pentachlorophenol	64	5
2,4-Dichlorophenol	2,4-D, dichloroprop, other	64	45

Source: Hill et al. (1995).

Breast Milk

Organochlorine levels in breast milk have generally declined dramatically since the 1960s; for instance, DDE levels decreased by over 90% in Canada between 1967 and the mid-1990s (Craan and Haines, 1998; Noren and Meironyte, 2000). Breast milk organochlorine levels vary by geographic region and maternal characteristics; DDE levels in breast milk decrease with lifetime months of lactation because of cumulative depletion of fat stores. Hexachlorobenzene, a fungicide, comprises 10%–60% of the total dioxin TEQ in human milk samples in most countries. Lactational intake of HCB, chlordane, dieldrin, and heptachlor epoxide may exceed WHO acceptable daily intakes.

RISK MANAGEMENT

Over 4.6 billion pounds of pesticide active ingredient chemicals were sold in the United States in 1997, including about 1 billion pounds of conventional pesticides (Table 7–3). Leading pesticides sold for domestic use included *p*-dichlorobenzene (used as a moth repellent and deodorizer), 2,4-D and glyphosate (herbicides), DEET (insect repellant), and chlorpyrifos (an insecticide). Total annual sales of pesticides for home and garden use in the United States decreased by 14% during 1979–1995, but sales of herbicides for home and garden use increased by 42%. By 1990, production of *p*-dichlorobenzene in the United States reached 70,000 tons, indicative of the widespread cosmetic uses of this known animal carcinogen.

Over 90% of current herbicide use occurs on just four crops—corn, soybeans, cotton, and wheat. By amount of active ingredient, atrazine and

TABLE 7–3. Pesticide Sales, United States, 1997

Pesticide Category	Millions of Lb	%
Herbicides	568	12
Insecticides	128	3
Fungicides	81	2
Other	198	4
Subtotal (conventional pesticides)	975	21
Sulfur, miscellaneous	256	6
Wood preservatives	665	15
Specialty biocides	272	6
Chlorine/hypochlorites	2459	54
Total	4627	100

Source: U.S. Environmental Protection Agency (1999a).

2,4-D, respectively, are the most widely used herbicides in the agricultural and nonagricultural sectors. By 1990, relatively nonpersistent OPs and carbamates had replaced most food uses of organochlorine pesticides in the United States but not in many other countries; OPs now comprise about half of the insecticides used in United States. The intensity of insecticide use on corn, soybeans, cotton, and wheat decreased after 1970 with the introduction of synthetic pyrethroids applied in much smaller quantities per acre. Fungicide use remained high because of increased acreage of fruits and vegetables.

Foods

Sources

Foods frequently consumed by children include apples, other fruits, and vegetables that often contain pesticide residues in the parts per billion range. Even the few countries that have conducted regular food consumption and food pesticide residue surveys to assess population exposure to pesticides from foods have not focused on exposures of infants and children. Canada, for instance, has not conducted a national nutrition survey including children and pregnant women since 1970–1972. Food consumption data by single year of age among children less than 5 years old are needed to estimate their pesticide exposures accurately (National Academy of Sciences, 1993).

The most intense pesticide applications include potatoes (43 lb of active ingredient per acre), apples and other vegetables (23 lb/acre), citrus fruit (10 lb/acre), corn (2.9 lb/acre), soybeans (1.2 lb/acre), and wheat

(0.4 lb/acre) (National Academy of Sciences, 2000). The 10 most frequently detected pesticide or pesticide metabolite residues in U.S. baby foods and some of their characteristics are shown in Table 7–4; three of the five leading pesticides were moderate to strong neurotoxins (endosulfan, chlorpyrifos, carbaryl). Apples were the most important food source of ingested chlorpyrifos, followed by tomatoes and grapes.

Despite heavy use of herbicides early in the growing season, food residues of insecticides and fungicides are generally higher because these are applied directly to food closer to or even after its harvest. Even when average daily pesticide ingestion levels can be estimated, these are insufficient for assessing the potential toxicity of peak exposures. Incidents of food-related OP poisoning during the 1980s and early 1990s were linked

TABLE 7–4. Ten Most Frequent Pesticide Residues Found in Selected Baby Foods in 1999

Pesticide or Metabolite	% of Foods[a]	Toxicity[b]
Endosulfan	26	Organochlorine insecticide; potent neurotoxin, fetal resorption and skeletal defects at high maternal doses in rats, mutagenic, unknown carcinogenicity
Iprodione	21	Dicarboximide fungicide; toxicity studies mostly negative
Chlorpyrifos	14	OP insecticide; moderately strong neurotoxin on acute exposure
Carbaryl	13	Carbamate insecticide; moderate to potent neurotoxin on acute exposure, possible teratogen at high doses, weak mutagen but can react with nitrite to produce N-nitrosocarbaryl, a potent mutagen
Permethrin	13	Pyrethroid insecticide; low mammalian toxicity
Chlorpyrifosmethyl	12	OP insecticide; equivocal evidence of delayed neurotoxicity, inadequate developmental toxicity database[c]
Malathion	12	OP insecticide; neurotoxic, mutagenic
Thiabendazole	12	Benzimidazole fungicide; toxicity seen only at high doses
Dimethoate	6	OP insecticide; potent neurotoxin, fetal deaths, reduced fetal growth rate, teratogenic, mutagenic, possible carcinogen
Ethylene thiourea	4	Metabolite of ethylene bisthiocarbamate fungicides, possible human carcinogen[d]

[a]U.S. Food and Drug Administration (2000).

[b]EXTOXNET (Extension Toxicology Network), (2000).

[c]U.S. Environmental Protection Agency (2000).

[d]IARC (1987).

to aldicarb, a carbamate insecticide used on fruits, nuts, potatoes, and other vegetables. Aldicarb is not removable by peeling or washing because it is a systemic agent, that is, it is taken up by roots into the plant itself. Although aldicarb levels in blended samples of banana were within the legal limit, individual bananas had up to ten times this limit. The manufacturer agreed to stop selling aldicarb for use on bananas since they are commonly eaten by children at levels up to fivefold those of adults (on a body weight basis).

The FDA tests about 40 food samples per day for a limited number of pesticides, a rate that precludes careful monitoring of the residues of the many registered pesticides and the many suppliers of food products. The FDA program has detected pesticide residues in 56% of fruit, 41% of grain, 32% of fish/shellfish, and 31% of vegetable products. Levels above FDA maximum residue levels (MRLs) occurred on 5% or more of domestic strawberries, spinach, red beets, head lettuce, and other leaf and stem vegetables. The most frequently detected pesticides or metabolites in animal fat and hen eggs were PCP (35%) and DDE (21%). Whole milk was the main source of DDE for persons in the upper decile of estimated daily intake (MacIntosh et al., 1996).

Intervention
Pesticide active ingredients for use on foods must each receive a registration and a tolerance from the EPA. Tolerances, the most important means by which the EPA limits pesticide residues in foods, are the legal limits of pesticides allowed in raw or processed foods and are the highest levels likely to occur with normal agricultural pesticide uses. Until the 1993 report *Pesticides in the Diets of Infants and Children* was published, tolerances had generally been based on good agricultural practice, not risk to human health; this report strongly recommended that tolerances be set to safeguard infant and child health (National Academy of Sciences, 1993).

The FQPA requires an additional tenfold uncertainty factor in risk assessments for pesticide residue tolerances if there is evidence of special sensitivities of infants and children or if data on toxicity and exposures are incomplete. The FQPA and the 1996 Safe Drinking Water Act both require assessment of chemicals for hormonal activity. In setting tolerances, the EPA now considers (1) RfDs based on animal toxicity tests including developmental toxicity, developmental neurotoxicity, and two-generation reproductive tests and (2) data on pesticide residues in foods and age-specific food consumption patterns of children and other population subgroups.

Based on evidence that young children may ingest methyl parathion, one of the most toxic OPs, at levels up to eight to nine times the RfD, the

EPA in 1999 accepted voluntary cancellation of its use on fruit and vegetable crops representing 90% of the dietary risk to children. The EPA also accepted voluntary measures in 1999 to reduce use of the OP azinphos-methyl because of an unacceptable dietary risk to young children and agricultural workers. Ten years after Sweden initiated pesticide risk-reduction programs during the mid-1980s, the weight of pesticide active ingredients sold annually decreased by about two-thirds. Pesticide residues exceeded Swedish MRLs in 3%–5% of imported fruits and vegetables compared to 0.5%–1% of domestically grown products. Food preparation such as washing, peeling, and cooking appears to reduce the prevalence of detectable pesticide residues in foods by about half, results varying by food and pesticide; for example, endosulfan residues were almost completely removed from apples and pears by peeling but persisted on spinach after washing.

Indoor and Home Environment

Methods to assess pesticide exposures of young children include measurements of pesticide concentrations in indoor air, carpet dust, outdoor soil, and handwipes. Children's exposures can be estimated using time-location-activity diaries, videotaped activity studies, probability distributions of measured surface residues and exposure factors, and pharmacokinetic rate constants. Personal air sampling has shown that indoor airborne pesticide exposure may exceed dietary doses for pesticides used mainly in the home. Exposure to airborne insecticides tends to be higher in warmer climates because of increased indoor use (e.g., for termite control) and higher evaporation of semivolatile compounds.

Urban Homes

Six million urban children living in poverty in the United States are at risk of exposure to pesticides used extensively in schools, homes, and day-care centers (Landrigan et al., 1999). Pesticide products are used indoors in over 90% of U.S. households, the main types being insecticide bombs, broadcast applications, crack and crevice treatments, no-pest strips, pet shampoos, and flea collars. Pesticide use was reported in over 70% of households with pregnant women or infants less than 6 months of age. The most frequently detected pesticides in dust and surface wipe samples from U.S. homes were chlorpyrifos, atrazine, malathion, chlordane, DDT/DDE, methoxychlor, propoxur, carbaryl, permethrin, o-phenylphenol, PCP, and 2,4-D. Tracking of pesticide-contaminated soil and dust into homes by pets and people is a major source of pesticide residues in house dust.

Young children may be exposed to pesticides through inhalation, dermal absorption, or ingestion of pesticides in rugs, furniture, stuffed toys, other absorbent surfaces, dust, or soil. Exposure is enhanced by behaviors common among young children including hand–mouth and object–mouth behaviors and playing barefoot indoors and outdoors. After application to residential lawns, 2,4-D can be detected in indoor air and on surfaces throughout homes (Nishioka et al., 2001; U.S. Environmental Protection Agency, 1999b). The main sources of indoor 2,4-D deposition were track-in by pets and people and settling of resuspended floor dust on tables and sills; the estimated exposure of young children to 2,4-D was 1–40 μg/kg/day (the EPA chronic oral RfD for 2,4-D is 10 μg/kg/day). On occasion, insecticides are applied indoors in entire communities, particularly in endemic malaria regions, where large amounts of DDT continue to be used; in 1993, over 1 million kg of DDT was used to spray house walls in the Western Hemisphere alone. In 2000 the EPA banned some indoor uses of chlorpyrifos including broadcast spraying and direct uses on pets; crack and crevice treatment is still allowed.

Agricultural Area Homes
In agricultural areas, children may be more exposed to pesticides because of higher environmental levels in their indoor and outdoor environments and maternal breast milk. In rural California, ten pesticides were detected in house dust and hand-wipe samples from young children; the most exposed toddlers could ingest diazinon doses above the EPA chronic RfD. The highest house dust OP levels in Washington State occurred in homes with at least one farm worker and in those close to apple or pear orchards.

Schools
There have been few studies of pesticide contamination in school environments, but school kitchens, cafeterias, classrooms, offices, athletic fields, and playgrounds are often treated with a variety of pesticides. Incidents involving illness of students and staff in some U.S. schools have been attributed to unwitting exposure to excessive levels of pesticides including resmethrin, chlorpyrifos, diazinon, and chlordane. In its first statewide survey of pesticide use in public schools, New York State found that 87% of schools used pesticides and usually took few precautions. The Attorney General of New York recommended that schools should adopt and communicate written pest management policies and practices and select the least toxic pesticides when their use is deemed necessary. Other recommendations included notification of school staff, students, and parents, use of warning signs around treated areas, application only by certified personnel, maintenance of detailed records on pesticide use, and avoidance

of pesticides containing known or probable carcinogens (Attorney General of New York, 1996). The EPA noted a health concern for use of chlorpyrifos in crack and crevice treatment in schools, day-care centers, or other rooms that children may occupy for extended periods of time.

Other Sources
Automatic insecticide dispensers are registered by the EPA for use in restaurants, schools, supermarkets, hospitals, day-care centers, and other facilities to control indoor flying insects in food service or work areas (Centers for Disease Control and Prevention, 2000). These automatically dispense a fine mist of pyrethrin or resmethrin (a pyrethroid) along with other active and inert ingredients at frequent intervals (e.g., every 15 minutes). Data for the period 1993–1996 from the TESS, based on poisoning reports from 85% of U.S. poison control centers, showed 54 cases of illness (age 3 to 73 years) associated with automatic insecticide dispensers. The CDC recommended that automatic insecticide dispensers be installed according to manufacturers' labeling instructions, that warning stickers be placed on the dispensers, that installation near air ducts be avoided, and that timers be set to dispense insecticide during nonbusiness hours. There appears to be no ongoing monitoring of pesticide exposure in commercial, institutional, day-care, and other indoor areas accessible to children.

Water

Drinking water is a minor source of pesticide exposure for children or adults in the general population but may be important for subgroups such as farm families. At least 130 pesticides and metabolites have been detected in groundwater, particularly aldicarb, atrazine, DDE, dieldrin, and soil fumigants including ethylene dibromide, dichloropropane, and DBCP. The median total herbicide concentration in Iowa municipal well water increased about tenfold with inclusion of their breakdown products, some of which have toxicity similar to that of their parent compounds. Drinking water guidelines and standards for individual pesticides vary by factors of up to 10 between the WHO and the EPA (Table 7–5). In contrast, the European Union Drinking Water Directive sets maximum limits of 0.1 μg/L for any individual pesticide, 0.03 μg/L for certain specific pesticides, and 0.5 μg/L for total pesticides (European Union, 1998).

General Issues

Pesticide Toxicity Testing
Child health protection requires societal targets for reduction of pesticide use, monitoring of pesticide exposures, and sophisticated premarket de-

TABLE 7–5. Drinking Water Guidelines and Standards for Selected Pesticides

Pesticide	WHO[a]	EPA[b]
Alachlor	20 μg/L	2 μg/L
Atrazine	2 μg/L	3 μg/L
Aldrin/dieldrin	30 ng/L	—
DDT	2 μg/L	—
2,4-D	30 μg/L	70 μg/L
Pentachlorophenol	9 μg/L	1 μg/L

[a]World Health Organization (1998).
[b]U.S. Environmental Protection Agency (2001a).

velopmental toxicity testing (Landrigan et al., 1999). Governments must balance public and scientific concerns about pesticide safety against the benefits of pesticides, especially increased, affordable, and high-quality food supplies. In developed countries, the main control of pesticides is the registration process; this generally includes evaluation of standardized information provided by the manufacturer on efficacy, toxicity, environmental fate and dispersion, and potential ecologic effects. The herbicide 2,4-D was introduced during the 1940s and has been one of the most widely used pesticides for several decades, including applications in areas where children may be exposed. The IARC has designated chlorophenoxy herbicides as possible human carcinogens, but both the IARC and the EPA concluded that animal carcinogenicity tests of 2,4-D were inadequate for evaluation.

The report *Pesticides in the Diets of Infants and Children* recommended that pesticide evaluations include developmental neurotoxicity data; at present, however, only adult neurotoxicity test data are available for most of the 900 pesticide active ingredients in use. The EPA developmental neurotoxicity testing guideline has been criticized for failing to require studies that expose developing animals during all vulnerable periods, assess delayed effects, and use standard neurobehavioral and neuropathology test methods (Claudio et al., 2000). The EPA recently requested developmental neurotoxicity data from manufacturers on about 140 pesticides considered to be neurotoxic.

Inert ingredients are considered trade secrets, and the EPA does not require disclosure except for highly toxic compounds. Unless an inert ingredient is determined to be highly toxic, it does not have to be identified by name or percentage on the label, but the total percentage of such ingredients must be declared. In what appears to be a precedent, the New York City mosquito control program for prevention of West Nile virus infections included both active and inert ingredients in its environmental impact assessment (New York City Department of Health, 2001).

Child-Oriented Interventions

The FQPA required the EPA to evaluate pesticide safety in light of aggregate exposures from nondietary and dietary routes. The insecticide chlorpyrifos illustrates some of the key pesticide risk management issues relevant to child health protection, including cumulative risks from multiple agents sharing a common mechanism and aggregate exposure from multiple environmental media. After the banning of heptachlor and chlordane, chlorpyrifos rapidly became one of the most widely used OPs in the United States. By 2000, about 800 chlorpyrifos-containing products were registered in the United States for use on food crops, lawns, playgrounds, parks, and pets (flea collars) and in homes, schools, day-care centers, and many other settings. Broadcast application of chlorpyrifos indoors appears to cause accumulation in polyurethane foam in pillows, toys, bedding, and mattresses, potentially causing uptake of over 200 μg/kg bw/day among young children (40% from dermal and 60% from oral contact), far higher than the EPA RfD for chronic exposure of 3 μg/kg bw/day from all sources (Gurunathan et al., 1998).

In a reevaluation of chlorpyrifos, concern was raised by new evidence including the following:

- Neonatal rats were more sensitive than adults to inhibition of cholinesterase in frontal cortex, plasma, and red blood cells after acute chlorpyrifos exposure.
- Lack of a NOAEL for developmental neurotoxicity in rats based on structural changes in the developing brains of offspring.

The EPA decided to implement a phased partial ban of chlorpyrifos that will eliminate its uses in and around homes and nonresidential settings (mainly for termite control) and on tomatoes and restrict its use on apples. This action should reduce total chlorpyrifos use by up to 50% when fully implemented in 2004.

Persistent Organochlorine Pesticides

Extensive use of DDT, mainly to control malaria in tropical countries, remains an issue more than 30 years after it was banned in Canada and other countries. Transmission of malaria is enhanced by changes in land use that provide suitable habitats for malaria-transmitting mosquitoes close to human populations, such as, road building, mining, logging, agricultural, and irrigation projects in the Amazon Basin and Southeast Asia. The WHO malaria vector control efforts now favor pyrethroid-treated protective nets for beds, nonpersistent insecticides with minimal impact on nontarget organisms, and limitation of house spraying to specific high-risk and epidemic-prone areas. Although DDT use has decreased sharply in countries such as Mexico (from 25,000 tons in 1970 to about 300 tons in 1998), illegal use of DDT and other persistent organochlorine pesticides continues in parts of Asia. The United Nations Economic Commission for Europe (UN-ECE) has a protocol that legally binds Canada, the United States, Europe, Russia, and several other countries to ban production and use of eight organochlorine pesticides (aldrin, chlordane, dieldrin, endrin, hexabromobiphenyl, chlordecone, mirex, and toxaphene). The protocol will also limit the production and/or use of DDT, heptachlor, lindane, and HCB.

Exposure to Pesticides Sharing a Common Mechanism
The National Academy of Sciences evaluated the risk of exposure to multiple pesticides with a common toxic mechanism by assessing five OPs (National Academy of Sciences, 1993). Although the Academy had to rely on scanty data, it concluded that some children have sufficient aggregate OP exposures to produce symptoms of acute poisoning.

Pesticide Benefits
A National Academy of Sciences expert committee recently reviewed the future role of pesticides in agriculture (National Academy of Sciences, 2000). Net benefits of pesticides on crop yields depend on crop type, weather conditions, types of pests controlled, and other factors. Fumigants, fungicides, and other pesticides appear to be effective in reducing loss and spoilage during storage, distribution, and marketing of crops and foodstuffs. Herbicides allow corn, wheat, and other cereal grains to be planted earlier in the growing season at high densities that raise productivity but preclude machine weed control. Several fungicides, soil fumigants, and insecticides control fungal and insect diseases that are major problems in potato production; up to half of vegetable and fruit produce could be lost to insects and fungi during storage and transportation without the use of pesticides. The expert committee concluded that chemical pesticides would continue to be important because reduced-risk chemical products are being registered and competitive alternatives are not available.

Conclusions

Proven Child Health Outcomes

- Poisonings—50,000 reports annually of U.S. children exposed to pesticide products in and around homes, with about 25% requiring health care services and about 3% causing moderate or severe symptoms
- Reduced sperm counts and infertility—among men occupationally exposed during production of chlordecone and DBCP

Unresolved Issues and Knowledge Gaps

- Developmental effects—limited evidence that periconceptual parental pesticide exposure may cause early and late fetal deaths, preterm delivery, IUGR, and birth defects (particularly orofacial and limb reduction defects)
- Neurotoxicity
    - Inadequate evidence to assess the role of perinatal pesticide exposure in brain development
    - Limited evidence that occupational exposure of older children (and adults) to OPs or carbamates can cause prolonged suppression of AChE, visual disturbances, and peripheral neuropathy
- Childhood cancer—limited evidence that parental exposures before or during pregnancy and childhood exposures may cause childhood cancers (brain cancer, leukemia, non-Hodgkin's lymphoma, Wilms' tumor, Ewing's sarcoma)
- Knowledge gaps—longitudinal studies needed beginning in the first trimester to assess the risk of subtle and delayed health effects of pesticides and other contaminants with known or suspected developmental toxicity

Risk Management Issues

- Prevention
    - Toxicity testing—need comprehensive testing of pesticide active ingredients and inert components for developmental toxicity
    - Exposure reduction—need to minimize occupational and domestic exposures of reproductive-age persons, pregnant women, and young children to pesticides, especially those known or suspected to be developmental toxins or carcinogens
    - Efficacy testing—need rigorous efficacy testing of pesticides to justify the explicit trade-off between benefits and harm in their risk management

- Biomonitoring—need to measure internal doses of pesticides periodically in representative samples of children and reproductive-age men and women to monitor progress in exposure reduction and to identify high-exposure groups

REFERENCES

Arbuckle TE, Lin Z, Mery LS. (2001). An exploratory analysis of the effect of pesticide exposure on the risk of spontaneous abortion in an Ontario farm population. Environ Health Perspect 109:851–7.

Arbuckle TE, Savitz DA, Mery LS, Curtis KM. (1999). Exposure to phenoxy herbicides and the risk of spontaneous abortion. Epidemiology 10:752–60.

Arbuckle TE, Sever LE. (1998). Pesticide exposures and fetal death: a review of the epidemiologic literature. Crit Rev Toxicol 28:229–70.

Attorney General of New York. (1996). Pesticides in schools: reducing the risks. Located at http://www.oag.state.ny.us/environment/schools96.html.

Bell EM, Hertz-Picciotto I, Beaumont JJ. (2001a). A case-control study of pesticides and fetal death due to congenital anomalies. Epidemiology 12:148–56.

Bell EM, Hertz-Picciotto I, Beaumont JJ. (2001b). Case-cohort analysis of agricultural pesticide applications near maternal residence and selected causes of fetal death. Am J Epidemiol 154:702–10.

Bell EM, Hertz-Picciotto I, Beaumont JJ. (2001c). Pesticides and fetal death due to congenital anomalies: implications of an erratum. Epidemiology 12:595–6.

Briassoulis G, Narlioglou M, Hatzis T. (2001). Toxic encephalopathy associated with use of DEET insect repellents: a case analysis of its toxicity in children. Hum Exp Toxicol 20:8–14.

Centers for Disease Control and Prevention. (2000). Illnesses associated with use of automatic insecticide dispenser units—selected states and United States, 1986–1999. MMWR 49:492–5.

Centers for Disease Control and Prevention. (2001). National report on human exposure to environmental chemicals: dimethylphosphate. Atlanta: Centers for Disease Control and Prevention.

Chen WL, Sheets JJ, Nolan RJ, Mattsson JL. (1999). Human red blood cell acetylcholinesterase inhibition as the appropriate and conservative surrogate endpoint for establishing chlorpyrifos reference dose. Regul Toxicol Pharmacol 29:15–22.

Claudio L, Kwa WC, Russell AL, Wallinga D. (2000). Testing methods for developmental neurotoxicity of environmental chemicals. Toxicol Appl Pharmacol 164:1–14.

Cordier S, Mandereau L, Preston-Martin S, Little J, Lubin F, Mueller B, Holly E, Filippini G, Peris-Bonet R, McCredie M, and others. (2001). Parental occupations and childhood brain tumors: results of an international case-control study. Cancer Causes Control 12:865–74.

Craan AG, Haines DA. (1998). Twenty-five years of surveillance for contaminants in human breast milk. Arch Environ Contam Toxicol 35:702–10.

Daniels JL, Olshan AF, Savitz DA. (1997). Pesticides and childhood cancers. Environ Health Perspect 105:1068–77.

Daniels JL, Olshan AF, Teschke K, Hertz-Picciotto I, Savitz DA, Blatt J, Bondy ML,

Neglia JP, Pollock BH, Cohn SL, and others. (2001). Residential pesticide exposure and neuroblastoma. Epidemiology 12:20–7.

Darvill T, Lonky E, Reihman J, Stewart P, Pagano J. (2000). Prenatal exposure to PCBs and infant performance on the Fagan Test of Infant Intelligence. Neurotoxicology 21:1029–38.

Dich J, Zahm SH, Hanberg A, Adami HO. (1997). Pesticides and cancer. Cancer Causes Control 8:420–43.

Dimich-Ward H, Hertzman C, Teschke K, Hershler R, Marion SA, Ostry A, Kelly S. (1996). Reproductive effects of paternal exposure to chlorophenate wood preservatives in the sawmill industry. Scand J Work Environ Health 22:267–73.

Engel LS, O'Meara ES, Schwartz SM. (2000). Maternal occupation in agriculture and risk of limb defects in Washington State, 1980–1993. Scand J Work Environ Health 26:193–8.

Eskenazi B, Castorina R. (1999). Association of prenatal maternal or postnatal child environmental tobacco smoke exposure and neurodevelopmental and behavioral problems in children. Environ Health Perspect 107:991–1000.

European Union. (1998). Council directive 98/83/EC on the quality of water intented for human consumption. Located at http://europa.eu.int/comm/environment/water/water-drink/index_en.html.

EXTOXNET (Extension Toxicology Network). (2000). Pesticide active ingredient profiles. Located at http://pmep.cce.cornell.edu/profiles/extoxnet/index.html.

Fenske RA, Kedan G, Lu C, Fisker-Andersen JA, Curl CL. (2002). Assessment of organophosphorus pesticide exposures in the diets of preschool children in Washington State. J Expo Anal Environ Epidemiol 12:21–8.

Fenske RA, Kissel JC, Lu C, Kalman DA, Simcox NJ, Allen EH, Keifer MC. (2000). Biologically based pesticide dose estimates for children in an agricultural community. Environ Health Perspect 108:515–20.

Feychting M, Plato N, Nise G, Ahlbom A. (2001). Paternal occupational exposures and childhood cancer. Environ Health Perspect 109:193–6.

Garcia AM. (1998). Occupational exposure to pesticides and congenital malformations: a review of mechanisms, methods, and results. Am J Ind Med 33: 232–40.

Gocmen A, Peters HA, Cripps DJ, Bryan GT, Morris CR. (1989). Hexachlorobenzene episode in Turkey. Biomed Environ Sci 2:36–43.

Goldman LR, Koduru S. (2000). Chemicals in the environment and developmental toxicity to children: a public health and policy perspective. Environ Health Perspect 108(Suppl 3):443–8.

Gunier RB, Harnly ME, Reynolds P, Hertz A, Von Behren J. (2001). Agricultural pesticide use in California: pesticide prioritization, use densities, and population distributions for a childhood cancer study. Environ Health Perspect 109: 1071–8.

Gurunathan S, Robson M, Freeman N, Buckley B, Roy A, Meyer R, Bukowski J, Lioy PJ. (1998). Accumulation of chlorpyrifos on residential surfaces and toys accessible to children. Environ Health Perspect 106:9–16.

Hill RH Jr, Head SL, Baker S, Gregg M, Shealy DB, Bailey SL, Williams CC, Sampson EJ, Needham LL. (1995). Pesticide residues in urine of adults living in the United States: reference range concentrations. Environ Res 71:99–108.

Hosie S, Loff S, Witt K, Niessen K, Waag KL. (2000). Is there a correlation between organochlorine compounds and undescended testes? Eur J Pediatr Surg 10:304–9.

Infante-Rivard C, Labuda D, Krajinovic M, Sinnett D. (1999). Risk of childhood leukemia associated with exposure to pesticides and with gene polymorphisms. Epidemiology 10:481–7.

International Agency for Research on Cancer. (1987). Overall evaluations of carcinogenicity: an updating of IARC Monographs Volumes 1 to 42 (Supplement 7). Lyon, France: International Agency for Research on Cancer.

Jarrell J, Gocmen A, Foster W, Brant R, Chan S, Sevcik M. (1998). Evaluation of reproductive outcomes in women inadvertently exposed to hexachlorobenzene in southeastern Turkey in the 1950s. Reprod Toxicol 12:469–76.

Karmaus W, Asakevich S, Indurkhya A, Witten J, Kruse H. (2002). Childhood growth and exposure to dichlorodiphenyl dichloroethene and polychlorinated biphenyls. J Pediatr 140:33–9.

Karmaus W, Kuehr J, Kruse H. (2001). Infections and atopic disorders in childhood and organochlorine exposure. Arch Environ Health 56:485–92.

Karmaus W, Wolf N. (1995). Reduced birthweight and length in the offspring of females exposed to PCDFs, PCP, and lindane. Environ Health Perspect 103: 1120–5.

Korrick SA, Chen C, Damokosh AI, Ni J, Liu X, Cho SI, Altshul L, Ryan L, Xu X. (2001). Association of DDT with spontaneous abortion: a case-control study. Ann Epidemiol 11:491–6.

Krajinovic M, Sinnett H, Richer C, Labuda D, Sinnett D. (2002). Role of NQO1, MPO and CYP2E1 genetic polymorphisms in the susceptibility to childhood acute lymphoblastic leukemia. Int J Cancer 97:230–6.

Kristensen P, Irgens LM, Andersen A, Bye AS, Sundheim L. (1997). Gestational age, birth weight, and perinatal death among births to Norwegian farmers, 1967–1991. Am J Epidemiol 146:329–38.

Landrigan PJ, Claudio L, Markowitz SB, Berkowitz GS, Brenner BL, Romero H, Wetmur JG, Matte TD, Gore AC, Godbold JH, and others. (1999). Pesticides and inner-city children: exposures, risks, and prevention. Environ Health Perspect 107:431–7.

Litovitz TL, Klein-Schwartz W, White S, Cobaugh DJ, Youniss J, Omslaer JC, Drab A, Benson BE. (2001). 2000 Annual report of the American Association of Poison Control Centers Toxic Exposure Surveillance System. Am J Emerg Med 19:337–95.

Loffredo CA, Silbergeld EK, Ferencz C, Zhang J. (2001). Association of transposition of the great arteries in infants with maternal exposures to herbicides and rodenticides. Am J Epidemiol 153:529–36.

Longnecker MP, Klebanoff MA, Brock JW, Zhou H, Gray KA, Needham LL, Wilcox AJ. (2002). Maternal serum level of 1,1-dichloro-2,2-*bis*(*p*-chlorophenyl)ethylene and risk of cryptorchidism, hypospadias, and polythelia among male offspring. Am J Epidemiol 155:313–22.

Longnecker MP, Klebanoff MA, Zhou H, Brock JW. (2001). Association between maternal serum concentration of the DDT metabolite DDE and preterm and small-for-gestational-age babies at birth. Lancet 358:110–4.

Lu C, Fenske RA, Simcox NJ, Kalman D. (2000). Pesticide exposure of children in an agricultural community: evidence of household proximity to farmland and take home exposure pathways. Environ Res 84:290–302.

Ma X, Buffler PA, Gunier RB, Dahl G, Smith MT, Reinier K, Reynolds P. (2002). Critical windows of exposure to household pesticides and risk of childhood leukemia. Environ Health Perspect 110:955–60.

MacIntosh DL, Spengler JD, Ozkaynak H, Tsai L, Ryan PB. (1996). Dietary exposures to selected metals and pesticides. Environ Health Perspect 104:202–9.

Michalek JE, Rahe AJ, Boyle CA. (1998). Paternal dioxin, preterm birth, intrauterine growth retardation, and infant death. Epidemiology 9:161–7.

National Academy of Sciences. (1993). Pesticides in the diets of infants and children. Washington, DC: National Academy Press.

National Academy of Sciences. (2000). The future role of pesticides in U.S. agriculture. Washington, DC: National Academy Press.

National Academy of Sciences. (2001). Veterans and agent orange. Update 2000. Washington, DC: National Academy Press.

New York City Department of Health. (2001). Adult mosquito control programs. Final environmental impact statement. New York: New York City Department of Health.

Nishioka MG, Lewis RG, Brinkman MC, Burkholder HM, Hines CE, Menkedick JR. (2001). Distribution of 2,4-D in air and on surfaces inside residences after lawn applications: comparing exposure estimates from various media for young children. Environ Health Perspect 109:1185–91.

Nordstrom M, Hardell L, Lindstrom G, Wingfors H, Hardell K, Linde A. (2000). Concentrations of organochlorines related to titers to Epstein-Barr virus early antigen IgG as risk factors for hairy cell leukemia. Environ Health Perspect 108:441–5.

Noren K, Meironyte D. (2000). Certain organochlorine and organobromine contaminants in Swedish human milk in perspective of past 20–30 years. Chemosphere 40:1111–23.

Nurminen T. (1995). Maternal pesticide exposure and pregnancy outcome. J Occup Environ Med 37:935–40.

Savitz DA, Arbuckle T, Kaczor D, Curtis KM. (1997). Male pesticide exposure and pregnancy outcome. Am J Epidemiol 146:1025–36.

Shaw GM, Wasserman CR, O'Malley CD, Nelson V, Jackson RJ. (1999). Maternal pesticide exposure from multiple sources and selected congenital anomalies. Epidemiology 10:60–6.

Sinnett D, Krajinovic M, Labuda D. (2000). Genetic susceptibility to childhood acute lymphoblastic leukemia. Leuk Lymphoma 38:447–62.

Thomas DC, Petitti DB, Goldhaber M, Swan SH, Rappaport EB, Hertz-Picciotto I. (1992). Reproductive outcomes in relation to malathion spraying in the San Francisco Bay Area, 1981–1982. Epidemiology 3:32–9.

U.S. Environmental Protection Agency. (1999a). Pesticide industry sales and usage: 1996 and 1997 market estimates (EPA733-R-99-01). Washington, DC: U.S. Environmental Protection Agency.

U.S. Environmental Protection Agency. (1999b). Transport of lawn-applied 2,4-D from turf to home: assessing the relative importance of transport mechanisms and exposure pathways (EPA 600-R-99-040). Washington, DC: U.S. Environmental Protection Agency.

U.S. Environmental Protection Agency. (2000). Chlorpyrifos methyl: toxicology section of the RED chapter. Located at http://www.epa.gov/pesticides/op/chlorpyrifosmethyl/rev_toxicology.pdf.

U.S. Environmental Protection Agency. (2001a). Current drinking water standards. Located at http://www.epa.gov/safewater/mcl.html.

U.S. Environmental Protection Agency. (2001b). Lists of other (inert) pesticide ingredients. Washington, DC: Located at http://www.epa.gov/opprd001/inerts/lists.html.

U.S. Food and Drug Administration. (2000). Pesticide program: residue monitoring 1999. Washington DC: U.S. Food and Drug Administration.

Weidner IS, Moller H, Jensen TK, Skakkebaek NE. (1998). Cryptorchidism and hypospadias in sons of gardeners and farmers. Environ Health Perspect 106: 793–6.

Whyatt RM, Barr DB. (2001). Measurement of organophosphate metabolites in postpartum meconium as a potential biomarker of prenatal exposure: a validation study. Environ Health Perspect 109:417–20.

World Health Organization. (1998). Guidelines for drinking water quality, 2nd edition, Vol. 2, Health criteria and other supporting information, 1996 (p 940–949) and Addendum to Vol. 2, 1998 (p 281–283). Located at http://www.who.int/water_sanitation_health/GDWQ/index.html.

Zahm SH, Ward MH. (1998). Pesticides and childhood cancer. Environ Health Perspect 106(Suppl 3):893–908.

8

Hormonally Active Agents

In multicellular organisms, cell signaling through the nervous, immune, and endocrine systems is essential for coordinating metabolic functions among all cells. Signals range from nutrient and metabolite levels in extracellular fluids to specialized systems including chemical messengers, storage and transportation mechanisms, and receptors. Specialized endocrine cells produce chemical messengers (hormones) that interact with receptors in local and distant target cells. There are intimate links between the endocrine and nervous systems such as the hypothalamic–pituitary gland complex in which specialized neurons produce hormones.

Depending on the hormone, target cells may be confined to a specific organ or may be more widespread. By binding to receptors and influencing intracellular signaling systems, hormones control many processes at the molecular level during gestation and postnatal life. Major endocrine glands include the pituitary gland, thyroid gland, parathyroid glands, pancreatic islets, adrenal glands, testes, and ovaries. When activated by a hormone, receptors on or in target cells trigger a cascade of intracellular reactions. An agonist is a hormone or chemical that binds to a receptor and induces specific biochemical effects; antagonists compete for binding to a receptor but do not induce the biochemical effects associated with the receptor.

Endocrine disruptors have been defined as exogenous agents that interfere with the synthesis, secretion, transport, binding, action, or elimination of natural hormones in the body and may cause adverse effects at the level of an organism, progeny, and populations. As recommended by the National Academy of Sciences, the term *hormonally active agents* (HAAs) is used here to describe substances with hormone-like activity, regardless of the mechanism (National Academy of Sciences, 1999). Although there has been concern during recent years about environmental HAAs, especially in relation to apparent estrogenic effects in wildlife, the ability of DDT/DDE to inhibit testicular and secondary sexual development in roosters was reported several decades earlier (Burlington and Lindeman, 1950). Experience with the potent synthetic estrogen, diethylstilbestrol (DES), showed that prenatal exposure of women to an HAA, albeit a therapeutic product and not an environmental contaminant, could cause early and delayed adverse developmental, reproductive, and carcinogenic effects in offspring; use of other drugs including estrogens, androgens, and progestins during pregnancy has also been linked to abnormal reproductive development. Wildlife and experimental animal studies have shown important adverse effects of HAAs at high doses on reproductive system development, sexual behavior, fertility, and immune function (Vos et al., 2000).

Several studies indicate that incidence rates of birth defects of the penis (hypospadias) and testes (cryptorchidism) and testicular cancer in humans have increased during recent decades, while sperm quality has declined. The validity of these trends and the possible role of environmental HAAs as potential causes remain uncertain and controversial. On the one hand, the increased testicular cancer incidence rates, particularly among young men, are supported by high-quality population-based incidence data from several countries (see, e.g., Power et al., 2001; Weir et al., 1999). These data indicate that testicular cancer incidence rates increased twofold or more during the past three to four decades, especially among more recent birth cohorts. On the other hand, cryptorchidism birth prevalence rates from the late 1960s to the late 1990s have varied considerably among countries and irregularly over time within countries (Paulozzi, 1999). Prevalence rates of cryptorchidism are influenced by diagnostic efficiency and age at examination; in about 70% of affected neonates, testes spontaneously descend by age 3 months. Increased clinical surveillance and intervention, especially soon after birth, tend to detect many cases that would otherwise have resolved spontaneously.

Birth prevalence rates of hypospadias, a birth defect in which the urethra opens on the ventral surface of the penis, also vary substantially among countries (e.g., 0.26 per 1000 male births in Mexico and 2.11 in

Hungary); even in countries with high reported rates, there was a 30%–40% underascertainment of cases later treated surgically (Kallen et al., 1986). Hypospadias rates approximately doubled in the United States during 1968–1993; rates of severe hypospadias and the ratio of severe to mild cases both increased over time, findings suggestive of a true increase (Paulozzi et al., 1997). Increases have been reported by surveillance systems in Alberta (Canada), Norway, and Israel but not in several other developed countries. In Finland, where all children are examined at birth by a pediatrician, the cumulative prevalence of hypospadias to age 8 years remained constant during 1970–1986 (Aho et al., 2000). Variable case detection and reporting over time and place may explain the inconsistent hypospadias incidence trends.

Available evidence suggests that average sperm concentrations (number of sperm per unit volume) and semen volumes both declined substantially during 1938–1991 (Carlsen et al., 1992). These trends occurred in several but not all countries for which data were available, and most of the apparent decrease occurred before 1970. A recent reanalysis concluded that changes in counting methods and population characteristics such as abstinence time did not explain the observed trends (Swan and Elkin, 1999). A survey of semen quality in four European cities, using standardized measurement methods, showed that the range of average sperm concentrations across centers was 98–132 million/ml (Jorgensen et al., 2001). There appear to have been no population-based studies in which semen quality and exposures to nonoccupational environmental HAAs were measured at the individual level.

There is continuing controversy about the reality of declining sperm production and potential environmental links. A review of available evidence concluded that estrogenic environmental HAAs play only a minor role in the trends noted above and that further research is needed on other endocrine mechanisms including thyroid and androgen-dependent processes (Foster, 1998). The National Research Council also concluded that there is insufficient toxicologic and epidemiologic evidence to attribute changes in hypospadias, cryptorchidism, testicular cancer, and sperm counts to environmental HAAs (National Academy of Sciences, 1999). The potential for exposure to environmental HAAs and evidence of the sensitivity of the developing reproductive tract from studies in animals and humans, as well as the many knowledge gaps, support continuing concern about this issue.

This chapter can do little more than introduce the reader to the complexities of the endocrine system and the known or potential impacts of environmental HAAs on animal and human health. The objective is to describe current knowledge and uncertainties in this field, particularly in relation to the limited human evidence and the more definitive animal evidence of developmental, reproductive, and carcinogenic effects. The focus is on areas where much of the animal research has been done, that is, the effects of environmental HAAs on the normal functioning of endogenous estrogens, androgens, and thyroid hormones. The ability of anthropogenic environmental HAAs to act through both hormonal and nonhormonal mechanisms is described. The chapter closes with a discussion of the need for improved risk management including bioassays to detect HAAs, biomonitoring, and research on major knowledge gaps.

NORMAL ENDOCRINE FUNCTION

The concentrations of hormones at receptor sites in target cells relate to rates of synthesis and secretion, delivery, degradation, and elimination. The strongest controls are feedback loops, usually negative feedback, at the level of hormone synthesis and secretion. The two main categories of hormone receptors are cell surface and nuclear receptors:

- Cell surface receptors—protein and peptide hormones usually bind to cell surface receptors, activating intracellular second messengers that modulate the activity of enzymes and other intracellular targets; second messengers and examples of hormones that activate them include cyclic adenosine monophosphate (AMP) (LH, FSH, TSH[1]), protein kinase (insulin, growth hormone, prolactin, several growth factors), and calcium and/or phosphoinositides (gonadotropin-releasing hormone, TRH[1]).
- Nuclear receptors—steroids and thyroid hormones bind to nuclear receptors that are ligand-dependent transcription factors; the hormone–nuclear receptor complexes bind to promoter regions of hormone-responsive genes and stimulate or inhibit their transcription

Through either type of receptor, the effect of small hormone concentrations is greatly amplified to produce biologic effects.

Gonadal Development

The Y chromosome gene *SRY* and other regulator genes control development of the male gonadal ridge into a testis with seminiferous cords con-

---

[1]LH = luteinizing hormone, FSH = follicle-stimulating hormone, TSH = thyroid-stimulating hormone, TRH = thyrotropin-releasing hormone.

taining Sertoli and primordial germ cells and interstitial tissue containing Leydig cells. During early pregnancy, *SRY* directs embryonic bipotential gonadal ridge cells to produce Mullerian inhibitory hormone (MIH) and testosterone (T) and to downregulate expression of *CYP19*, a gene that encodes the aromatase enzyme that converts T to estradiol-17β (E2). Mullerian inhibitory hormone causes regression of the Mullerian ducts that form the fallopian tubes, uterus, and upper vagina in females. Testosterone and MIH induce the differentiation of the mesonephric (Wolffian) ducts into the epididymis, seminal vesicles, and prostate. During early infancy, testicular volume increases rapidly, reflecting Sertoli cell division and growth in the length of the seminiferous cords; thyroid hormones regulate the duration of infant Sertoli cell proliferation, affecting adult Sertoli cell number and sperm-producing capacity.

At puberty, pulsatile release of hypothalamic gonadotropin-releasing hormone stimulates similar pulsatile release of LH and FSH from the anterior pituitary gland. Luteinizing hormone binds to receptors on target cells (testicular Leydig cells in boys and, in girls, ovarian theca interna, theca lutein, and granulosa lutein cells) and stimulates T production in boys and sustained follicle growth, E2 production, inhibin A production, granulosa cell luteinization, ovulation, luteal formation, and progesterone production in girls (Table 8–1). Follicle-stimulating hormone binds to receptors on ovarian granulosa cells and testicular Sertoli cells, stimulating proliferation and differentiation of granulosa cells (including inhibin B secretion and *CYP19* induction) in girls, and Sertoli cell inhibin B secretion and spermatogenesis in boys.

Testosterone stimulates Sertoli cell differentiation, spermatogenesis, growth in seminiferous tubule diameter, and further testicular growth and has anabolic effects, that is, it stimulates growth of nonreproductive tissues including muscle, kidney, liver, and salivary gland. Sertoli cells produce several hormones of the transforming growth factor (TGF-β) family, including MIH, inhibin, and activin. Production of MIH occurs in the fetus and child until about age 8–10 years; at puberty, Sertoli cells develop androgen receptors, and increased T levels suppress MIH production. The peptide hormones inhibin A and B, produced by Sertoli and ovarian granulosa cells, provide negative feedback signals to suppress pituitary FSH synthesis.

In the early female fetus, primordial germ cells migrate to the bipotential gonadal ridge and are incorporated in the developing ovary as oogonia that divide by mitosis initially and then enter meiosis. It appears that female fetal reproductive tract development requires signals to maintain the Mullerian duct, repress the Wolffian duct, suppress Leydig cell development, and maintain meiotic oocytes. Meiosis is halted during

TABLE 8–1. Functions of Selected Endogenous Hormones

Hormone, Main Site of Production	Function
LH; anterior pituitary gland	Binds to LH receptors on testicular Leydig cells and ovarian theca interna, theca lutein, and granulosa lutein cells; stimulates T production in males and stimulates sustained follicle growth, E2 production, inhibin A production, granulosa cell luteinization, ovulation, luteal formation, and progesterone production in females
FSH; anterior pituitary gland	Binds to FSH receptors on testicular Sertoli cells and ovarian granulosa cells; stimulates proliferation and differentiation of granulosa cells (including inhibin A production and *CYP19* induction) and Sertoli cell inhibin B production and spermatogenesis
Human chorionic gonadotropin (hCG)—fetal form is produced in fetal liver and kidney	Fetus—little maternal hCG crosses the placenta; fetal hCG may control fetal androgen synthesis, go nadal steroid production, and brain growth and differentiation
Estradiol (E2); ovarian theca interna, theca lutein, and granulosa lutein cells (and small amounts in testicular Leydig cells)	Binds to estrogen receptors in target tissues (ovary, breast, uterus, cervix, liver, bone, other) and stimulates transcription of estrogen-responsive genes; exerts positive feedback on frequency and amplitude of hypothalamic gonadotropin-releasing hormone and LH during the late follicular phase of the menstrual cycle but negative feedback at other times

T; testicular Leydig cells	Male fetus—fetal Leydig cells produce T that stabilizes Wolffian ducts and stimulates growth and development of the epididymis, vasa deferentia, and seminal vesicles Adolescent boys and men—Leydig cells produce T that stimulates spermatogenesis; T is converted to DHT in prostate, liver, kidney, skin, and muscle; adolescent girls and women—T serves as precursor for E2 synthesis; exerts negative feedback on frequency and amplitude of hypothalamic gonadotropin-releasing hormone and LH; stimulates growth of nonreproductive tissues including muscle, kidney, liver, salivary gland
Dihydrotestosterone (DHT); fetal external genitalia	Male fetus—differentiation of penis, scrotum, prostate, Cowper glands
Inhibin; Sertoli and granulosa cells	Exerts negative feedback on FSH secretion
TSH; anterior pituitary gland	Binds to TSH receptor on thyroid follicular epithelial cells; stimulates all aspects of thyroid hormone production except storage, that is, production of thyroglobulin, endocytosis of thyroglobulin, proteolytic cleavage of thyroglobulin to release T4, deiodination of T4 to T3, and secretion of T4 and T3 into blood
Thyroid hormones—triiodothyronine (T3), thyroxine (T4); thyroid gland	Bind to receptors (TRα, TRβ, and their isoforms); TRβ2 mediates negative feedback of T4 on pituitary TSH secretion; other TR isoforms are ubiquitously expressed and mediate the effects of T3 and T4 needed for normal function of every organ system

Source: Darlington and Dallman (2001).

prophase of the first meiotic division of oogonia, yielding primordial follicles, that is, primary oocytes enclosed in single layers of follicular cells. The primordial follicles in each fetal ovary decrease during later life until relatively few remain at menopause. Follicle-stimulating hormone binds to ovarian granulosa cell FSH receptors and stimulates proliferation and differentiation; the follicle(s) most responsive to FSH express the LH receptor to which LH binds and stimulates sustained follicle growth and E2 production. Pituitary LH surges cause further granulosa cell differentiation (luteinization) and ovulation.

Hormone Synthesis

Steroid synthesis in the gonads and adrenals is subject to acute and chronic regulation, the latter occurring at the level of gene transcription. The steroidogenic acute regulatory protein (StAR) controls the rate-limiting step in steroid hormone synthesis; by activating a regulated channel, it allows translocation of cholesterol from the outer to the inner mitochondrial membrane and rapid increases in steroid synthesis. Expression of StAR in gonads is controlled by LH and FSH. Most steroidogenic enzymes belong to the cytochrome P450 family encoded by *CYP* genes, several of which are controlled by LH and FSH (see Fig. 8–1):

- LH—controls several genes including
  - *CYP11A1*—encodes the enzyme P450scc (cholesterol-20,22-desmolase), which converts cholesterol to pregnenolone
  - *CYP17*—encodes P450c17, which has 17α-hydroxylase and 17,20-lyase activities and acts at key branch points in steroidogenesis
  - 3β-Hydroxysteroid dehydrogenase—converts pregnenolone to progesterone in ovarian thecal cells
  - 17β-Hydroxysteroid dehydrogenase—converts 4-androstenedione to T and E2 to estrone and vice versa
- Follicle-stimulating hormone increases expression of *CYP19* in ovarian granulosa cells; this gene encodes P450arom, an enzyme with aromatase activity that converts T to E2 and 4-androstenedione to estrone
- 5α-Reductase—this enzyme converts T to DHT, which has about 2.5 times more potency than T as an androgen receptor agonist; occurs in Leydig cells, prostate, and skin; expression in skin is influenced by genetic factors, transforming growth factor, insulin-like growth factor, and circulating androgens

Thyroid hormones control growth, development, differentiation, and metabolism in vertebrates. Hypothalamic neurons produce TRH, which, in

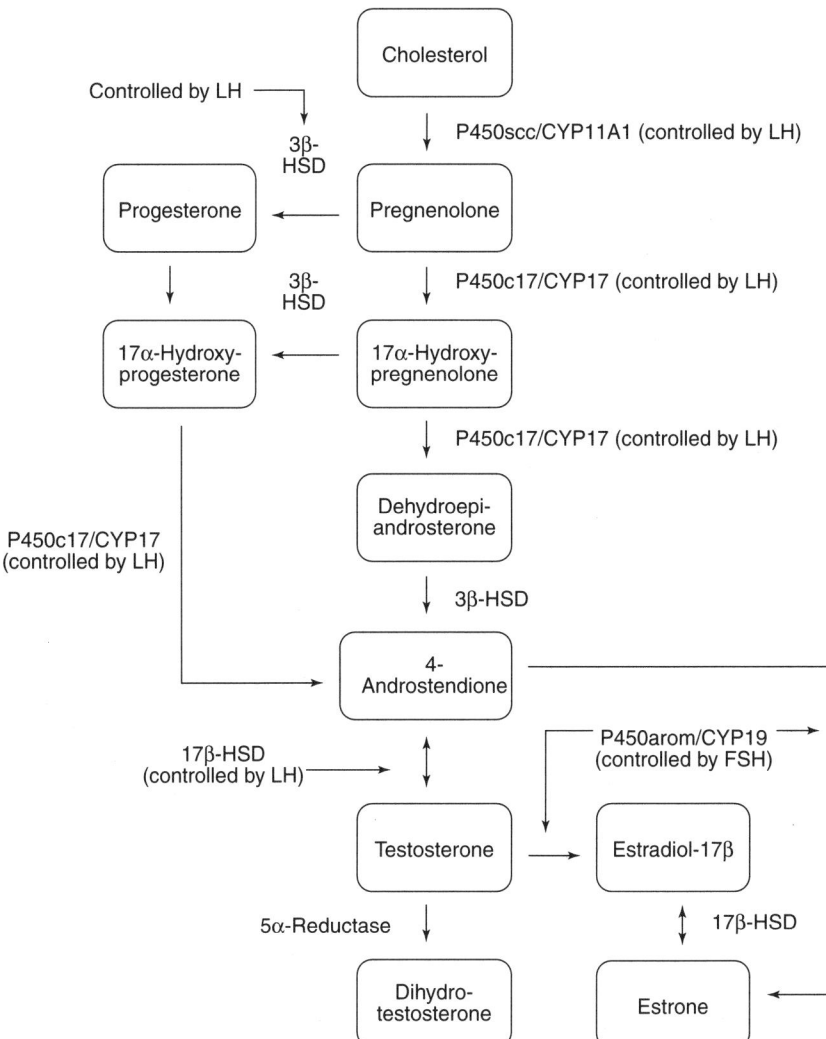

FIGURE 8–1. Androgen and estrogen biosynthesis, showing enzymes/genes that control each step.

turn, stimulates cells in the anterior pituitary gland to secrete TSH; the latter binds to thyroid epithelial cell receptors, activates a G-protein-linked signaling system, and stimulates all aspects of thyroid hormone synthesis (except storage): production, endocytosis, and proteolytic cleavage of thyroglobulin, deiodination of T4 to T3, and secretion of T4 and T3 into blood. At high circulating levels, T3 and T4 inhibit secretion of TRH by hypothalamic neurons; this inhibition is reversed when T3 and T4 levels are low. Triiodothyronine and T4 bind to ubiquitously expressed receptors (TRα, TRβ, and their isoforms); TRβ2 mediates negative feedback of T4 on pituitary TSH secretion. The various TR isoforms mediate the essential roles of T3 and T4 in the normal function of every organ system.

Hormone Receptors

Several small, lipid-soluble hormones (T, E2, T3, T4) and signaling molecules (vitamin D_3, retinoic acid, retinoids, and certain fatty acids) bind to nuclear receptors coded by genes of the nuclear receptor superfamily. The best-known effects of sex steroid hormones are delayed because of the time required for their interaction with nuclear receptors in target tissues, activation of gene transcription, and impacts on phenotype arising from cell division and cell differentiation.

Estrogen Receptors

There are two known estrogen receptor (ER) subtypes in rodents and humans, ERα and ERβ, having tissue-specific patterns of expression and reacting differently to the same ligand. A wide variety of chemical ligands can bind to ERs with variable affinities and half-lives and with effects ranging from full agonist to full antagonist. E2 binds to either receptor with similar affinities, and the resulting complexes interact with short DNA promoter sequences known as *estrogen-response elements* (EREs) and induce expression of several genes (Kuiper et al., 1998). In contrast, the affinities of the phytoestrogens genistein and coumestrol for ERβ substantially exceed those for ERα.

The relative expression of ERα and ERβ appears to be a key determinant of cell responses to ER ligands; for instance, antiestrogens such as the drug tamoxifen show some agonistic activity with ERα but not with ERβ. Human ERβ decreases cell sensitivity to E2 and modulates ERα transcriptional activity. Estrogen receptor β is expressed in human Sertoli, Leydig, and peritubular myoid cells, variably in germ cells, and in epithelial and stromal cells throughout other parts of the male reproductive tract; ERα is expressed in seminal vesicles. The presence of ERs in fetal and adult male germ and Sertoli cells suggests that estrogen influences testicular development and spermatogenesis.

During embryogenesis, ERs are also expressed in many nonreproductive tissues including the fetal rodent brain, suggesting a role for estrogen in early brain development. In human brain, ERα appears to dominate in the hypothalamus and amygdala, while ERβ is prominent in the hippocampal formation, entorhinal cortex, and thalamus. In rodents, T induces *CYP19* expression in cortical and hypothalamic neurons during fetal development, enabling such neurons to convert T to E2. Despite low ER levels, bone responds strongly to estrogen, possibly through an ER-related receptor (ERRα).

Androgen Receptors

A member of the nuclear receptor gene superfamily on the X chromosome encodes the androgen receptor (AR). The ARs are expressed ubiquitously in genital and nongenital tissues in both sexes including ovarian granulosa cells, skin, eccrine glands, sebocytes, hair follicle root sheath, liver, prostate, oral mucosa, breast, and muscle. By mediating the biologic actions of T and DHT, AR controls the growth, differentiation, and function of the male urogenital tract. In addition, AR modulates transcription of androgen-responsive genes (e.g., sex-limited protein, probasin, and prostate-specific antigen). Also, AR interacts with other signaling pathways. Gene polymorphisms and mutations of AR may cause up to 10% of human male infertility.

Progesterone Receptors

Progesterone, produced in the ovary during the latter half of the menstrual cycle and early pregnancy and by the placenta during later gestation in humans, targets two types of progesterone receptors, PR-A and PR-B, encoded by one gene with two distinct estrogen-regulated promoter sites. Although the distinct functions of the PR subtypes are unknown, knockout mice missing the *PR* gene display anovulation, uterine hyperplasia, and lack of mammary gland development. Progesterone signaling through PRs is essential for lobulo-alveolar breast development during pregnancy but not for ductal growth at puberty. E2 increases responsiveness to progesterone by inducing PRs in neural and uterine tissues. Progesterone also plays important roles in brain function; for example, it inhibits the neuronal nicotinic acetylcholine receptor and stimulates glial cell myelin production.

Thyroid Hormone Receptors

Thyroid hormone receptors (TRs) and T4-activating enzymes are expressed in the human fetal brain during early gestation, consistent with the important role of T4 in perinatal brain development. When taken up by tissues, T4 may undergo outer-ring monodeiodination to active T3 or inner-ring monodeiodination to inactive T3 (reverse T3 or rT3). Nuclear receptors TRα and TRβ each have two isoforms and mediate most thyroid hormone actions. When activated by T3, TR promotes transcription of several genes, facilitated by coactivators that acetylate histones, loosening the chromatin structure and facilitating access of TR and other key transcription factors. Independent of TR, T3 and T4 have important effects on calcium, sodium, and glucose transport across cell membranes, enzyme activity, mitochondrial respiration, and actin polymerization. Acute effects of T3 on mitochondrial respiration may be mediated by T3 receptors on the inner mitochondrial membrane; T3 also stimulates transcription of mitochondrial genes through both TR-mediated and mitochondrial-mediated mechanisms including p43 (Wrutniak-Cabello et al., 2001). Functions of thyroid hormone and its receptors during development include:

- Development of brain and other systems—severe mental deficits and multiple birth defects accompany fetal hypothyroidism.
- Auditory development—TRβ2 is an essential transcription factor for auditory development
- Thyroid hormone-dependent differentiation of Sertoli cells.
- Astrocyte structure and function—astrocytes comprise nearly 40% of cells in the human brain and are distinguished by their content of glial fibrillary acidic protein (GFAP), a component of their cytoskeleton essential for myelination, cell adhesion, and signaling pathways; thyroid hormone modulates expression of GFAP.

Hormone Transport and Inactivation

Protein-bound hormones provide a reservoir of hormone that can be released quickly as plasma levels of free hormone fall. Transport proteins also protect hormones from peripheral metabolism, especially by liver enzymes, thus increasing their half-lives. E2 and T bind to sex hormone binding globulin (SHBG) and albumin; thyroid hormones bind to thyroxine-binding globulin, transthyretin, and albumin. The purpose of SHBG is to regulate the concentration of free androgens and estrogens in plasma; about 98% of endogenous E2 is bound to plasma proteins, leaving about 2% free to enter target cells. Complexes of SHBG bind to SHBG receptors on sex steroid responsive cell membranes, activating an adenyl cyclase/ cyclic AMP second messenger cascade that may modulate the effects of sex steroids; for instance, SHBG inhibits E2-induced proliferation of human breast cancer cells in vitro.

Cytochrome P450 enzymes in liver and kidney hydroxylate sex steroids to more hydrophilic forms, thus aiding urinary and biliary excretion. In breast tissue, various progestins stimulate the activity of sulfotransferase, an enzyme that converts E2 to inactive estrogen sulfates. Luteinizing hormone stimulates sulfotransferase activity and inhibits sulfatase enzymes in testicular Leydig cells, thereby inactivating E2. Human sulfotransferase also sulfates T3, T4, and reverse T3, contributing to thyroid hormone processing and iodide recycling.

MECHANISMS OF ENVIRONMENTAL
HORMONALLY ACTIVE AGENTS

Bioassays for Hormonally Active Agents

Hormonal and other effects of selected HAAs are shown in Table 8–2 and discussed below. No internationally recognized methods exist for quantifying the hormonal activity of pure or mixed substances. Of 17 chemicals tested in eight different short-term bioassays, only 3 had above-background ER-binding affinities (bisphenol A, nonylphenol, o,p'-DDT), with bisphenol A having the highest estrogenic activity in all the bioassays (Andersen et al., 1999). Based on results of three in vitro screening tests and one in vivo bioassay of estrogenic activity, the National Academy of Sciences concluded that (1) several chemicals were positive in all four assays (e.g., o,p'-DDT, methoxychlor, bisphenol A), while others reacted in only one or two assays (e.g., toxaphene, dieldrin, diphenylphthalate), and (2) a few were positive in all three in vitro tests but negative in vivo (e.g., chlordecone, α-endosulfan, butylbenzyl phthalate) (National Academy of Sciences, 1999).

A systematic examination of selected HAAs in mammalian species by peer-review panels concluded that definite low-dose effects included (Melnick et al., 2002)

- Estrogenic—E2, DES, genistein, methoxychlor, nonylphenol
- Immunologic—genistein, methoxychlor, nonylphenol

HAAs with possible low-dose effects included bisphenol (estrogenic) and vinclozolin (antiandrogenic).

Estrogen Modulators

Estrogen Receptor Agonists

The synthetic estrogen drug DES was used in the 1950s and 1960s for treatment of threatened miscarriage, causing an unusual type of vaginal cancer among exposed daughters about 20 years later; it also causes cancer in experimental animals. It is discussed here to show the potential human health effects of high-dose prenatal exposure to a potent HAA. Diethylstilbestrol readily crosses the placenta and differs from maternal E2 in that it is not inactivated by placental enzymes and has weak affinity

TABLE 8–2. Mechanisms of Selected Environmental HAAs[a]

Compound	Mechanisms of Hormonal Activity	Genotoxicity	Developmental and Reproductive Toxicity of Perinatal Exposures	Carcinogenicity[b]
p,p'-DDE (main metabolite of the organochlorine insecticide, DDT)	AR antagonist	+ in vitro	Animals—males had retained nipples, reduced anogenital distance, delayed puberty, reduced sperm production, reduced testicular and accessory sex organ weight	Humans—DDT is a probable carcinogen Animals—DDT causes liver and thyroid tumors
o,p-DDT (DDT isomer; 15–21% of technical grade DDT)	ER agonist	+ in vitro	Animals—females had increased uterine weight, premature vaginal opening	See above
Chlordecone (Kepone)	ER agonist	+ in vitro	Humans—occupationally exposed men developed reduced sperm concentration and infertility Animals—females: neonatal exposure caused earlier vaginal opening and persistent vaginal estrus in adulthood	Animals—liver tumors
Vinclozolin (fungicide)	AR antagonist—vinclozolin binds fairly weakly to AR; its metabolites, M1 and M2, are stronger antiandrogens	+ in vitro	Animals—males had reduced anogenital distance, hypospadias, agenesis of sex accessory tissues, retained nipples and areolas, cryptorchidism, epididymal agenesis	Not available

	Mechanism	Genotoxicity	Developmental/reproductive effects	Carcinogenicity
TCDD	Aryl hydrocarbon receptor (AhR) agonist; decreased AR and ER expression; disruption of cell differentiation; interference by TCDD-AhR-Arnt (aromatic hydrocarbon receptor nuclear translocator) complex with binding of ER to enhancer elements of estrogen-responsive genes	+ in vivo; genotoxicity appears to be an indirect effect; for example, induction of CYP1A1 by TCDD may activate other endogenous and exogenous substances to reactive metabolites capable of damaging DNA	Humans—men: increased LH and FSH levels, decreased T levels. Animals—fetal death, low birth weight, cleft palate, hydronephrosis of the kidneys (caused by hyperplasia of the epithelium of the ureters), hypomineralization of teeth, thymic atrophy, and immunosuppression; males had hypospadias, cryptorchidism, delayed puberty, feminized sexual behavior, reduced size of testes and male accessory sex glands (especially ventral prostate), reduced anogenital distance; females had ovarian atrophy, cleft phallus	Humans—known carcinogen. Animals—tumors at multiple sites
PCBs	Coplanar PCBs—see TCDD above; hydroxylated PCBs compete with T4 for binding to transthyretin and inhibit E2 metabolism	+ in vitro and in vivo (Schiestl et al., 1997); commercial PCB mixtures not potent genotoxins	Humans—IUGR, perinatal mortality, small head circumference (after high-level prenatal exposure). Animals—early and late fetal deaths, reduced fetal growth rate, hydronephrosis, cleft palate	Humans—probable carcinogen. Animals—liver, bile duct, thyroid tumors
Benzo[a]pyrene (example of a PAH)	AhR agonist—see TCDD above	+ in vitro and in vivo	Animals—early and late fetal deaths, birth defects, reduced growth rates prenatally and postnatally, reduced fertility of offspring	Humans—probable carcinogen; animals—skin, lung, forestomach tumors

(continued)

TABLE 8–2. Mechanisms of Selected Environmental HAAs[a] (continued)

Compound	Mechanisms of Hormonal Activity	Genotoxicity	Developmental and Reproductive Toxicity of Perinatal Exposures	Carcinogenicity[b]
Diesel exhaust (contains PAHs, other toxins)	AhR agonist—see PAHs	+ in vitro and in vivo	Animals—increased anogenital distances (both sexes), reduced ovarian primary follicles and Sertoli cells	Humans—probable carcinogen Animals—lung tumors
Bisphenol A (plastic monomer)	hERα and hERβ agonist	+ in vitro	Animals—males had increased anogenital distance, increased prostate size, decreased epididymal weight, persistent increased prostate AR levels; females had increased weight and earlier onset of puberty	Animals—equivocal carcinogen, with males being more susceptible; leukemia, testicular tumors
Di(2-ethylhexyl) phthalate (DEHP)	Main testicular target appears to be Sertoli cells that proliferate during the neonatal period in humans	Chromosome aberrations in vitro	Animals—decreased fertility, degeneration of seminiferous tubules, fetal death, birth defects; females had normal reproductive development, consistent with DEHP as an antiandrogen	Humans—probable carcinogen; animals—liver tumors

[a]Toxicological Profiles, Agency for Toxic Substances and Disease Registry, unless otherwise indicated.

[b]International Agency for Research on Cancer.

for α-fetoprotein and SHBG, allowing free DES to access ERs in fetal tissues. In the presence of α-fetoprotein or SHBG, a much greater proportion of DES remains free and able to bind to human ER (hER), compared to E2. Diethylstilbestrol has about two-fold higher affinity than E2 for hERs (hERα and hERβ) in vitro (Table 8–3), modulates ER-dependent DNA transcription, causes reduced and mutated transcripts of DNA polymerase-β (a DNA repair gene), stimulates mammary gland proliferation, and causes persistently altered expression of several *HOX* genes involved in patterning of the fetal mouse reproductive tract (Block et al., 2000).

TABLE 8–3. Relative Activities of Sex Steroids, DES, Suspected Environmental Hormonally Active Agents, and Phytoestrogens for Human ERs (hERα and hERβ)

Compound	Relative Binding Affinity[a]		Relative Transactivation Activity[b]	
	hERα	hERβ	hERα	hERβ
Estradiol-17β (E2)	100	100	100	100
Progesterone	<0.01	<0.01	NA	NA
Testosterone	<0.01	<0.01	NA	NA
DES	236	221	117	69
o,p'-DDT	0.01	0.02	54	10
p,p'-DDE	<0.01	<0.01	NA	NA
2',4',6'-Trichloro-4-biphenylol[c]	2.4	4.7	77	62
2',3',4',5'-tetrachloro-4-biphenylol[c]	3.4	7.2	68	41
p-Octylphenol	0.02	0.07	61	57
p-Nonylphenol	0.05	0.09	62	34
Bisphenol A	0.01	0.01	50	41
Methoxychlor	<0.01	<0.01	9	2
Endosulfan	<0.01	<0.01	6	1
Chlordecone	0.06	0.1	27	1
Genistein	4	87	198	182
Coumestrol	20	140	102	98
Zearalenone	7	5	91	27
Daidzein	0.1	0.5	97	80

[a] Affinity for hER relative to estradiol-17β.

[b] Ratio of luciferase reporter gene induction values of each compound relative to estradiol-17β at concentrations of 1 μM each.

[c] Hydroxylated PCB congeners.

NA = not available in this source (Kuiper et al., 1998).

Although phytoestrogens are not environmental contaminants, some are hormonally active and are ubiquitous in plant foods commonly eaten by children, including soy-based infant formula, fruits, and vegetables. About 200 naturally occurring phytoestrogens have been identified, the main categories being lignans and isoflavones. Phytoestrogens occur at particularly high levels in flaxseeds and soybeans. Soy-based infant formulas contain isoflavones (mainly glycosides of genistein and daidzein) at levels far higher than those in human breast milk. Phytoestrogens vary widely in their affinity for hERα and hERβ; genistein, coumestrol, and zearalenone have the highest relative binding affinities for both hERβ and ERα, but their rank order varies for the two subtypes (Table 8–4). Genistein has much higher affinity for ERβ than for ERα, suggesting that it may influence tissues high in ERβ (e.g., human vascular smooth muscle, prostate epithelial cells, testicular Leydig and Sertoli cells). Hydroxylation by P450 enzymes increases the ability of some phytoestrogens to bind to and activate ERs. Although diets high in fruits and vegetables appear to reduce the risk of cardiovascular disease, cancer, and other chronic diseases, there is no convincing evidence that these benefits are attributable to phytoestrogens per se.

The relative hER binding affinities and ER-dependent gene expression activities of selected sex steroids, suspected environmental HAAs, and phytoestrogens are shown in Tables 8–3 and 8–4. Important features include the following: (1) potencies span at least four orders of magnitude, (2) ER binding affinity is weakly correlated with the ability to activate ER-dependent gene expression, (3) o,p'-DDT, certain hydroxylated PCB metabolites, and several phytoestrogens are relatively potent inducers of ER-dependent gene expression, and (4) the test substances behave similarly with ERα and ERβ. Other ER agonists include *tris*(4-chlorophenyl)methane (TCPM—a recently identified global contaminant of

TABLE 8–4. Relative Binding Affinity of Estradiol-17β and Selected Phytoestrogens for hERα and hERβ

Hormone or Phytoestrogen	hERα	hERβ
Estradiol-17β (E2)	100	100
Genistein	1.6	100
Coumestrol	12	34
Zearalenone	22	75
Daidzein	0.2	1.8

Note: Relative affinity, compared to E2 set at 100, based on concentration of competitor needed to displace half of ER-bound E2 (Nikov et al., 2000).

unknown origin but structurally related to DDT), brominated bisphenol A compounds, and metabolites of methoxychlor, polybrominated diphenylethers, and TCPM. Reported findings of extreme synergism between pairs of weakly estrogenic organochlorine pesticides in a human ER-dependent *in vitro* assay were not confirmed in subsequent studies, and the original paper was withdrawn (McLachlan, 1997).

Other Mechanisms
The complexities of environmental HAAs are illustrated by considering some of their known or suspected mechanisms:

- Mixed effects—some methoxychlor metabolites are agonists of ERβ and antagonists of ERβ and AR.
- Altered expression of ER—prenatal exposure of swine to TCDD caused increased testicular ERα levels.
- Aryl hydrocarbon receptor agonists—TCDD and dioxin-like compounds bind to AhR and trigger a cascade of biochemical responses in rodents including:
  - Upregulation of *CYP1A1* and *CYP1B1*—this may increase hydroxylation and inactivation of E2 and hydroxylation and activation of xenobiotics (e.g., some hydroxylated PAH metabolites are ER agonists in vitro).
  - Tissue-specific downregulation of ER protein and ER mRNA in reproductive tissues and liver.
- Unknown mechanisms—triazine herbicides are estrogenic in rodents in vivo; while the mechanism is unknown, it may involve modulation of hypothalamic control of LH secretion and/or induction of aromatase (the enzyme that catalyzes conversion of androgens to estrogens).

Androgen Modulators

Androgen Receptor Agonists/Antagonists
Certain isomers of DDT and DDE and some PAHs such as dibenzo[a,h] anthracene are weak agonists of human AR (hAR) in vitro. ρ,ρ'-DDE (the major DDT metabolite found in human tissues), vinclozolin and procymidone (fungicides), linuron (a herbicide), fenitrothion (an insecticide), and some PAHs inhibit human and/or animal AR-dependent transcriptional activity. Vinclozolin binds fairly weakly to AR, but two of its metabolites (M1, M2) are stronger antiandrogens.

Other Mechanisms
- Sertoli cell toxicants—aphthalate metabolite (mono-(2-ethylhexyl) phthalate) inhibits neonatal rat Sertoli cell division at submicromolar

concentrations in vitro; the fungicide benomyl and its main metabolite (carbendazim) interfere with microtubules and intermediate filaments of Sertoli and germ cells, causing germ cell death and abnormal spermatid development.

- Steroid synthesis and catabolism
  - The phthalates DEHP and di-*n*-butyl phthalate (DBP) reduce fetal and neonatal T production, possibly by inhibiting expression of StAR and genes encoding steroidogenic enzymes.
  - TCDD reduces testicular levels of *CYP11A*, thereby reducing T production; it may also increase inactivation of T in liver and testicles.
  - Tributyltin inhibits aromatase (reducing conversion of androgens to estrogens) and reduces the conjugation and excretion of androgens.
  - Altered AR expression—prenatal exposure of animals to TCDD or DES causes decreased AR levels in testes, prostate, and accessory sex glands.

Thyroid Modulators

Chemicals known to interfere with thyroid hormone function inhibit the synthesis, transport, or catabolism of thyroid hormones. TCDD induces the enzyme UDP-glucuronosyltransferase-1, triggering increased glucuronidation and excretion of T4, increased TSH levels, and thyroid hyperplasia. Hydroxylated metabolites of PCBs, dioxins, and furans bind strongly to human transthyretin, the only thyroid hormone-binding protein synthesized in the brain, with affinities up to several times those of T4; by binding to transthyretin in brain, some hydroxylated PCBs, dioxins, and furans may alter brain free T4 levels and interfere with brain development and function. Neonatal cord plasma free T4 levels are inversely associated with cord plasma hydroxylated PCB levels but not with individual or total PCBs (Sandau et al., 2002).

Health Effects

Multiple male reproductive system abnormalities may comprise a testicular dysgenesis syndrome (Boisen et al., 2001). The syndrome of male genital tract birth defects, testicular cancer, poor semen quality, and subfertility may all involve disruption by HAAs of embryonic programming and fetal gonadal development in genetically susceptible individuals. There is considerable animal evidence to support this hypothesis and some evidence from the few directly relevant epidemiologic studies.

Developmental Effects

Animal studies indicate that prenatal exposure to environmental HAAs can cause abnormal development of the male and female reproductive tracts through mechanisms including germ cell toxicity and steroid hormone receptor modulation. Developmental exposure of animals to germ cell toxicants generally reduces fertility without causing malformations of external genitalia and accessory glands. In contrast, prenatal exposure to antiandrogenic agents causes male reproductive tract malformations (hypospadias, cryptorchidism, vaginal pouches, agenesis of the ventral prostate, and nipple retention) while generally having less effect on the testes. There is a marked dearth of epidemiologic studies on the potential role of environmental HAAs in reproductive tract developmental abnormalities in humans.

Reproductive Tract Birth Defects

Final testicular descent in humans appears to require a T surge just before birth, suggesting that antiandrogens could cause cryptorchidism. Only a few studies of cryptorchidism have assessed environmental exposures, providing limited evidence of links to prenatal parental pesticide exposure (Hosie et al., 2000; Kristensen et al., 1997; Weidner et al., 1998), increased free E2 and decreased T levels in maternal blood during early gestation (Bernstein et al., 1988; Key et al., 1996), maternal smoking (Akre et al., 1999; McBride et al., 1991), and maternal use of exogenous estrogens during pregnancy (Depue, 1984). A small case-control study of cryptorchidism in Germany showed associations with heptachlor and hexachlorobenzene levels in fat samples (Hosie et al., 2000). In another of the few epidemiologic studies to measure internal doses of environmental HAAs, there were weak, nonsignificant associations between elevated maternal serum DDE levels and cryptorchidism and hypospadias, as well as a borderline association with accessory nipples among male infants (OR = 1.9, CI 0.9–4.0) (Longnecker et al., 2002). This study took advantage of stored, frozen maternal serum samples collected during the Collaborative Perinatal Project (1959–1966), a time when human serum DDT/DDE levels were much higher than they are currently.

Hypospadias has been associated with low birth weight (Akre et al., 1999; Weidner et al., 1999), proximity of residence to landfill sites (Dolk et al., 1998), and prenatal DES exposure (Beral and Colwell, 1981). In the first human evidence of a transgenerational effect of DES, the sons of women exposed to DES in utero (i.e., the grandsons of women who took DES during pregnancy) had a substantially increased risk of hypospadias (RR = 21, CI 6.5–70) (Klip et al., 2002). The daughters of women who consumed DES during pregnancy had increased risks of vaginal adenosis, cervical ectropion, transverse cervical and vaginal ridges, and hypoplastic uterus (Swan, 2000). In addition, DES produced similar abnormalities in prenatally exposed male and female rodents and monkeys.

Feminization of Males

Although maternal serum DDE has been linked to accessory nipples in male infants (see above), most evidence linking HAA exposures to developmental feminization comes from animal studies. Developmental abnormalities among male rodents prenatally exposed to pesticidal AR antagonists (vinclozolin, procymidone, linuron, and DDT/DDE) include feminization (reduced anogenital distance, retained nipples/areolas), reproductive tract birth defects (agenesis of sex accessory tissues, cryptorchidism, hypospadias), and sexual dysfunction (inability after puberty to mate with sexually receptive females) (Gray et al., 2001). The timing of exposure is critical; the fetal male rat is most susceptible on gestational days 14 through 19.

The antiandrogenic effects of phthalates appear to relate to Sertoli cell toxicity and inhibition of fetal T synthesis. Expert review panels concluded that prenatal exposure of experimental animals to high doses of the plasticizers butylbenzyl phthalate (BBP), DEHP, DBP, diisononyl phthalate (DINP), or di-*n*-hexyl phthalate (DnHP) can cause feminization of males, reproductive tract birth defects, and various abnormalities of testes (reduced Sertoli cells, seminiferous tubular atrophy, reduced weight) and accessory glands (reduced prostate weight) (Agency for Toxic Substances and Disease Registry, 2000a). The sensitivity of testes to phthalates appears to be greatest prenatally, intermediate among juvenile animals, and lowest among adults. As noted above, bisphenol A and nonylphenols have estrogenic activity in in vitro systems. Low-dose prenatal exposure of male mice to bisphenol A caused feminization, increased prostate size, and persistent increased prostate AR levels. There is mixed evidence of estrogenic effects in male and female offspring after perinatal exposure to high-dose nonylphenol.

Male rats exposed prenatally to single low doses of TCDD had reduced ventral prostate weight and reduced anogenital distance. Prenatal exposure of swine to TCDD caused male reproductive tract abnormalities including cryptorchidism and reduced testicular germ cell populations. See Chapter 6 (PCBs, Dioxins, and Related Compounds) for further discussion of developmental effects of TCDD and dioxin-like chemicals.

Other Developmental Abnormalities

Prenatal exposure of rodents to DEHP at high doses caused eye, neural tube, skeletal, and cardiac birth defects, but it is not known if these involved hormonal mechanisms; DEHP is a structural isomer of the anticonvulsant valproic acid that is known to cause similar birth defects in humans. Female mice prenatally exposed to low-dose bisphenol A were heavier and had earlier onset of puberty than controls. Female rats exposed prenatally to single low doses of TCDD had genital clefting with hypospadias and vaginal threads, effects that can also be produced by prenatal exposure to DES or E2. Rats prenatally exposed to diesel exhaust or filtered diesel exhaust had increased anogenital distance (both sexes) and reduced ovarian primary follicles and Sertoli cells, possibly from inhibition of *CYP19* activity and synthesis, causing reduced conversion of T to E2 and accumulation of T (Watanabe and Kurita, 2001).

Reproductive Effects

The average age at menarche may have decreased during recent decades in the United States and other countries (see, e.g., de Muinck Keizer and Mul, 2001). This apparent trend may reflect improved nutrition and other factors; the possible role of environmental HAAs remains undefined. Premature breast development among young Puerto Rican girls was associated with serum levels of phthalates (especially DEHP) and their metabolites (Colon et al., 2000); this potentially important finding needs verification. Breast-fed daughters of women with high serum polybrominated biphenyl (PBB) levels had earlier menarche than daughters of women with low serum PBB levels or formula-fed girls (Blanck et al., 2000). Daughters of women who consumed DES during pregnancy had increased risks of menstrual irregularity, infertility, ectopic pregnancy, spontaneous abortion, and preterm delivery (Goldberg and Falcone, 1999). Epidemiologic studies that measured internal doses of environmental contaminants and sperm quality have shown inverse associations between PCBs and DDE in serum or semen specimens and sperm concentration, motility, and morphology (Bush et al., 1986; Hauser et al., 2002). The EPA reviewed 63 pesticides and identified 8 that have effects on reproduction (see Chapter 7 for further discussion of reproductive effects of pesticides).

Endocrine System

There is good evidence in experimental animals and limited evidence in humans and wildlife that PCBs and other dioxin-like compounds inhibit thyroid function. Polychlorinated biphenyl or total TCDD toxic equivalent (TEQ) levels in breast milk, maternal blood, or cord blood were generally associated with reduced plasma thyroid hormone and elevated TSH levels in mothers during late pregnancy, in neonates, and in older children (see, e.g., Osius et al., 1999). Because untreated congenital hypothyroidism causes severe cognitive deficits and because the severity of maternal hypothyroidism during pregnancy has been linked to cognitive deficits at age 8 years, modestly reduced thyroid hormone levels in the mother and/or the fetus may have adverse neurobehavioral effects on the developing child. Several brominated fire retardants (tetrabromobisphenol A, pentabromophenol, and hydroxylated metabolites of polybrominated diphenyl ethers) have high affinity for human transthyretin in vitro. Occupational and environmental TCDD exposures have been linked to diabetes in adults, but no studies of children have been reported. In experimental animals, TCDD causes profound reductions in glucose transport into tissues (Kern et al., 2002).

Immune System

TCDD and many other organochlorine chemicals are immunotoxic in animals, but there have been few studies of their potential effects in humans. Evidence of the potential for HAAs to interfere with immune system development and function includes the following:

- Genes regulated by nuclear thyroid hormone receptors appear to determine the B-cell pool size in mice; hypothyroid mice have reduced numbers of pro-B, pre-B, and B cells in bone marrow, an effect reversible by treatment with T4.
- E2 reduces T cell–dependent immune function but enhances B-cell antibody production; androgens suppress both T-cell and B-cell immune responses.
- Prenatal DES exposure in rodents causes persistent deficits in T-cell, B-cell, and natural killer cell function, as well as increased susceptibility to transplanted and carcinogen-induced cancers.
- A systematic examination of low-dose effects of selected HAAs in mammalian species by peer-review panels concluded that exposure (prenatal to puberty) to genistein, methoxychlor, and nonylphenol has definite low-dose immunologic effects including (Melnick et al., 2002)
  - Genistein—increased splenic T-lymphocyte proliferation after anti-CD3 stimulation
  - Methoxychlor—decreased percentage of CD4+/CD8− thymocytes and decreased antibody plaque-forming cell response in males
  - Nonylphenol—increased relative thymus weight and splenic T-lymphocyte proliferation after anti-CD3 stimulation

Cancer

Discovery of clear cell adenocarcinoma of the vagina and cervix among teenage girls and young adult women exposed in utero to DES provided the first clear evidence of adverse effects from prenatal exposure to a synthetic estrogen in humans (Herbst et al., 1971). Exposed women had increased risks of clear cell cervicovaginal cancer and breast cancer; exposed men had a marginally increased risk of testicular cancer (Strohsnitter et al., 2001). The mechanism by which DES causes vaginal cancer is not known but may involve activation of ERα, genotoxic effects, or both. Diethylstilbestrol and its metabolites bind to DNA and tubulin, increasing the rate of aneuploidy and nondisjunction in dividing cells.

Incidence rates of testicular cancer, the most common cancer among young men in most developed countries, are increasing in many countries; for example, Canadian men born during 1959–1968 are twice as likely to develop testicular cancer as those born during 1904–1913 (Liu et al., 1999). Risk factors for testicular cancer include persistent cryptorchidism, early birth order, low birth weight, prenatal exposure to exogenous estrogen, and delayed puberty (protective). Correction of cryptorchidism early in life does not reduce the risk of testicular cancer, and men with unilateral cryptorchidism have an increased risk of contralateral testicular cancer, suggesting that these conditions have a common cause. Given the strong animal evidence that environmental AR antagonists can cause cryptorchidism, it is possible that some human testicular cancers may be attributable to such agents.

Thyroid cancer incidence rates, especially papillary thyroid cancers, increased markedly in the United States and Canada during the late twentieth century (see, e.g., Liu et al., 2001). Birth cohort analysis of the Connecticut data indicate that the increase occurred among persons born during 1915–1945, a period when radiation was used to treat benign conditions of the head and neck region of children (see Chapter 9, Radiation). Pooled analyses of thyroid cancer studies in several countries showed associations with current oral contraceptive use (especially with papillary thyroid carcinomas), a history of exposure to fertility drugs, and lactation suppression treatment but not with postmenopausal hormone replacement treatment or fish consumption (Bosetti et al., 2001; La Vecchia et al., 1999).

No epidemiologic studies have been done on prenatal exposures to environmental HAAs and cancer risks later in life. Epidemiologic studies of hormone-sensitive cancers (breast, ovarian, endometrial, prostate, testicular) and blood or tissue concentrations of HAAs during adulthood (e.g., PCB, DDT, and DDE) showed inconsistent evidence of associations.

EXPOSURES

Data from NHANES III on urinary phthalate metabolite levels in representative samples of the U.S. population are the only population-based phthalate exposure measurements for any country (Table 8–5). Metabolites of diethylphthalate (DEP) and DBP occurred at highest concentrations; this result was surprising, as these phthalates are produced in much lower quantities than DEHP and DINP. Urinary DBP and DEHP metabolite levels were higher among low-income groups (Koo et al., 2002). Reproductive-age women had average urinary DBP metabolite levels 50% higher than those of other subgroups (Blount et al., 2000). Diethylphthalate and DBP are used extensively in products with volatile components such as perfumes, nail polishes, and hair sprays. The CDC has initiated additional studies to identify the sources of exposure to DEP and DBP.

The highest lipid-adjusted PCB concentrations occur in placenta, where they can exceed 5 μg/g fat or almost three times those in breast milk. Organochlorines including α-hexachlorocyclohexane, p,p'-DDE, and PCBs were detected in one-third of human amniotic fluid samples in Los Angeles (Foster et al., 2000). The median concentration of p,p'-DDE in human serum, on a molar basis, is about 100-fold greater than that of E2 in premenopausal women and about the same level as T in men. Tris(4-chlorophenyl)methane (TCPM) and TCPM-OH were detected at levels of about 1–20 ng/g lipid in all human adipose samples tested in Japan. See also Chapters 6 (PCBs, Dioxins, and Related Compounds) and 7 (Pesticides) for further details on population exposure levels of potential HAAs.

Infants raised on soy-based formula ingest about 5–8 mg/kg/day of total isoflavones and have average plasma isoflavone levels of about

TABLE 8–5. Urinary Phthalate Metabolites, United States

Urinary Phthalate Metabolite (parent phthalate)	50th Percentile Urinary Concentration (μg/g creatinine)[a]	50th Percentile Urinary Concentration (μg/g creatinine)[b]
Mono-ethyl (DEP)	280	134
Mono-butyl (DBP)	33	22
Mono-benzyl (BBP)	20	14
Mono-2-ethylhexyl (DEHP)	3	3
Mono-isononyl (DINP)	<LOD	<LOD

[a]U.S. population aged 20–60 years, NHANES III, 1988–1994 (Blount et al., 2000).

[b]U.S. population aged 6 years and older, 1999 (Centers for Disease Control and Prevention, 2001).

LOD = limit of detection.

1 mg/L, that is, more than three orders of magnitude higher than E2 concentrations in early life (Setchell et al., 1998). Average plasma levels of isoflavones among infants fed breast or cow's milk are about 5 μg/L. Isoflavone exposures among formula-fed infants are six- to elevenfold higher (on a body weight basis) than those that have hormonal effects on adults consuming soy foods, that is, such exposures may be sufficient to produce biologic effects in infants (Setchell et al., 1997).

RISK MANAGEMENT

The 1996 FQPA and the Safe Drinking Water Act require screening tests for HAAs in food and source drinking water. An EPA advisory committee recommended evaluation of pesticides, commercial chemicals, and environmental contaminants for effects on estrogen, androgen, and thyroid hormone function. The EPA must prioritize more than 87,000 chemicals including 75,500 in the Toxic Substances Control Act Inventory, 900 active pesticide ingredients, 2500 pesticide inerts, and 8000 cosmetic ingredients, food additives, and nutritional supplements for endocrine disruption screening and testing. The EPA has also committed to test six mixtures representative of contaminants in human breast milk, phytoestrogens in soy-based infant products, chemicals commonly found in hazardous waste sites, pesticide/fertilizer mixtures, drinking water disinfection by-products, and gasoline (U.S. Environmental Protection Agency, 1998).

The EPA adopted a tiered approach that will prioritize chemicals for evaluation based on existing information on exposure and hormonal activity (U.S. Environmental Protection Agency, 2000a). Evaluation will require the validation of existing in vitro and animal tests and the development of new methods. The EPA decided to use a two-tiered approach and is collaborating with the Office of Economic Cooperation and Development and the National Toxicology Program to standardize and validate Tier 1 and 2 bioassays of effects on male and female reproductive systems and behaviors and thyroid function.

The European Commission in 1999 decided to address HAAs by prioritizing substances for testing when appropriate test methods become available, to identify HAAs covered by existing European Community legislation, to expand epidemiologic studies of cause–effect relations, and to consider policies for vulnerable groups including children. The Commission identified 564 HAAs with various levels of evidence, among which 146 were high production and/or highly persistent chemicals (BKH Consulting Engineers and TNO Nutrition and Food Research, 2000). Information on production and use of selected HAAs is shown in Table 8–6.

TABLE 8-6. Production and Use of Selected HAAs

Chemical	Uses (Past and/or Present)[a]	Production	Major Source of Human Exposure[a]
PCBs	Dielectrics, flame retardants, hydraulic fluids, electrical equipment, pigments, others	Banned in USA in 1977; annual production in USA 42,500 tons (1970), 2 million tons produced globally since the 1930s[b]	Food (especially fatty foods), breast milk
DDT	Insecticide	Banned in the USA in 1973; peak annual production was 90,000 tons (USA, 1962); estimated cumulative global production about 2 million tons[c]	Food (especially fatty foods), breast milk
Bisphenol A	Monomer for production of polycarbonate polymers, epoxy resins, dyes, flame retardants, dental sealants	2.6 million tons, 1999 (USA, South America, Europe, Asia)[d]	Food (especially fatty foods)
Nonylphenol (accounts for about 85% of alkylphenol production)	Surfactants—nonylphenol ethoxylates used in surfactants for industrial and institutional formulations, household liquid detergents; used in antioxidants such as tris(nonylphenol)phosphite	120,000 tons (USA, 2000)[e]	Water, food
Diethylphthalate (DEP)—monoester metabolite had highest urinary level in a CDC study	Toothbrushes, automobile parts, tools, toys, food packaging, cosmetics, insecticides, aspirin	USA—production 13,000 tons (1988)[f]	Food in plastic packaging, contaminated fish and shellfish, contaminated water near waste sites and landfills, certain consumer products

Di-*n*-butyl phthalate (DBP)—monoester metabolite had second highest urinary level in a CDC study	Plastics, paints, glue, hair spray, and other chemical products	USA—production 13,000 tons (1988)[g]	Fish, shellfish, cosmetic use
Di(2-ethylhexyl) phthalate (DEHP)	Polyvinyl chloride (PVC) plastics may contain up to 40% DEHP—toys, vinyl upholstery, adhesives, coatings; DEHP also used in inks, pesticides, cosmetics, and vacuum pump oil	USA—one U.S. company produced 143,000 tons of DEHP and ocytlphthalates in 1998[h]	Medical products packaged in plastic (e.g., blood products, dialysis fluids), foods packaged in plastics (especially fatty foods like milk products, fish/seafood, oils), groundwater near waste sites, workplace or indoor air where DEHP is released from plastic materials, coatings, flooring

[a]Agency for Toxic Substances and Disease Registry (2001a).

[b]National Academy of Sciences (1999).

[c]Agency for Toxic Substances and Disease Registry (2000b).

[d]Bisphenol A global industry group (2002).

[e]Chemical Market Reporter (2001).

[f]Agency for Toxic Substances and Disease Registry (1995).

[g]Agency for Toxic Substances and Disease Registry (2001b).

[h]Agency for Toxic Substances and Disease Registry (2000c).

Water

Nonylphenol ethoxylates, a subgroup of nonionic surfactants known as *alkylphenol ethoxylates*, are high-volume chemicals (over 300,000 tons per year produced globally). These chemicals have been used for over 40 years as cleaners, degreasers, detergents, and emulsifiers in domestic and industrial products (textiles, pulp and paper, paints, resins and protective coatings, pesticides, and cosmetics). Microbial biodegradation of the parent compounds during sewage treatment releases estrogenic alkylphenols, primarily nonylphenol and octylphenol.

Relatively high amounts of nonylphenol ethoxylates and their degradation products (particularly nonylphenol, nonylphenol ethoxylate, and nonylphenol diethoxylate) occur in municipal wastewater treatment plant effluents, often at levels exceeding 1 mg/L. Nonylphenol occurs at high concentrations in some sewage sludges applied to agricultural lands and is relatively persistent in groundwater. Although nonylphenol ethoxylate has been detected in human urine, there are no population-based data on the prevalence of exposure. Other HAAs potentially present in water include the natural hormones E2 and estrone and the synthetic hormone ethynyl estradiol-17α (from municipal wastewater discharges) and organotin compounds (may leach from PVC pipes).

Food

Foods are potential sources of exposure to certain HAAs including phytoestrogens, phthalates, dioxins, PCBs, certain pesticides, and organotin compounds. The synthetic estrogen zeranol, used as a growth promoter in beef production, has potency similar to that of DES and E2 in inducing estrogen-dependent gene expression in human MCF7 cells in vitro. Although zeranol is not an environmental contaminant, its potency shows the need for integrated risk management of HAAs.

Phytoestrogens
Soy protein is relatively cheap, and about 60% of processed foods contains soy derivatives. Although diets high in phytoestrogens are associated with reduced risks of certain cancers among adults, it is not known whether exposure during infancy and early childhood has any adverse effects.

Phthalates
Global phthalate production appears to be about 5–6 million tons per year. Phthalates are used to make flexible polyvinyl chloride products with smaller amounts being used as components in consumer products includ-

ing soaps, lotions, perfumes, insect repellants, and other products applied to skin. Phthalates can migrate from polyvinyl chloride food packaging in contact with foods; such migration is increased by heat and fat content. Foods wrapped in plastic film contained di(2-ethylhexyl) adipate (DEHA) at levels up to 310 mg/kg (cheese). Di(2-ethylhexyl) phthalate from plastic tubing used in commercial milking equipment can leach into milk. Dairy products from the United Kingdom contained average total phthalate levels of 0.06–0.32 mg/kg in milk, 1.8–19 mg/kg in cream, 4.8–56 mg/kg in butter, and 2.4–114 mg/kg in various types of cheese; similar levels occurred in Norway and Spain. After Denmark banned the use of DEHP-plasticized milk tubing, average DEHP levels in whole milk fell to less than 50 μg/L within 6 months.

Average adult human daily phthalate intakes, mainly from foods, are generally far lower than the estimated NOAELs in rodents. Infants and toddlers, however, may be exposed to relatively high DEHP levels from mouthing plastic toys and objects (National Institute of Environmental Health Sciences, 2000). During the 1980s, toy manufacturers voluntarily phased out the use of DEHP in soft toys for children; DINP became the predominant phthalate used to soften the polyvinyl chloride used in some children's products until its use was voluntarily restricted in 1998 because of evidence that it causes liver cancer in rodents. Although the U.S. Consumer Produce Safety Commission (CPSC) concluded that few if any children are at risk from DINP because of low absorbed doses, it asked industry to remove phthalates from soft rattles and teethers, and most manufacturers agreed to comply by early 1999 (U.S. Consumer Product Safety Commission, 1998). The CPSC also asked industry to find a substitute for phthalates in other products intended for children aged 3 years or less that are likely to be mouthed or chewed. Canada and the European Union (EU) have acted to stop using DEHP and DINP and to limit the use of certain other phthalates (e.g., di-*n*-octyl phthalate) in toys intended for mouthing (nipples, teethers, pacifiers, and rattles) but not in larger toys designed for older children.

Persons receiving intensive treatment including parenteral fluids (e.g., premature infants or very ill children) may have high DEHP exposures (because of leaching from plastic medical devices). United States and Canadian expert panels have identified serious health concerns about DEHP (Health Canada, 2002; National Institute of Environmental Health Sciences, 2000). The Canadian panel concluded that DEHP exposure from medical devices in infants, toddlers, critically ill children, and pregnant and lacatating women may cause reproductive and developmental risks and recommended that alternatives to DEHP in medical devices be assured. Whereas most previous research and regulatory attention to phthalates has focused on DEHP and DINP, the results of the CDC survey of urinary phthalate levels noted above indicate the need to control exposures to DEP, DBP, and other phthalates (Blount et al., 2000).

Other Sources

Bisphenol A is a monomer precursor used in production of polycarbonate plastic (used in baby bottles, household appliances, food and drink containers, and many other products) and epoxy resins. Total bisphenol A production in the United States, Western Europe, and Japan was about 2 million tons in 1999, with annual growth of about 7% during the period 1996–1999. Cans for preserved foods are often lined with organosol (polyvinylchloride type) or epoxy lacquers. Bisphenol A diglycidyl ether (BADGE) is used in organosol lacquers, and it and related derivatives can migrate into canned foods, especially fatty foods, at levels of up to several milligrams per kilogram, exceeding the limit of 1 mg/kg proposed by the European Commission Scientific Committee for Food. Bisphenol A has been found in the liquid phase of preserved vegetables in lacquer-coated cans at levels capable of inducing proliferation of MCF-7 human breast cancer cells in vitro. *Tris*(nonylphenyl) phosphite is used in some plastic food wrap products and can release nonylphenol into foods.

Other Products

Pesticides

Many pesticides are applied after harvesting to fruits and vegetables to extend their lives and preserve their quality during storage, transport, and marketing. Persistence and distribution of pesticide residues in the edible portions of produce have been reported for foods, including fruits and vegetables, commonly eaten by children and pregnant women. Vinclozolin is registered as a fungicide for use on fruits and vegetables in the United States and Europe; its metabolites include two potent antiandrogens (see above) and 3,5-dichloroaniline, a genotoxin that is structurally similar to a known animal carcinogen (parachloroaniline). The EPA was concerned about ground and surface water 3,5-dichloroaniline levels and about the fact that this metabolite is also formed from the related dicarboximide fungicides, iprodione and procymidone. Under the FQPA, the EPA has assessed the cumulative hazard of these fungicides, which have a common antiandrogenic toxic mechanism. In what appears to be the first pesticide regulatory action arising in part from concern about hormonal activity, phased restrictions on some food crop and ornamental uses of the fungicide vinclozolin in the United States were implemented because of concerns about its antiandrogenic and carcinogenic effects (U.S.

Environmental Protection Agency, 2000b). After 2004, predicted annual use of this pesticide on canola, nondomestic wine grapes, and turf will be reduced by about half from the current 141,000 pounds.

Others

Brominated flame-retardants, including polybrominated diphenyl ethers (PBDEs), pentabromophenol, and tetrabromobisphenol A, are used in large quantities in electronic equipment, plastics, fabrics, and building materials. Tributyltin bioaccumulates in crabs, oysters, and salmon, particularly those grown in captivity and exposed to organotin used as an antifouling agent. In Japan and the United Kingdom, organotin levels in marine products decreased after the introduction of legal controls during 1987-1990. Several sunscreens had estrogen agonist activity in bioassays (Schlumpf et al., 2001).

Diethylstilbestrol was used as a pregnancy medication in North America and several European countries from the 1940s to the 1970s in the mistaken belief that it would prevent miscarriage. It was also used to prevent lactation in women who wished to bottle-feed, as a postcoital contraceptive, and as a growth promoter for livestock. In the United States alone, at least 3–5 million pregnant women were given DES and related synthetic estrogens, which are now known to be carcinogens and teratogens. Although DES is not an environmental HAA, the experience with it illustrates the potential for harm in using therapeutic HAAs without proven efficacy and the value of modern regulatory practices.

General Considerations

Although there is strong evidence of the adverse developmental and reproductive effects of environmental HAAs at high doses in animals, few studies have been done in humans and the results to date are largely inconclusive. The dearth of human evidence should not be interpreted as evidence of no risk. Rather, the large-scale epidemiologic studies with good exposure and outcome assessment needed to detect the potential risks of multiple low-level environmental HAA exposures in humans have not been done. The planned U.S. longitudinal study of children is the type of study needed to fill this important knowledge gap (National Institute of Child Health and Human Development, 2001).

In assessing animal or epidemiologic studies of environmental HAAs and developmental and reproductive outcomes, it is important to consider that (1) these processes can be disrupted not only by hormonal mechanisms but also by toxic effects of the same agents, (2) results from high-dose testing of single agents in animal systems must be interpreted with caution because human exposures are usually much lower and there are many other uncertainties in extrapolating from animals to humans, and (3) humans are exposed to multiple low-level HAAs and other toxicants during critical prenatal and childhood development periods.

CONCLUSIONS

Proven Health Outcomes

- Although DES is not an environmental HAA, past experience has shown that prenatal exposure to this potent synthetic estrogen causes reproductive tract abnormalities (hypospadias, hypoplastic testicles, epididymal cysts) and vaginal cancer in offspring.

Unresolved Issues and Knowledge Gaps

- Developmental effects—despite considerable animal evidence, the potential roles of prenatal parental exposure to environmental HAAs in human fetal deaths, growth deficits, and birth defects are unknown; for example, only two epidemiologic studies of cryptorchidism have measured internal doses of environmental HAAs, and none have measured biomarkers of susceptibility to HAAs.
- Reproductive system development and function
  ○ There is limited, inconclusive evidence that the average age at menarche has decreased in several countries during recent decades; the validity of these trends and the potential roles of environmental HAAs and other factors remain undefined.
  ○ Limited evidence suggests that the ability of the pesticide chlordecone to cause severely reduced sperm concentrations among occupationally exposed men may involve a hormonal mechanism, that is, ER agonist activity.
  ○ Some pesticides have antiandrogenic activity in animals and in in vitro bioassays, but their role in human subfertility is unknown.
  ○ Internal HAA doses have rarely been measured in studies of human sperm quality.
- Cancer
  ○ Testicular cancer—incidence rates have increased substantially in several countries during recent decades; definitive epidemiologic studies of the possible role of HAAs have not been done.
  ○ Thyroid cancer—incidence rates have increased in several countries during recent decades, especially among young women; the potential role of environmental HAAs remains unknown.

- Knowledge gaps
  - Longitudinal studies of children beginning in the first trimester of pregnancy (or earlier) are needed to assess the risk of subtle and delayed health effects of HAAs and other contaminants with known or suspected developmental toxicity.
  - It is necessary to identify the exposure sources of the phthalates DEP and DBP in reproductive-age women and to assess potential developmental and child health effects (see "Biomonitoring" below).

Risk Management Issues

- Prevention
  - Toxicity testing—ongoing efforts to implement tiered toxicity testing for hormonal activity on a prioritized set of chemicals to which reproductive-age women and children are most exposed should be encouraged.
  - Exposure reduction—it is necessary to minimize exposures of reproductive-age women, pregnant women, and young children to environmental HAAs identified in screening tests.
- Biomonitoring—NHANES III detected relatively high urinary levels of metabolites of the phthalates DEP and DBP in a representative sample of the U.S. population, with reproductive-age women having average DBP metabolite levels about 50% higher than those of other age/sex groups; it is necessary to initiate biomonitoring for HAAs in other countries, with a focus on reproductive-age women and children.
- Disease tracking—the limited, inconclusive evidence of increasing incidence rates of hypospadias and cryptorchidism and increasing prevalence of reduced sperm quality shows the need for tracking systems to enable population-based monitoring of these conditions.

REFERENCES

Agency for Toxic Substances and Disease Registry. (1995). Toxicological profile for diethyl phthalate. Atlanta: Agency for Toxic Substances and Disease Registry.
Agency for Toxic Substances and Disease Registry. (2000a). Final phthalate expert panel reports (Center for the Evaluation of Risks to Human Reproduction). Located at http://cerhr.niehs.nih.gov/news/index.html
Agency for Toxic Substances and Disease Registry. (2000b). Toxicological profile for DDT, DDE, DDD. Atlanta: Agency for Toxic Substances and Disease Registry.
Agency for Toxic Substances and Disease Registry. (2000c). Toxicological profile for di(2-ethylhexyl)phthalate. Atlanta: Agency for Toxic Substances and Disease Registry.

Agency for Toxic Substances and Disease Registry. (2001a). ToxFAQS. Located at http://atsdr1.atsdr.cdc.gov/toxfaq.html

Agency for Toxic Substances and Disease Registry. (2001b). Toxicological profile for di-n-butyl phthalate. Atlanta: Agency for Toxic Substances and Disease Registry.

Aho M, Koivisto AM, Tammela TL, Auvinen A. (2000). Is the incidence of hypospadias increasing? Analysis of Finnish hospital discharge data 1970–1994. Environ Health Perspect 108:463–5.

Akre O, Lipworth L, Cnattingius S, Sparen P, Ekbom A. (1999). Risk factor patterns for cryptorchidism and hypospadias. Epidemiology 10:364–9.

Andersen HR, Andersson AM, Arnold SF, Autrup H, Barfoed M, Beresford NA, Bjerregaard P, Christiansen LB, Gissel B, Hummel R, and others. (1999). Comparison of short-term estrogenicity tests for identification of hormone-disrupting chemicals. Environ Health Perspect 107(Suppl 1):89–108.

Beral V, Colwell L. (1981). Randomised trial of high doses of stilboestrol and ethisterone therapy in pregnancy: long-term follow-up of the children. J Epidemiol Commun Health 35:155–60.

Bernstein L, Pike MC, Depue RH, Ross RK, Moore JW, Henderson BE. (1988). Maternal hormone levels in early gestation of cryptorchid males: a case-control study. Br J Cancer 58:379–81.

Bisphenol A global industry group. (2002). Bisphenol A home page. Located at http://www.bisphenola.org/

BKH Consulting Engineers and TNO Nutrition and Food Research (for the European Commission DG ENV). (2000). Towards the establishment of a priority list of substances for further evaluation of their role in endocrine disruption—preparation of a candidate list of substances as a basis for priority setting. (M0355008/1786Q/10/11/00). Located at http://europa.eu.int/comm/environment/docum/bkh_main.pdf.

Blanck HM, Marcus M, Tolbert PE, Rubin C, Henderson AK, Hertzberg VS, Zhang RH, Cameron L. (2000). Age at menarche and tanner stage in girls exposed in utero and postnatally to polybrominated biphenyl. Epidemiology 11:641–7.

Block K, Kardana A, Igarashi P, Taylor HS. (2000). In utero diethylstilbestrol (DES) exposure alters Hox gene expression in the developing mullerian system. FASEB J 14:1101–8.

Blount BC, Silva MJ, Caudill SP, Needham LL, Pirkle JL, Sampson EJ, Lucier GW, Jackson RJ, Brock JW. (2000). Levels of seven urinary phthalate metabolites in a human reference population. Environ Health Perspect 108:972–82.

Boisen KA, Main KM, Rajpert-De Meyts E, Skakkebaek NE. (2001). Are male reproductive disorders a common entity? The testicular dysgenesis syndrome. Ann NY Acad Sci 948:90–9.

Bosetti C, Kolonel L, Negri E, Ron E, Franceschi S, Dal Maso L, Galanti MR, Mark SD, Preston-Martin S, McTiernan A, and others. (2001). A pooled analysis of case-control studies of thyroid cancer. VI. Fish and shellfish consumption. Cancer Causes Control 12:375–82.

Burlington H, Lindeman VF. (1950). Effect of DDT on testes and secondary sex chacters of white leghorn cockerels. Proc Soc Exp Biol Med 74:48–51.

Bush B, Bennett AH, Snow JT. (1986). Polychlorobiphenyl congeners, p,p'-DDE, and sperm function in humans. Arch Environ Contam Toxicol 15:333–41.

Carlsen E, Giwercman A, Keiding N, Skakkebaek NE. (1992). Evidence for decreasing quality of semen during past 50 years. BMJ 305:609–13.

Centers for Disease Control and Prevention. (2001). National report on human exposure to environmental chemicals. Atlanta: Centers for Disease Control and Prevention.

Chemical Market Reporter. (2001). Chemical Market Reporter. Located at http://www.aperc.org/nonylphenol.pdf

Colon I, Caro D, Bourdony CJ, Rosario O. (2000). Identification of phthalate esters in the serum of young Puerto Rican girls with premature breast development. Environ Health Perspect 108:895–900.

Darlington DN, Dallman MF. (2001). Feedback control in endocrine systems. Principles and practice of endocrinology and metabolism. New York: Lippincott Williams & Wilkins.

de Muinck Keizer SM, Mul D. (2001). Trends in pubertal development in Europe. Hum Reprod Update 7:287–91.

Depue RH. (1984). Maternal and gestational factors affecting the risk of cryptorchidism and inguinal hernia. Int J Epidemiol 13:311–8.

Dolk H, Vrijheid M, Armstrong B, Abramsky L, Bianchi F, Garne E, Nelen V, Robert E, Scott JE, Stone D, and others. (1998). Risk of congenital anomalies near hazardous-waste landfill sites in Europe: the EUROHAZCON study. Lancet 352:423–7.

Foster W, Chan S, Platt L, Hughes C. (2000). Detection of endocrine disrupting chemicals in samples of second trimester human amniotic fluid. J Clin Endocrinol Metab 85:2954–7.

Foster WG. (1998). Endocrine disruptors and development of the reproductive system in the fetus and children: is there cause for concern? Can J Public Health 89(Suppl 1):S37–41, S52, S41–6.

Goldberg JM, Falcone T. (1999). Effect of diethylstilbestrol on reproductive function. Fertil Steril 72:1–7.

Gray LE, Ostby J, Furr J, Wolf CJ, Lambright C, Parks L, Veeramachaneni DN, Wilson V, Price M, Hotchkiss A, and others. (2001). Effects of environmental antiandrogens on reproductive development in experimental animals. Hum Reprod Update 7:248–64.

Hauser R, Altshul L, Chen Z, Ryan L, Overstreet J, Schiff I, Christiani DC. (2002). Environmental organochlorines and semen quality: results of a pilot study. Environ Health Perspect 110:229–33.

Health Canada. 2002. Health Canada Expert advisory panel on DEHP in medical devices. Located at http://www.hc-sc.gc.ca/hpb-dgps/therapeut/zfiles/english/advcomm/eap/dehp/eap-dehp-final-report-2002-jan-11_e.pdf.

Herbst AL, Ulfelder H, Poskanzer DC. (1971). Adenocarcinoma of the vagina. Association of maternal stilbestrol therapy with tumor appearance in young women. N Engl J Med 284:878–81.

Hosie S, Loff S, Witt K, Niessen K, Waag KL. (2000). Is there a correlation between organochlorine compounds and undescended testes? Eur J Pediatr Surg 10:304–9.

Jorgensen N, Andersen AG, Eustache F, Irvine DS, Suominen J, Petersen JH, Andersen AN, Auger J, Cawood EH, Horte A, and others. (2001). Regional differences in semen quality in Europe. Hum Reprod 16:1012–9.

Kallen B, Bertollini R, Castilla E, Czeizel A, Knudsen LB, Martinez-Frias ML, Mastroiacovo P, Mutchinick O. (1986). A joint international study on the epidemiology of hypospadias. Acta Paediatr Scand Suppl 324:1–52.

Kern PA, Dicker-Brown A, Said ST, Kennedy R, Fonseca VA. (2002). The stimulation of tumor necrosis factor and inhibition of glucose transport and lipoprotein lipase in adipose cells by 2,3,7,8-tetrachlorodibenzo-*p*-dioxin. Metabolism 51:65–8.

Key TJ, Bull D, Ansell P, Brett AR, Clark GM, Moore JW, Chilvers CE, Pike MC. (1996). A case-control study of cryptorchidism and maternal hormone concentrations in early pregnancy. Br J Cancer 73:698–701.

Klip H, Verloop J, van Gool JD, Koster ME, Burger CW, van Leeuwen FE. (2002). Hypospadias in sons of women exposed to diethylstilbestrol in utero: a cohort study. Lancet 359:1102–7.

Koo JW, Parham F, Kohn MC, Masten SA, Brock JW, Needham LL, Portier CJ. (2002). The association between biomarker-based exposure estimates for phthalates and demographic factors in a human reference population. Environ Health Perspect 110:405–10.

Kristensen P, Irgens LM, Andersen A, Bye AS, Sundheim L. (1997). Birth defects among offspring of Norwegian farmers, 1967–1991. Epidemiology 8:537–44.

Kuiper GG, Lemmen JG, Carlsson B, Corton JC, Safe SH, van der Saag PT, van der Burg B, Gustafsson JA. (1998). Interaction of estrogenic chemicals and phytoestrogens with estrogen receptor beta. Endocrinology 139:4252–63.

La Vecchia C, Ron E, Franceschi S, Dal Maso L, Mark SD, Chatenoud L, Braga C, Preston-Martin S, McTiernan A, Kolonel L, and others. (1999). A pooled analysis of case-control studies of thyroid cancer. III. Oral contraceptives, menopausal replacement therapy and other female hormones. Cancer Causes Control 10:157–66.

Liu S, Semenciw R, Ugnat AM, Mao Y. (2001). Increasing thyroid cancer incidence in Canada, 1970–1996: time trends and age-period-cohort effects. Br J Cancer 85:1335–9.

Liu S, Wen SW, Mao Y, Mery L, Rouleau J. (1999). Birth cohort effects underlying the increasing testicular cancer incidence in Canada. Can J Public Health 90:176–80.

Longnecker MP, Klebanoff MA, Brock JW, Zhou H, Gray KA, Needham LL, Wilcox AJ. (2002). Maternal serum level of 1,1-dichloro-2,2-*bis*(*p*-chlorophenyl) ethylene and risk of cryptorchidism, hypospadias, and polythelia among male offspring. Am J Epidemiol 155:313–22.

McBride ML, Van den Steen N, Lamb CW, Gallagher RP. (1991). Maternal and gestational factors in cryptorchidism. Int J Epidemiol 20:964–70.

McLachlan JA. (1997). Synergistic effect of environmental estrogens: report withdrawn. Science 277:462–3.

Melnick R, Lucier G, Wolfe M, Hall R, Stancel G, Prins G, Gallo M, Reuhl K, Ho SM, Brown T, and others. (2002). Summary of the National Toxicology Program's report of the endocrine disruptors low-dose peer review. Environ Health Perspect 110:427–31.

National Academy of Sciences. (1999). Hormonally active agents in the environment. Washington, DC: National Academy Press.

National Institute of Child Health and Human Development. (2002). The National Children's Study. Located at http://nationalchildrensstudy.gov/about/042002.cfm.

National Institute of Environmental Health Sciences. (2000). Expert panel review of phthalates. Research Triangle Park. Located at http://cerhr.niehs.nih.gov.

Nikov GN, Hopkins NE, Boue S, Alworth WL. (2000). Interactions of dietary estrogens with human estrogen receptors and the effect on estrogen receptor–

estrogen response element complex formation. Environ Health Perspect 108: 867–72.

Osius N, Karmaus W, Kruse H, Witten J. (1999). Exposure to polychlorinated biphenyls and levels of thyroid hormones in children. Environ Health Perspect 107:843–9.

Paulozzi LJ. (1999). International trends in rates of hypospadias and cryptorchidism. Environ Health Perspect 107:297–302.

Paulozzi LJ, Erickson JD, Jackson RJ. (1997). Hypospadias trends in two U.S. surveillance systems. Pediatrics 100:831–4.

Power DA, Brown RS, Brock CS, Payne HA, Majeed A, Babb P. (2001). Trends in testicular carcinoma in England and Wales, 1971–99. BJU Int 87:361–5.

Sandau CD, Ayotte P, Dewailly E, Duffe J, Norstrom RJ. (2002). Pentachlorophenol and hydroxylated polychlorinated biphenyl metabolites in umbilical cord plasma of neonates from coastal populations in Quebec. Environ Health Perspect 110:411–7.

Schiestl RH, Aubrecht J, Yap WY, Kandikonda S, Sidhom S. (1997). Polychlorinated biphenyls and 2,3,7,8-tetrachlorodibenzopdioxin induce intrachromosomal recombination in vitro and in vivo. Cancer Res 57:4378–83.

Schlumpf M, Cotton B, Conscience M, Haller V, Steinmann B, Lichtensteiger W. (2001). In vitro and in vivo estrogenicity of UV screens. Environ Health Perspect 109:239–44.

Setchell KD, Zimmer-Nechemias L, Cai J, Heubi JE. (1997). Exposure of infants to phyto-oestrogens from soy-based infant formula. Lancet 350:23–7.

Setchell KD, Zimmer-Nechemias L, Cai J, Heubi JE. (1998). Isoflavone content of infant formulas and the metabolic fate of these phytoestrogens in early life. Am J Clin Nutr 68:1453S–61S.

Strohsnitter WC, Noller KL, Hoover RN, Robboy SJ, Palmer JR, Titus-Ernstoff L, Kaufman RH, Adam E, Herbst AL, Hatch EE. (2001). Cancer risk in men exposed in utero to diethylstilbestrol. J Natl Cancer Inst 93:545–51.

Swan SH. (2000). Intrauterine exposure to diethylstilbestrol: long-term effects in humans. APMIS 108:793–804.

Swan SH, Elkin EP. (1999). Declining semen quality: can the past inform the present? Bioessays 21:614–21.

U.S. Consumer Product Safety Commission. (1998). The risk of chronic toxicity associated with exposure to diisononyl phthalate (DINP) in children's products. Bethesda, MD: U.S. Consumer Product Safety Commission.

U.S. Environmental Protection Agency. (1998). Endocrine disruptor screening and testing advisory committee (EDSTAC) final report. Located at http://www.epa.gov/oscpmont/oscpendo/history/finalrpt.htm

U.S. Environmental Protection Agency. (2000a). Endocrine disruptor screening program report to Congress. Located at http://www.epa.gov/scipoly/oscpendo/reporttocongress0800.pdf.

U.S. Environmental Protection Agency. (2000b). Reregistration eligibility decision. Vinclozolin (EPA 738-R-00-023). Washington, DC: U.S. Environmental Protection Agency.

Vos JG, Dybing E, Greim HA, Ladefoged O, Lambre C, Tarazona JV, Brandt I, Vethaak AD. (2000). Health effects of endocrine-disrupting chemicals on wildlife, with special reference to the European situation. Crit Rev Toxicol 30: 71–133.

Watanabe N, Kurita M. (2001). The masculinization of the fetus during pregnancy due to inhalation of diesel exhaust. Environ Health Perspect 109:111–9.

Weidner IS, Moller H, Jensen TK, Skakkebaek NE. (1998). Cryptorchidism and hypospadias in sons of gardeners and farmers. Environ Health Perspect 106: 793–6.

Weidner IS, Moller H, Jensen TK, Skakkebaek NE. (1999). Risk factors for cryptorchidism and hypospadias. J Urol 161:1606–9.

Weir HK, Marrett LD, Moravan V. (1999). Trends in the incidence of testicular germ cell cancer in Ontario by histologic subgroup, 1964–1996. CMAJ 160: 201–5.

Wrutniak-Cabello C, Casas F, Cabello G. (2001). Thyroid hormone action in mitochondria. J Mol Endocrinol 26:67–77.

9

Radiation

The electromagnetic spectrum ranges from ionizing radiation through ultraviolet light, visible light, infrared light, microwaves, and radio waves (Figure 9–1). Ionizing radiation comprises very short wavelength/high frequency electromagnetic waves and particles with sufficient energy to remove electrons from atoms or molecules, thereby creating ions. At the other extreme, transmission and use of electricity that cycles 50 or 60 times per second (i.e., 50 or 60 Hz) produces distinct electric and magnetic waves in the extremely long wavelength/low frequency range of the electromagnetic spectrum.

The known and potential health effects of electromagnetic radiation vary markedly by wavelength/frequency. Prenatal and early childhood high-level ionizing radiation exposure can cause severe neurotoxicity and delayed effects including cancer; such effects arise from the ability of ionizing radiation to damage DNA. Intense childhood sun exposure, especially among genetically susceptible subgroups (e.g., fair-skinned Caucasians), is a major cause of malignant melanoma of skin; although UV light is less energetic than ionizing radiation, it causes photochemical and oxidative DNA damage. There is some evidence (albeit inconsistent) of an association between childhood exposure to relatively high-level power-frequency magnetic fields and childhood acute lymphoblastic leukemia.

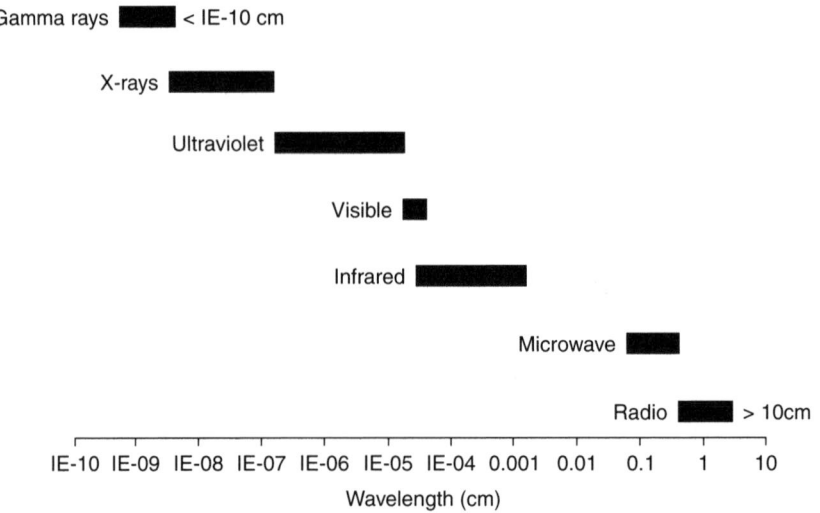

FIGURE 9–1. Electromagnetic spectrum.

The potential biologic mechanism remains unknown; power-frequency radiation at intensities found in the general population appears to be nongenotoxic. Despite much concern about the safety of wireless phones, there is no convincing evidence that radiofrequency radiation exposure at levels found among humans is genotoxic or carcinogenic. This chapter explores these and other potential health effects of prenatal or childhood radiation exposure.

I. IONIZING RADIATION

All persons are continually exposed to ionizing radiation from natural sources including cosmic rays from the sun and outer space and natural radionuclides in the earth's crust, air, water, and foods. Important anthropogenic sources include medical X-rays, radionuclide emissions from nuclear reactor accidents, and nuclear weapons detonations. Radionuclide emissions during a nuclear reactor incident in 1979 at Three Mile Island in Pennsylvania and a much larger release in 1986 at Chernobyl in the Soviet Union raised renewed public concern about radiation and health. Large increases in thyroid cancer among children living close to Chernobyl within a few years of exposure point to the vulnerability of children to radiation, whether through high exposures or because of age-related susceptibility. The biological effects of ionizing radiation (BEIR) V report concluded that the excess risk of cancer from radiation exposure during childhood is about twice that of adults but subject to uncertainties because of the limited follow-up of exposed children (National Academy of Sciences, 1990).

Radiation from radionuclides comprise α- and β-particles and high-energy photons (γ-rays). α-Particles are high-energy positively charged helium nuclei (emitted by heavier radionuclides such as uranium) that cause extensive damage over short distances in tissues. β-Particles are electrons (emitted by radionuclides such as tritium) that penetrate tissues further than α-particles but cause less damage per unit distance. Health risks from α- or β-particles are related mainly to inhaled or ingested radionuclides, for example, lung cancer from inhalation of radon, an α-emitter. γ-Rays are high-energy photons emitted by radionuclides; lacking charge and mass, they penetrate the body easily, causing tissue damage. X-rays are also photons but generally have lower energy than γ-rays and have a different source, that is, the bombardment of matter with charged particles causing X-ray emissions from extranuclear processes. Globally, average population exposure from medical uses of radiation is about half that from natural sources (United Nations Scientific Committee on the Effects of Atomic Radiation, 2000).

The objective of Part I of this chapter is to define the known and potential impacts of ionizing radiation on child health including genotoxicity, adverse pregnancy outcomes, neurotoxicity, and cancer. The discussion addresses the major categories of anthropogenic radiation exposure, particularly radioactive fallout from atmospheric nuclear weapons tests, preconceptual and prenatal parental exposure to diagnostic X-rays or occupational sources, and postnatal exposure of children to X-rays, radon, nuclear detonations, and nuclear power plant emissions. Radiation exposure levels, sources, and risk management issues are explored. The reader is referred to other sources for more detailed information on ionizing radiation hazards (Agency for Toxic Substances and Disease Registry, 1999; National Academy of Sciences, 1990, 1999; United Nations Scientific Committee on the Effects of Atomic Radiation, 2000).

Health Effects

The health effects of ionizing radiation depend on the type, dose, and duration of radiation exposure, time since exposure (or first exposure), tissue, age, sex, and other personal characteristics. Knowledge of radiation-related adult cancer risks comes mainly from epidemiologic studies of

Japanese atomic bomb survivors and persons exposed to relatively high doses of medical X-rays during diagnosis or treatment of diseases (tuberculosis, ankylosing spondylitis, cervical cancer, tinea capitis, and alleged thymus enlargement). Radiation exposure units include

- Gy (gray)—1 Gy equals 1 joule of energy deposited in 1 kg of a material; equivalent to 100 rads
- Sv (sievert)—the biologically effective dose, estimated by multiplying the absorbed dose in grays by a quality factor Q specific for the type of incident radiation; equivalent to 100 rem
- Bq (becquerel)—quantity of a radionuclide that will have one transformation in 1 second

Genotoxic Effects

By depositing energy directly in DNA or by creating free radicals, ionizing radiation can cause DNA base damage, single- and double-strand breaks, and DNA–protein cross-links. Nuclear DNA repair enzymes usually restore normal DNA structure and function, but unsuccessful, incomplete, or inaccurate repair can cause mutations, chromosomal aberrations (deletions, inversions, translocations), and cell death. Double-strand DNA breaks are prone to inaccurate repair (e.g., nonhomologous DNA end joining by DNA repair enzymes), causing mutations and chromosomal aberrations characteristic of leukemia and other cancers. Potential mechanisms for radiation-induced cancer include activation of oncogenes (e.g., *ras* and c-*myc*) and inactivation of tumor-suppressor genes such as *p53* and *Rb* (retinoblastoma gene). In cells with DNA damage, *p53* normally blocks cell division and may trigger apoptosis; inactivated *p53* allows cells with DNA damage to divide, increasing the risk of malignant transformation. Rapidly dividing fetal cells appear to be more prone to radiation-induced damage than more slowly dividing differentiated cells (Agency for Toxic Substances and Disease Registry, 1999).

Estimated genetic effects of exposure to low-level ionizing radiation are shown in Table 9–1. Radiation-induced heritable mutations, that is, germ cell mutations, have not been clearly demonstrated in humans. The BEIR V report concluded that the acute radiation dose required to double the spontaneous mutation rate in humans is likely to be at least that observed in mice (1 Sv) but noted considerable uncertainties; doubling dose estimates, for instance, do not include diseases related to multiple genes, the likely largest category of genetically related diseases (National Academy of Sciences, 1990).

Elevated indoor air radon levels in homes or schools have been linked to DNA damage, chromosomal abnormalities, and micronuclei in pe-

TABLE 9–1. Estimated Genetic Effects of 1 rem (10 mSv) per Generation[a]

Genetic Effect	Background Incidence per 10⁶ Live-Born Infants	Additional Cases per 10⁶ Live-Born Infants per Rem per Generation	
		First Generation	Equilibrium
Autosomal dominant disorder—			
clinically severe	2,500	5–20	25
clinically mild	7,500	1–15	75
X-linked disorder	400	<1	<5
Recessive disorder	2,500	<1	Very slow increase
Chromosomal—unbalanced translocations	600	<5	Very little increase
Chromosomal—trisomies	3,800	<1	<1
Birth defects	20,000–30,000	10	10–100
Disorders of complex etiology—			
heart disease	600,000	NA	NA
cancer	300,000	NA	NA

Source: National Academy of Sciences (1990).

[a]Risks are for an average population exposure of 10 mSv per generation with background gene mutation incidence rates and an assumed doubling dose for chronic exposure of 1 Sv.

NA = not available.

ripheral lymphocytes from exposed children. Compared to their parents and siblings born before the Chernobyl disaster, children conceived afterward by parents occupationally exposed in the cleanup had a sevenfold increase in new bands on multisite DNA fingerprinting, a finding suggestive of germ-cell mutations. Adults exposed as children or young adults to relatively high-dose X-rays had higher proportions of lymphocytes with stable chromosome aberrations.

Radiation-induced somatic cell mutations may also cause genetic instability. Several inherited conditions conferring increased cancer risks involve defects of genes encoding DNA repair enzymes needed to correct damage caused by ionizing radiation and other mutagens[1] and clastogens.[2] The genes *BRCA1*, *BRCA2*, and *ATM*, for instance, encode proteins

[1]Chemical or physical agents that produce heritable changes in nucleotide sequence (by causing base-pair substitutions or small additions or deletions of one or more base pairs in genetic material).

[2]Agents that can cause breaks in chromosomes that result in the gain, loss, or rearrangement of chromosomal segments or cause sister chromatid exchanges during DNA replication.

involved in homologously directed repair of double-strand DNA breaks; mutations in these genes are causally linked to an increased risk of breast and other cancers.

Developmental Effects

Japanese children prenatally exposed to atomic bomb radiation had increased risks of reduced head circumference, mental retardation, long-lasting complex chromosomal aberrations, and growth deficits at ages 9–19 years. Findings from the limited number of epidemiologic studies in other populations include

- Stillbirths—associations with self-reported exposure of either parent to ionizing radiation (Parker et al., 1999; Savitz et al., 1989; Zhang et al., 1992)
- Birth defects—associations between preconceptual parental or first trimester maternal exposure to occupational radiation or diagnostic X-rays and the risk of neural tube defects (Kallen et al., 1998; Parker et al., 1999; Sever et al., 1988; Zhang et al., 1992) and cardiac defects (Correa-Villasenor et al., 1993; Loffredo et al., 2001)
- Birth weight—IUGR associated with maternal periconceptual occupational radiation or paternal preconceptual gonadal exposure to diagnostic X-rays (Shea and Little, 1997; Zhang et al., 1992)

Animal studies indicate that preconceptual exposure of gametes to ionizing radiation (or chemical mutagens) causes pre- and peri-implantation deaths and growth retardation without birth defects; exposure of the embryo during early organogenesis causes fetal deaths, reduced body weight, and birth defects (Rutledge, 1997).

Cancer

Ionizing radiation is a known cause of cancer in humans and can produce cancer in virtually every tissue in animals and likely in humans (Agency for Toxic Substances and Disease Registry, 1999; International Agency for Research on Cancer, 2000). The risk of radiation-induced cancer depends on several factors including the total dose, dose rate, age at exposure, sex, time since first exposure, and tissue. Readily inducible malignancies include leukemia and thyroid, breast, stomach, and colon cancers. Prenatal exposure to diagnostic X-rays, especially during the last trimester of pregnancy, is associated with an increased risk of childhood cancer (Doll and Wakeford, 1997). Several generalizations about radiation carcinogenesis can be made:

- A single exposure is sufficient to elevate the cancer incidence many years later.
- Although body organs vary in sensitivity to radiation, the risks of most cancers increase after exposure.
- Age at exposure influences the subsequent cancer risk.
  - Short-term radiation exposure during childhood appears to double the lifetime excess risk of fatal cancer compared to the same exposure during adulthood.
  - Children exposed to ionizing radiation have an increased risk of leukemia and thyroid cancer that may develop as soon as 2–4 years after exposure.
  - Girls exposed to X-rays during or before adolescence have higher excess breast cancer risks as adults than those exposed at older ages.
- At the same dose, high linear energy transfer (LET) radiation (e.g., α-particles) is far more cytotoxic and oncogenic than low-LET radiation (e.g., X-rays) and can increase cell transformation rates at doses that have little effect on cell survival.

Atomic Bomb Survivors

Only two cases of cancer before age 15 years occurred among 1829 Japanese children prenatally exposed to atomic bomb radiation. Postnatally exposed Japanese children had increased risks of adult cancers including leukemia and breast cancer. The estimated lifetime risk of solid tumors per sievert for those exposed at age 10 years was 1.0–1.8 times that of persons exposed at age 30 years (Pierce et al., 1996).

Radioactive Fallout

Atmospheric nuclear detonations and nuclear reactor accidents have released iodine, cesium, strontium, and other radionuclides over wide areas. Findings from investigations of children exposed to radioactive fallout from nuclear testing in Nevada and the Marshall Islands and the Chernobyl nuclear reactor disaster include:

- Thyroid cancer—fairly consistent evidence of increased risks of benign and malignant thyroid tumors, particularly among persons exposed as children, with latent periods ranging from a few years to several decades
- Leukemia—limited evidence of increased risks, especially among children and persons exposed before age 20 years

The Chernobyl accident released large amounts of radionuclides including ^{131}I, ^{137}Cs, and ^{134}Cs in a plume that moved mainly north into Belarus, west into Ukraine, and to a lesser degree throughout the Northern Hemisphere. In the immediate surroundings there were 143 adult cases of acute radiation syndrome including 34 deaths. About 5%–8% of children in Belarus aged less than 15 years received estimated thyroid doses of at least 2 Gy. Childhood thyroid cancer incidence rates increased from 0.2 to 4.0 per 100,000 persons per year during 1987–1995. An intensive thyroid cancer screening survey of children within 150 km of the Chernobyl power plant and born before, during, or after the year of the accident showed a markedly increased risk among those born during the 3 years before the accident and exposed as young children (Shibata et al., 2001). Although thyroid screening likely contributed to the increased incidence rates, a case-control study showed a strong association between childhood thyroid cancer and estimated thyroid radiation dose from ground deposition of [131]I (Astakhova et al., 1998). Factors possibly contributing to the markedly increased risk of childhood thyroid cancer include relatively high thyroid doses from energy-rich, shorter-lived radioiodides and iodide deficiency in the region of the Chernobyl reactor.

The International Program on the Health Effects of the Chernobyl Accident, established by the WHO in 1991, concluded that childhood thyroid cancer increased significantly in Belarus and Ukraine beginning 3 years after the accident but there was no increase in leukemia or mental retardation among children exposed prenatally. It may be expected that radiation-induced thyroid cancer and adenomas will continue among those exposed as children well into their adult lives. Elevated childhood leukemia rates among children living near nuclear facilities have been reported, but other large studies have shown no association, justifying the conclusion that there is no convincing evidence that radiation released during normal operations of nuclear plants increases childhood cancer rates in surrounding populations.

Prenatal Exposure to Ionizing Radiation
Although medical X-rays are not part of the environment as defined here, they are a major source of radiation exposure during childhood, and studies of exposed children have provided insights into potential risks from environmental sources of ionizing radiation. The Oxford Survey of Childhood Cancers produced the first substantive evidence that prenatal exposure to diagnostic abdominal X-rays is associated with an increased risk of childhood cancer, especially leukemia (Stewart et al., 1958). The estimated radiation dose from prenatal X-rays (mainly to detect pelvic disproportion) was 0.46 cGy/film; 9% of pregnant women were exposed to five or more films, that is, to at least 2.3 cGy. A similar association was observed in a large U.S. study (MacMahon, 1962). These findings were in contrast to the apparent absence of excess childhood cancer among pre-

natally exposed Japanese atomic bomb survivors; there were, however, only about 1800 prenatally exposed Japanese children, substantially limiting the statistical power of the study. (Note: the childhood leukemia incidence rate in the United States is about 45 cases per million children per year; assuming the same risk in unexposed Japanese children, about two cases would be expected over a 30-year follow-up period).

A recent review of epidemiologic studies of childhood leukemia and prenatal maternal exposure to diagnostic X-rays, especially in the third trimester, concluded that there is strong evidence of an increased risk (pooled $RR = 1.38, 1.31–1.47$) (Doll and Wakeford, 1997); other reviewers reached a similar but less definitive conclusion (Boice and Miller, 1999). Negative results from recent studies of maternal X-ray exposure and childhood leukemia could reflect a true null association or differences from earlier studies, such as, reduced radiation doses of diagnostic X-rays (Meinert et al., 1999; Naumburg et al., 2001; Shu et al., 2002). Prenatal maternal X-ray exposure in a German study was associated with childhood lymphomas (Meinert et al., 1999). There is inadequate evidence of an association between childhood leukemia and preconceptual paternal exposure to X-rays or occupation-related radiation. The UNSCEAR estimated that the absolute excess risk of childhood cancer from prenatal maternal exposure to X-rays is about 5% per sievert (United Nations Scientific Committee on the Effects of Atomic Radiation, 2000).

Postnatal Exposure of Children to Therapeutic and Diagnostic Radiation
A pooled analysis of five cohort and two case-controls studies of thyroid cancer indicated a strong association with radiation exposure during childhood, a linear exposure–risk relationship extending to doses as low as 0.10 Gy, and higher absolute and relative excess risks for females compared to males (Ron et al., 1995). The UNSCEAR concluded that children are more susceptible to radiation-induced thyroid cancer than older persons; for example, the risk for children aged 0–5 years at exposure was fivefold that for those exposed at ages 10–14 years (United Nations Scientific Committee on the Effects of Atomic Radiation, 2000).

Children given radiotherapy for ringworm of the scalp or skin hemangiomas had substantially increased brain and thyroid cancer risks and strong exposure–risk relationships. In Connecticut, cohorts born during 1915–1945, the period when use of X-rays to treat benign conditions of the head and neck was common, had increased thyroid cancer risks (Zheng et al., 1996). Among three recent studies of childhood leukemia and postnatal diagnostic X-ray exposure, one showed an overall association (including interactions between X-ray exposure and polymorphisms in several DNA repair genes), another showed a link only to pre-B acute lymphatic leukemia, and the other showed no relationship (Infante-Rivard et al., 2000; Meinert et al., 1999; Shu et al., 2002).

Postnatal Exposure of Children to Environmental Radiation
Radon, a proven human carcinogen, is the most ubiquitous source of radiation exposure for the general population; residential radon may cause 6600–24,000 lung cancer deaths annually among adults in the United States, the risk being about tenfold higher for persons first exposed at age 15 compared to age 50. Polonium, a radon decay product, behaves like calcium in vivo and is taken up by bone, potentially causing significant radiation exposure of bone marrow cells of the fetus and child, but there is inadequate evidence of an association between radon exposure and childhood leukemia. There was a moderately strong association between CNS tumors and measured indoor radon levels (Kaletsch et al., 1999). The BEIR VI report concluded that the limited evidence linking general population radon exposure to nonlung cancers does not warrant consideration in setting radon standards and guidelines (National Academy of Sciences, 1999). Other sources of residential radiation exposure have been linked to childhood leukemia (γ-radiation from uranium-containing concrete) and bone sarcomas (drinking water radium levels) (Axelson et al., 2002; Finkelstein and Kreiger, 1996).

Neurotoxicity

Cases of reduced head circumference and mental retardation after prenatal exposure to therapeutic ionizing radiation were first reported in the 1920s. Children of mothers who received whole-body radiation from atomic bombs at Hiroshima and Nagasaki had an increased risk of microcephaly, mental retardation, and lower school performance. The risk of mental retardation was greatest for exposures during gestational weeks 8–15, the peak time of neuron proliferation and neuroblast migration to the cerebral cortex, processes that are disrupted by ionizing radiation. The average IQ deficit for exposure during early gestation was 21–29 points per gray (National Academy of Sciences, 1990). Children exposed to cranial radiation for treatment of tinea capitis had increased risks of IQ deficits, lower scores on high school aptitude tests, poor school performance, hospitalization for mental disorder (including a dose–response relationship), and a borderline increase in mental retardation. Among survivors of childhood cancer exposed to therapeutic whole-brain radiation, substantial cognitive deficits occurred mainly among those aged less than 3 years at exposure.

Exposures

The global average exposure to natural sources of radiation is about 2.4 mSv/year (Table 9–2). Other sources include the following (United Nations Scientific Committee on the Effects of Atomic Radiation, 2000):

- Atmospheric nuclear testing—global average exposure peaked at about 150 μSv/year in 1963, declining to about 5 μSv/year in 2000.
- Medical uses of radiation—the average annual dose in developed countries is about 1.2 mSv, but the range of individual exposures is very wide.
- Occupationally exposed persons—the average annual dose among monitored workers is about 0.6 mSv from anthropogenic sources and 1.8 mSv from enhanced natural sources (e.g., air crew, mining, mineral processing).

Nuclear Test and Reactor Emissions

Among the nuclear tests conducted in the Marshall Islands during 1946–1958, radioactive fallout was greatest after the large 1954 Bravo thermonuclear test, causing average absorbed thyroid doses of about 1 Gy in

TABLE 9–2. Average Annual Radiation Exposure (mSv) of General Population

Source	Worldwide Average Annual Dose (Range)
Cosmic rays	0.4 (0.3–1.0)
Terrestrial γ-rays	0.5 (0.3–0.6)
Inhalation (mainly radon)	1.2 (0.2–10)
Ingestion	0.3 (0.2–0.8)
Total natural sources	2.4 (1–10)
Medical uses of radiation	0.4 (<0.2–1.2)[a]
Atmospheric nuclear testing	0.005
Chernobyl accident	0.002
Nuclear power production	0.0002
Total anthropogenic	1.2

Source: United Nations Scientific Committee on the Effects of Atomic Radiation (2000).

[a] Varies by level of health-care resources per capita.

the most contaminated islands. Exposed children had a high prevalence of screen-detected thyroid nodules; iodine deficiency may have been a contributory factor. Average cumulated thyroid ^{131}I doses among persons most exposed to the Nevada atmospheric nuclear bomb tests during 1951–1958 were 12–16 cGy; a few persons, including young children, may have received thyroid doses of over 1 Gy. Early summer tests caused the greatest doses because of fallout when cows were on pasture and fresh local vegetables were used. The Chernobyl nuclear reactor accident released large amounts of radioisotopes, including several iodine and cesium radioisotopes. The estimated average thyroid ^{131}I dose among controls in a case-control study of childhood thyroid cancer in Belarus was 20 cGy.

Radon

Radioactive radon gas (^{222}Rn) and its decay products occur naturally in many homes and cause average doses of about 1.2 mSv per year, that is, about half of the average background radiation dose to the U.S. population. Average outdoor radon concentrations are about 10 Bq/m^3, whereas about 5%–10% of American homes have radon levels above 148 Bq/m^3 (the current remedial action level). Surveys of schools have detected occasional high radon levels. Average radon levels in drinking water from ground sources are about 20 Bq/L, much higher than those of surface sources.

RISK MANAGEMENT

Sources

Radon is released by the decay of naturally occurring thorium and uranium, elements present in rock and soil in highly variable concentrations. Radon decays into polonium isotopes (^{218}Po and ^{214}Po) that are α-particle emitters. Depending on the amount of radon in the underlying soil, building construction, and air exchange rates, indoor radon concentrations can reach relatively high levels. Radon can enter homes through exposed soil (e.g., crawl spaces), cracks in concrete floors and walls, floor drains, groundwater (e.g., sumps, showering), and building materials.

Atmospheric testing of nuclear weapons during 1945–1980 was the main anthropogenic environmental radiation source globally (United Nations Scientific Committee on the Effects of Atomic Radiation, 2000). These tests caused widespread dispersion of radionuclides such as ^{90}Sr, ^{137}Cs, and ^{131}I in the atmosphere; those with long half-lives (^{90}Sr and ^{137}Cs) remain widespread in ecosystems. ^{90}Sr mimics calcium and accumulates in bone, ^{131}I accumulates in thyroid, and ^{137}Cs emulates potassium and disperses throughout the body. Food is normally a minor source of radionuclides but radioactive iodine can be widely dispersed in air, deposit on pastureland, and enter the human food chain via fresh cow milk. Dairy products such as cheese are less hazardous, as they take time to prepare and the half-life of iodine radionuclides is quite short; for example, the half-life of ^{131}I is 8 days. Food crops and meat from wildlife and domestic animals may be contaminated by ^{137}Cs.

Intervention

The International Commission for Radiological Protection and national agencies such as the U.S. EPA have recommended radiation exposure limits for people and environmental media (Table 9–3). Cessation of atmospheric nuclear bomb detonations has reduced an important source of airborne radioactivity. Compliance with regulations on the design, operation, and maintenance of nuclear power plants must be monitored and enforced to protect the public from disasters such as that at Chernobyl. When large atmospheric releases of ^{131}I and other iodine radionuclides occur,

TABLE 9–3. Recommended Exposure Limits to Ionizing Radiation for the General Population

Exposure	Recommended Limit
Total exposure[a]	
Woman's abdomen	2 mSv/year
General public (whole body, 5 year average)	1 mSv/year
Radon in home indoor air[b]	
Remedial action level	148 Bq/m^3
Drinking water (MCLs)[c]	
α-Particles	0.555 Bq/L
β-Particles	0.04 mSv/year
^{226}Ra and ^{228}Ra combined[d]	0.185 Bq/L

[a] *Source:* International Commission on Radiological Protection (1991).

[b] *Source:* U.S. Environmental Protection Agency (1993).

[c] Maximum contaminant levels.

[d] Radium isotopes.

Source: U.S. Environmental Protection Agency (2001).

ingestion of iodide tablets reduces thyroid uptake of inhaled or ingested radioiodides but only if taken within hours after exposure (Zanzonico and Becker, 2000).

Control of radon exposure in homes, schools, and other buildings frequented by children also require monitoring, regulatory, and educational programs. Monitoring is important because radon levels vary enormously, with some buildings having very high levels. Only 43% of new single-family detached homes built in areas with high radon potential during 1998 incorporated radon-reducing features (U.S. Environmental Protection Agency 2002). The EPA advice to homeowners concerning radon includes the following: (1) conduct a short-term test (2–90 days) for radon levels, (2) if the result is 148 Bq/m^3 or higher, conduct a short- or long-term confirmatory test or, if the level is 370 Bq/m^3 or higher, conduct a second short-term test immediately, and (3) take remedial action if a long-term test result or the average of two short-term test results is 148 Bq/m^3 or higher. The EPA has proposed a standard for radon in public drinking water supplies that would limit radon to either 11.1 Bq/L or to 148 Bq/L with a requirement to develop indoor air radon programs.

Inappropriate radiotherapy for benign conditions subsided when the U.S. National Academy of Sciences and the U.K. Medical Research Council in 1956 recognized the health risks of ionizing radiation. There appear to be no population-based data on measured exposures of pregnant women or children to medical or dental diagnostic X-rays; although these are not environmental hazards as defined in this book, they are important sources of radiation exposure.

CONCLUSIONS

Proven Health Outcomes

- Microcephaly and mental retardation (high-dose first trimester exposure)
- Cancer
  - Low-dose prenatal exposure—childhood leukemia
  - High-dose childhood exposure—leukemia and thyroid, brain, and breast cancers in adulthood and childhood thyroid cancer

Unresolved Issues and Knowledge Gaps

- Developmental effects of parental preconceptual or first trimester exposure

- Inadequate evidence of an association between paternal preconceptual occupational exposure and childhood leukemia
  - Limited evidence of associations with birth defects (neural tube, cardiac)
  - Limited evidence of associations with IUGR
- Cancer related to low-dose radiation exposure during childhood
  - Limited evidence of associations between diagnostic X-ray exposure during childhood and childhood leukemia
  - Inadequate evidence of associations between environmental radiation exposure (radon in indoor air, radium in drinking water, other) and childhood cancers (leukemia and brain cancers, bone sarcomas)
- Knowledge development—need epidemiologic studies with improved exposure assessment and statistical power to assess childhood and delayed health effects of low-level, early-life exposures

Risk Management Issues

- Prevention—need to minimize exposure to occupational, medical, and environmental sources of ionizing radiation among children and reproductive-age persons, especially pregnant women
- Biomonitoring—need to measure ionizing radiation exposure among reproductive-age men and women and children in homes, schools, workplaces, and medical/dental applications (no population-based data available except for certain occupational exposures)

II. POWER FREQUENCY ELECTRIC AND MAGNETIC FIELDS AND RADIOFREQUENCY RADIATION

A 1979 report of an association between childhood cancer and residential electric wiring configurations in Denver, Colorado, raised concern about the potential health effects of electromagnetic fields (EMFs) and triggered substantial research (Wertheimer and Leeper, 1979). Electric field strength (volts/meter) depends on the voltage independent of current size. Magnetic fields are produced by moving electric charges and their strength (amps/meter) reflects the amount of current passing through a conductor, independent of voltage; most epidemiologic studies have measured magnetic flux density.[3] When electrical equipment is connected to a power

[3]Magnetic flux density units are gauss (G) or tesla (T); 1 μT = 10 mG.

supply, there is a 50 or 60 Hz electrical field along the power cord, and when the equipment is turned on, there is also a 50 or 60 Hz magnetic field. The strengths of electric and magnetic fields both decrease rapidly with distance from the source; common building materials and even shrubs shield against electric but not magnetic fields. Power-frequency EMFs have wavelengths of about 5,000 km, far greater than UV-light or ionizing radiation (Figure 9–1).

Radiofrequency (RF) radiation spans the frequency range 3 kHz to 300 GHz, that is, above EMFs and below visible light, with wavelengths of less than 1 cm to tens or hundreds of meters. Having much lower energy than shorter-wavelength electromagnetic radiation such as X-rays or γ-radiation, RF radiation has insufficient energy to ionize biologically important atoms but it can cause tissue heating. Microwave (MW) radiation comprises the subset of RF radiation at 300 MHz to 300 GHz (Figure 9–1). Exposure to RF radiation is ubiquitous and is increasing with the growing use of wireless phones and other communication systems. Existing safety codes for RF radiation are designed to protect the public and occupationally exposed persons from potential heat-induced adverse health effects. At distances more than several wavelengths from an RF emitter, RF radiation levels can be accurately estimated as power density (e.g., W/m^2).

The objective of Part II of this chapter is to describe the evidence relating environmental power-frequency magnetic fields and RF radiation to potential impacts on child health including biologic effects, reproductive outcomes, and childhood cancer. The discussion addresses parental and childhood exposure sources including proximity to high-voltage power lines, residential wire configuration, and use of electric devices, wireless phones, and radio/TV communication systems. Risk management issues are explored in light of the widespread exposure to potential hazards that are still poorly understood.

HEALTH EFFECTS

Epidemiologists face many obstacles in assessing potential health effects of EMF and RF radiation exposures. The relative rarity of serious health outcomes such as birth defects and childhood cancer, the low prevalence of high exposures to power-frequency magnetic fields, and the choice and accurate measurement of biologically relevant exposure indicators are among the most important challenges. Research to date has barely begun to address the numerous potentially relevant exposure parameters, susceptible population subgroups, and interactions with other factors.

Molecular Mechanisms and Biologic Effects

Power-Frequency Electromagnetic Fields

Power-frequency magnetic fields normally transmit negligible energy to tissues. The two main mechanisms by which biologic systems may interact with power-frequency EMFs are (International Radiation Protection Association, 1993) (1) induced electric currents, polarization of bound charge (formation of electric dipoles), and reorientation of existing electric dipoles in tissues and (2) induced electric fields and currents in tissues.

Electric and magnetic fields are independent entities for significant sources of human exposure. Unlike electric fields, magnetic fields can easily penetrate buildings and tissues. Power-frequency magnetic fields induce tissue currents of about 1 $\mu A/m^2$, three orders of magnitude lower than tissue currents associated with electrical activity in neurons and seven or eight orders of magnitude higher than those induced by external electric fields. The earth's static magnetic field does not induce tissue currents. The strength of both electric and magnetic fields is inversely proportional to a power function of the distance from the source that depends on the geometry of the source. Expert panel reviews of the potential biologic effects of power-frequency magnetic fields have concluded that (International Commission on Non-Ionizing Radiation Protection, 1998; National Academy of Sciences, 1997; National Institute of Environmental Health Sciences, 1998)

- Magnetic flux densities commonly experienced in residences (0.01–1 μT) have no reproducible in vitro biologic effects.
- Exposures above 50 μT have fairly consistent effects on intracellular calcium levels, signal transduction, and gene expression in experimental systems; exposures above 100 μT increase cell proliferation, disrupt signal transduction pathways, and inhibit differentiation, and exposures above 500 μT affect bone healing.
- Direct genotoxicity has not been consistently demonstrated at any magnetic flux density, but very strong magnetic fields may enhance mutation rates after initiation with ionizing radiation.
- There is no convincing evidence of adverse developmental effects or carcinogenicity in animals at relatively high magnetic flux densities, with the possible exception of enhanced growth of chemically induced mammary cancers in rodents exposed to magnetic flux densities in the range 0.01–30 mT.

The hormone melatonin appears to reduce the incidence and growth rate of chemically induced breast cancers in experimental animals. It has been hypothesized that power-frequency magnetic fields may reduce melatonin levels in humans and increase the breast cancer risk; a recent review, however, concluded that exposure to light at night profoundly suppressed blood melatonin levels, but magnetic fields had little or no effect (Graham et al., 2001).

Radiofrequency Electromagnetic Radiation
Absorption of RF and tissue heating are highest at frequencies near the body's resonant frequencies, for example, about 35 MHz for an ungrounded adult and 700 MHz for an infant's head. Animal studies have provided some evidence of genotoxicity and carcinogenicity at very high RF radiation levels; the weight of evidence from toxicologic studies, however, suggests that RF radiation is not directly mutagenic and that reported chromosomal abnormalities in experimental models are likely caused by tissue warming (Brusick et al., 1998). Reviews of the literature on the biologic effects of RF radiation at the frequencies used by wireless phones have concluded that (Expert panel on the potential health risks of RF fields from wireless telecommunication devices, 1999; International Commission on Non-Ionizing Radiation Protection, 1998)

- RF radiation penetrates tissues up to 1 cm, causing tissue heating.
- Ornithine decarboxylase activity and calcium efflux from neurons increase when the amplitude of RF radiation is modulated by EMFs; these effects are not known to cause adverse health effects and require further research.
- Reported effects of RF radiation on cell proliferation, genotoxicity, and increased permeability of the blood–brain barrier have been inconsistent.
- There is little evidence that RF radiation is carcinogenic in experimental animals.

Developmental Effects

Power-Frequency Magnetic Fields
A meta-analysis of nine case-control and cohort studies of pregnancy outcome and maternal exposure to video display monitors during pregnancy yielded pooled odds ratios of unity for spontaneous abortion and birth defects (Parazzini et al., 1993). A recent review of epidemiologic studies concluded that there were few associations and no consistent relationships between occupational or residential power-frequency magnetic field exposure and the risk of spontaneous abortion, birth defects, low birth weight, or preterm birth (Shaw, 2001). Nevertheless, two California cohort studies (one used a nested case-control design) demonstrated a doubling of the spontaneous abortion risk at dosimeter-measured personal

magnetic flux densities greater than 1.6 μT (Li et al., 2002) or 3.5 μT (Lee et al., 2002). Toxicologic evidence indicates that power-frequency magnetic fields are inconsistently teratogenic in chick embryos and generally have no effect on fetal growth, birth defects, fetal loss, and neurobehavioral development in other animal species.

Radiofrequency Radiation
The few epidemiologic studies of RF radiation and adverse pregnancy outcomes have shown no convincing relationships, that is, no strong and precise associations with quantitative exposure assessment, exposure–risk relationships, and control of confounders (Royal Society of Canada, 1999). Only a few RF radiation frequencies have been tested in experimental systems, and most have assessed acute high-dose exposure rather than the chronic low-level exposure typical of human populations; the most consistent high-dose effect was reduced fetal growth. Evidence of teratogenic effects is inconsistent and is seen only at RF radiation doses capable of causing substantial tissue heating.

Cancer

Childhood brain cancer and leukemia incidence rates have generally been stable or have increased slightly during recent decades. In the United States, most of the increase in childhood brain cancer and leukemia incidence rates occurred during the mid-1980s, suggestive of an artifact such as improved diagnosis or cancer registration (Linet et al., 1999). Despite extensive research into potential causes, including power-frequency magnetic fields, there are no known modifiable risk factors for childhood cancer with high attributable risks.

Power-Frequency Magnetic Fields
The first study of childhood cancer and high-current power line configurations in Denver, Colorado, showed a significant association and an exposure–risk relationship (Wertheimer and Leeper, 1979). An independent study in Denver confirmed this association and showed that the Wertheimer-Leeper wire code and a simplified version of it were both correlated with measured bedroom magnetic flux densities (Kaune and Savitz, 1994; Savitz and Kaune, 1993).

Leukemia. Leukemia has been associated with exposure to magnetic flux densities at home (childhood leukemia) and at work (especially adult chronic lymphocytic leukemia). Because childhood cancer is rare, almost all investigators have used case-control designs, estimating past exposures through parent-reported information, residential wire configuration, distance from electric power lines, and residential and personal exposure monitoring over very limited time periods (Savitz, 1995). Among the few studies focusing on electric fields, one reported a moderately strong exposure–risk relationship between measured nighttime bedroom electric fields and childhood leukemia (Coghill et al., 1996), but several larger studies, including two with personal electric field measurements, were negative (Green et al., 1999; London et al., 1991; McBride et al., 1999).

Key conclusions from several meta-analyses and expert panel reviews of childhood cancer and power-frequency magnetic flux density include (Ahlbom et al., 2000, 2001; International Agency for Research on Cancer, 2002; National Institute of Environmental Health Sciences, 1999) (see also Table 9–4):

- Childhood leukemia
  - Pooled odds ratios of 1.3 to 1.5 for residences within 50 m of power transmission and distribution lines
  - Pooled odds ratios of 1.3 to 1.7 for estimated high historic magnetic fields based on wire configuration; inconsistent odds ratios for present measured magnetic flux densities
  - An apparent concentration of risk among children with time-weighted average magnetic flux densities of 0.4 μT or greater; only 1.4% of cases and 0.6% of controls had such exposure (Ahlbom et al., 2000)
  - Inadequate evidence of an association with electric fields
- Other cancers—there were no consistent relationships between residential electric or magnetic fields and brain or other childhood cancers.
- Animal evidence—animal evidence of power-frequency magnetic field carcinogenicity was judged as inadequate; there were no data to assess the carcinogenicity of static magnetic fields or static or power-frequency electric fields or to support a specific exposure metric.

Of the individual studies of power-frequency magnetic fields and childhood leukemia, only two studies used personal exposure monitoring, one showing a positive association that was stronger among children aged less than 6 years (Green et al., 1999) and the other showing no relationship (McBride et al., 1999). Other reported associations with childhood leukemia include paternal but not maternal occupational exposure to power-frequency magnetic fields, residential power-frequency magnetic flux density at night, and time spent watching television or playing games connected to television sets (television sets produce very weak power-frequency magnetic fields but do produce stronger EMFs at certain frequencies).

TABLE 9–4. Meta-Analyses of Childhood Cancer and Power-Frequency Magnetic Fields

Reference	Studies Included	Pooled Estimates
Washburn et al. (1994)	13 studies of childhood cancer and residential proximity to electric power distribution equipment and risk of childhood leukemia, lymphoma, and CNS tumors	Pooled odds ratios based on residential distance from transmission and distribution wires included leukemia ($OR = 1.5$, CI 1.1–2.0), lymphoma ($OR = 1.6$, CI 0.9–2.8), and CNS tumors ($OR = 1.9$, CI 1.3–2.7); no association between pooled odds ratios and any of 15 indicators of epidemiologic quality
Miller et al. (1995)	7 case-control studies of childhood leukemia and wire code, distance to power distribution equipment, spot magnetic flux density measurements, and calculated indices based on distance and historic power load data	Pooled odds ratios by exposure index were wire codes ($OR = 1.6$, CI 1.3–2.0), distance ($OR = 2.1$, CI 1.2–3.7), spot measures ($OR = 1.1$, CI 0.7–1.7), and calculated index ($OR = 2.5$, CI 1.0–6.0)
Meinert and Michaelis (1996)	13 studies of childhood cancer and wire code, distance to power distribution equipment, spot magnetic flux density measurements; note: each OR based on pooling of 2 to 6 studies	Two-level wire code: all cancers combined ($OR = 1.4$, CI 0.9–2.0), leukemia ($OR = 1.7$, CI 1.1–2.5), CNS tumors ($OR = 1.5$, CI 0.7–3.3), and lymphomas ($OR = 1.3$, (CI 0.5–3.4) Distance odds ratios for leukemia for distances of <100 m, <50 m, and <25 m, respectively, were 1.1 (0.8–1.6), 1.3 (0.9–1.9), and 1.9 (1.0–3.5) Measured magnetic flux densities: odds ratios for leukemia for exposures >0.1 μT, >0.2 μT, and >0.3 μT, respectively, were 1.6 (0.9–2.7), 1.9 (1.1–3.3), and 1.3 (0.3–5.8)
National Academy of Sciences (1997)	Pooled analyses of 11 case-control studies of childhood leukemia in relation to wire codes and distance	Pooled odds ratios for high exposure: wire code ($OR = 1.5$, CI 1.1–2.1), distance ($OR = 1.4$, CI 1.1–1.8)

(continued)

TABLE 9–4. Meta-Analyses of Childhood Cancer and Power-Frequency Magnetic Fields (continued)

Reference	Studies Included	Pooled Estimates
Wartenberg (2001)	19 studies of childhood leukemia and magnetic flux density and distance to power distribution equipment	Pooled odds ratios for high exposure: calculated and measured magnetic flux density ($OR = 1.3$, CI 1.1–1.7), distance to power distribution equipment ($OR = 1.2$, CI 1.0–1.6)
Angelillo and Villari (1999)	Pooled analysis of 1 cohort and 14 case-control studies of childhood leukemia and wire codes, proximity to power distribution equipment, and spot and 24-hour measures of magnetic flux density	Pooled odds ratio for high exposure: wire code ($OR = 1.5$, CI 1.1–2.0), 24-hour measured magnetic flux densities ($OR = 1.6$, CI 1.1–2.2)
Ahlbom et al. (2000)	Pooled analysis of 9 epidemiologic studies of childhood leukemia and measured or estimated magnetic flux density and wire code	Pooled odds ratio for estimated magnetic flux densities of 0.4 µT or greater (versus less than 0.1 µT) was 2.0 (CI 1.3–3.1); adjustment for potential confounders made little difference; among North American subjects, the odds ratio for the highest wire code category was 1.2 (CI 0.8–1.9)
Greenland et al. (2000)	Pooled analysis of 15 epidemiologic studies of childhood leukemia and magnetic flux density and wire codes	Pooled odds ratios: magnetic flux density above 0.3 µT, relative to ≤0.2 µT, $OR = 1.7$ (CI 1.2–2.4); very high current wire configuration, relative to lowest wire code, ORs varied from 0.7 to 3.0 across studies and authors decided not to include summary estimate because of heterogeneity

Personal exposures depend on activity patterns and power-frequency magnetic flux densities that vary substantially over time and place; short-term exposure measures are likely poor proxies for lifetime dose or frequency of exposure to peak levels. Given the modest strength of the association in positive studies, ignorance about the etiology of childhood leukemia, the complexity of power-frequency magnetic field exposures, and the potential modifying effects of other environmental and socioeconomic factors, continuing uncertainty about the relation between magnetic fields and childhood leukemia seems inevitable (Savitz and Poole, 2001). The National Institute of Environmental Health Sciences (NIEHS) expert panel concluded that power-frequency magnetic fields should be considered a possible human carcinogen, noting that positive associations with childhood leukemia are consistent with the limited evidence of increased chronic lymphocytic leukemia risk among occupationally exposed adults.

Brain tumors. Meta-analyses of studies of childhood brain tumors and power-frequency magnetic fields yielded pooled odds ratios of 1.9 (CI 1.3–2.7) for proximity to high-voltage wires (Washburn et al., 1994) and 1.5 (CI 0.7–3.3) for high wire code configuration (Meinert and Michaelis, 1996). More recent reviews, however, concluded that there was no consistent evidence of associations with exposure of parents or children to power-frequency magnetic fields based on wire code, distance, measured or estimated magnetic flux density, or electrical appliance use (Ahlbom et al., 2001; Kheifets et al., 1999).

Radiofrequency Radiation

Epidemiologic studies of cancer and RF radiation from proximity to television/radio transmitters or occupational exposures have produced inadequate evidence to conclude that RF radiation is a likely cause of human cancer (Elwood, 1999). Among four studies published since this review, three showed no associations between RF radiation related to cell phone use or occupation and the risk of adult CNS tumors or leukemia. One study revealed an association between brain gliomas, but not meningiomas or salivary gland cancers, and exposure to analog but not digital wireless phones (Auvinen et al., 2002). Wireless phone use was also linked to a three- to fourfold increased risk of adult uveal melanoma (Stang et al., 2001). A large case-control study of childhood neuroblastoma showed a borderline association with maternal occupational RF radiation exposure (De Roos et al., 2001). The question of a role for RF radiation in childhood cancer will remain open until further large analytical studies with adequate exposure assessment are conducted.

EXPOSURES

Power-Frequency Magnetic Field Measurement

The exposure metrics that best indicate biologically relevant exposure to power-frequency magnetic fields or RF radiation are unknown. Epidemiologic studies of power-frequency magnetic fields and child health have used (1) indirect indices including job-exposure matrices, self-reported use of electrical appliances, proximity to power lines, and residential electric wire configuration coding, (2) spot and time-weighted measures of residential power-frequency magnetic flux densities, and (3) personal magnetic flux density exposures measured by wearing personal dosimeters for up to several days.

The Wertheimer-Leeper wire coding system and a simplified derivative were developed as low-cost, nonintrusive methods to assess long-term residential exposure to power line magnetic fields. Wire codes are thought to be less likely than short-term measurements to misclassify exposure because they depend on relatively constant characteristics, while measured power-frequency magnetic flux density varies substantially over time. Power lines strongly influence background magnetic fields over long time periods, while currents in residential electrical grounding systems cause the largest variations over shorter time periods. In homes where the electrical system is grounded to plumbing, appliances can transmit imperceptible contact currents to a person in contact with the appliance and produce stronger electric fields in target tissues compared to magnetic or electric fields (Kavet et al., 2000). The geometry of a source influences the rate of decline of magnetic field strength with distance; for example, magnetic field strength declines more rapidly with distance from a point source such as an electric motor than it does with distance from an extended source like a power line. Children receive geometric mean extremely low frequency (ELF) and very low frequency (VLF) magnetic flux densities of about 0.002–0.02 μT while watching TV or playing video games, very close to background levels.

Radiofrequency Radiation Measurement

Most RF radiation in the environment comes from commercial radio and television broadcasting and telecommunications facilities. There have been very few studies of population RF exposure levels. The average background RF power density in large U.S. cities is about 50 μW/m^2, with about 1% of persons having exposures exceeding 10 mW/m^2. Within homes, exposures from appliances (MW ovens, video display units, television sets) contribute a few tens of microwatts per square meter, much

TABLE 9–5. Reference Levels for the General Public for Electromagnetic Fields and Radiofrequency Radiation

Exposure	Guideline or Standard
Power-frequency (50–60 Hz) electromagnetic fields[a]	
Electric fields	5 kV/m (50 Hz)
	4.2 kV/m (60 Hz)
Power-frequency magnetic fields	0.1 μT
Radiofrequency radiation	
100 kHz to 10 GHz (e.g., wireless phones, radio, television, microwave ovens), specific absorption rates[a]	0.08 W/kg (whole body average)
	2 W/kg (localized, head and trunk)
	4 W/kg (localized, limbs)
	Non-essential or prolonged calls by children age <16 years should be discouraged[b]

[a]International Commission on Non-Ionizing Radiation Protection (1998).
[b]Department of Health (2000).

lower than international reference levels for ambient RF power density for such frequencies (Table 9–5).

Wireless phones are RF transmitters with maximum power of 0.2–0.6 W and expose the head at very close range, with peak energy specific absorption rates in the head of 0.12-2.8 W/kg, near the International Commission on Non-Ionizing Radiation Protection (ICNIRP) specific absorption rate limit for hand-held wireless phones (2.0 W/kg partial body) (Table 9.5). Wireless telecommunication base stations operate at power levels far lower than those of radio and TV broadcast antennas; ground-level RF power densities near wireless base stations are on the order of 10 mW/m^2 but can be much higher if multiple antennas are clustered at a site (Royal Society of Canada, 1999). At the frequency of wireless phone base stations (1850–1990 MHz), the FCC limits for RF power density for the general public is 10 W/m^2 (Federal Communications Commission, 1999).

RISK MANAGEMENT

Sources

Although wire code categories are correlated with measured magnetic flux densities, they explain only 10%–20% of the variance in spot, 24-hour stationary, and personal dosimetry measurements. The main determinants of personal magnetic flux densities measured by dosimetry appear to be electric appliances, grounding to metallic water lines, and currents in nearby power lines (mainly low-voltage distribution lines). Power-frequency magnetic flux density from household electrical appliances (hair dryers, vacuum cleaners, MW ovens, electric blankets, televisions, air conditioners, and computers) decreases rapidly with distance. Young children spend about 70% of their time at home, over half of which is in their bedrooms; magnetic flux densities measured by personal dosimetry of children are strongly correlated with 24-hour average bedroom levels. Median 24-hour magnetic flux densities above 0.2 μT occurred in only 1.4% of children's bedrooms in Germany (Schuz et al., 2000).

Radiofrequency radiation produced by anthropogenic sources, by ascending frequencies, includes AM and FM radio, VHF and ultrahigh frequency (UHF) television, two-way radios, base stations for transmitting wireless phone and MW communication signals, MW ovens, radar, and satellite communications. Other RF radiation sources include magnetic resonance imaging systems, video display monitors, and antitheft and security devices. There are now more wireless than fixed-line phone users globally and the former will grow to about 1.6 billion by 2005, driven by deployment of the lower-cost wireless systems in developing countries (Repacholi, 2001). Wireless phones, used increasingly by children and adolescents, continually transmit RF signals to base stations when turned on (Royal Society of Canada, 1999).

Intervention

No national body in the United States has recommended a precautionary policy to reduce power-frequency EMF exposure. The NIEHS concluded that there is insufficient evidence of adverse health effects upon which to base a regulatory limit, but it would be prudent to limit children's exposure by requiring a minimum distance between power lines and homes, schools, and day-care centers. The Australian government recommended that new electric power transmission lines be routed away from schools and that power line loads be phased to reduce nearby magnetic fields. The ICNIRP guidelines for general population exposure to EMF in the power-frequency range are 10 V/m for electric fields and 0.1 μT for magnetic flux density (International Commission on Non-Ionizing Radiation Protection, 1998).

The ICNIRP reviewed health issues related to the use of hand-held radiotelephones and base transmitters and concluded that (1) there is no substantive evidence that adverse health effects, including cancer, are caused by exposure to RF radiation levels at or below the ICNIRP specific absorption rate limits, and (2) neither the epidemiologic nor the toxicologic studies reported to date provide a basis for health hazard assessments of RF radiation exposure or for setting quantitative restrictions on human exposure. The ICNIRP guidelines for limiting EMF and RF radiation exposure, based on established health effects, include (International Commission on Non-Ionizing Radiation Protection, 1998)

- 1 Hz to 10 MHz—restrictions on current density (mA/m^2) to prevent effects on nervous system function
- 100 kHz to 10 GHz—restrictions on specific absorption rates (W/kg) to prevent whole-body heat stress and excessive localized tissue heating
- 10–300 GHz—restrictions on power density (W/m^2) to prevent excessive heating in tissue at or near the body surface

The ICNIRP guidelines address neither the potential for increased susceptibility during childhood nor the possibility of health outcomes other than tissue heating and acute effects on nervous system function. This approach, however, is consistent with the recent position of other agencies. Existing RF radiation exposure standards for the 100 kHz to 10 GHz range are all based on biologic data and a safety factor but vary because of different interpretations of the biologic data, magnitude of the safety factor, consideration of averaging times, and dependence on frequency (Erdreich and Klauenberg, 2001).

The Royal Society of Canada recently reviewed the evidence of health effects from RF radiation and concluded that the Canadian Safety Code 6 limits for specific energy absorption rates for RF and MW frequencies 100 kHz to 10 GHz generally protect the general public from adverse health effects related to tissue warming (Royal Society of Canada, 1999). The expert panel noted that biologic effects may occur at nonthermal exposure levels but concluded that there is insufficient evidence to assess whether these may cause adverse health effects. The U.K. Department of Health recommended that nonessential and prolonged calls on wireless phones by children below age 16 years be discouraged; it adopted this precautionary approach because of evidence that changes in brain activity occur at RF radiation levels below current guidelines, the significant gaps in scientific knowledge, and the possibility that the developing brains of children and teenagers may be susceptible to unknown health risks of RF radiation (Department of Health UK, 2000).

CONCLUSIONS

Proven Health Effects

- Tissue heating—at very high RF exposure levels not encountered in normal daily living

- Cell proliferation—increased at very high power-frequency magnetic field levels not encountered in daily life

Unresolved Issues and Knowledge Gaps

- Childhood cancer—limited evidence that exposure to relatively high power-frequency magnetic fields may cause childhood leukemia and inadequate evidence for an association with brain tumors; inadequate evidence to assess role of RF radiation
- Spontaneous abortion—inadequate evidence of an association with maternal magnetic field exposure
- Knowledge gaps—need epidemiologic studies with improved exposure assessment and statistical power to detect potential health effects of low-level exposures to power-frequency magnetic fields and RF radiation

Risk Management Issues

- Exposure reduction—prudent to minimize exposure to environmental sources of power-frequency magnetic fields and RF radiation, particularly among pregnant women and children
- Biomonitoring—need to monitor power-frequency magnetic fields and RF radiation exposure among children in homes and other settings to measure progress in reducing exposure levels and to identify high-risk groups for targeted actions including research and intervention

III. SUNLIGHT

Solar ultraviolet (UV) radiation has been subdivided into UVA (320–400 nm), UVB (290–320 nm), and UVC (200–290 nm). Over 90% of total ground-level UV radiation is UVA because UVC and about 90% of UVB are absorbed by ozone, water vapor, oxygen, and carbon dioxide as sunlight passes through the earth's atmosphere. Ground-level UVA radiation is most intense in the early morning and afternoon, passes through glass, penetrates skin to the dermis, and causes modest tanning and wrinkling (Ferrini et al., 1998). Ultraviolet B radiation is most intense at midday and causes sunburn and tanning but cannot penetrate glass. Concern about sun exposure and child health comes from evidence of rapidly increasing incidence rates of malignant melanoma (3%–7% per year from the mid-1960s to the mid-1980s in many Caucasian populations), discovery of the importance of intense sunlight exposures during childhood and youth as causes of melanoma, and evidence of thinning of the earth's stratospheric ozone layer. About 80%–90% of melanomas and nonmelanomas are caused by exposure to sunlight (International Agency for Research on Cancer, 2001).

The objective of Part III of this chapter is to define the importance of sun exposure during childhood and adolescence on the risk of benign nevi (moles) and skin cancer, with a focus on malignant melanoma. The genotoxic effects of UV light, the role of intermittent intense sun exposure and host factors in skin cancer, and risk management strategies are explored.

HEALTH EFFECTS

Small amounts of UV radiation are beneficial for dermal activation of vitamin D, but intense exposure to sunlight during childhood can cause sunburn, common and atypical nevi (moles), and freckling and can increase the risk of delayed effects including melanoma and basal cell skin cancers, other skin changes, and possibly cataracts.

Molecular Mechanisms

Ultraviolet A, UVB, and UVC all induce DNA damage including chromosomal aberrations, sister chromatid exchange, and mutations in human cells in vitro and can induce or enhance cell and viral gene expression. Ultraviolet B, a direct genotoxin, stimulates photochemical reactions in DNA that produce cyclobutane pyrimidine dimers and pyrimidine-pyrimidone (6-4) photoproducts. In human volunteers, UVA exposure caused increased urinary excretion of 8-oxo-2'-deoxyguanosine and cyclobutane thymine dimers, which peaked 3–4 days after exposure; the former metabolite indicates oxidative DNA damage, probably from UVA-induced free radicals, and the latter metabolite indicates thymidine dimer formation, possibly due to interaction of UVA with endogenous sensitizers (Cooke et al., 2001). The importance of DNA repair systems in reducing the genotoxicity of UV radiation is illustrated by the genetic disease xeroderma pigmentosum; affected persons have greatly increased risks of melanoma and other skin cancers because of defects in either of two DNA repair systems.

Inactivation of the *p53* tumor suppressor gene is a key molecular change in skin cancer and many other types of cancer. Molecular studies of human melanoma cells indicate that *p53* activation in response to UV damage is diminished and the regulation of its target genes is disrupted. About a third of *p53* mutations in human sun-related skin cancers occur at trinucleotide sequences containing the rare base 5-methylcytosine; experimental studies show that simulated sunlight preferentially causes mutations involving dimers at dipyrimidine sequences with 5-methylcytosine.

Precancerous Skin Lesions

Although benign, nevi are important because at least 20%–30% of melanomas appear to arise in preexisting common or dysplastic nevi. Epidemiologic studies of nevi have shown the importance of a low latitude of residence, recreational sun exposure, and frequent sunburns during childhood and youth. The prevalence of large numbers of nevi per person is associated with frequent intense sun exposure and sunburn. Atypical (or dysplastic) nevi are generally bigger than a pencil eraser and have irregular shapes and pigmentation; these lesions appear to be most closely associated with intense sun exposure and sunburns during childhood. Other risk factors for nevi include fair skin and hair color, freckling, and difficult tanning. Density (number per unit area of skin) of nevi less than 5 mm in diameter tends to be highest on frequently exposed skin (face, back, shoulders, and dorsal surfaces of arms), while density of larger nevi is higher on intermittently exposed areas, especially the trunk.

Skin Cancer

The IARC concluded that (1) solar radiation is a known cause of cancer in humans (melanoma and nonmelanoma skin cancers), (2) there is inadequate evidence for carcinogenicity due to fluorescent lighting in humans, (3) sunlamps, sunbeds, and UVA, UVB, and UVC are each probable human carcinogens, and (4) solar radiation, broad-spectrum UV light, UVA, UVB, and UVC are each known causes of cancer in animals (International Agency for Research on Cancer, 1992).

Malignant Melanoma
Because of its rarity during childhood, most epidemiologic studies of melanoma have involved adults. One of the few studies of childhood melanoma showed associations with a family history of melanoma, inability to tan, and indirect markers of sun exposure (number of nevi, facial freckling) (Whiteman et al., 1997). Important findings from systematic reviews of epidemiologic studies of melanoma and sun exposure include (Elwood and Jopson, 1997)

- Strong associations with a history of intermittent intense sun exposure and sunburns during childhood, adolescence, and adulthood and with skin changes related to childhood sun exposure (freckling, nevi)
- A propensity to occur on intermittently exposed body sites (trunk and limbs)
- Associations with evidence of genetic susceptibility including inability to tan and lightly colored hair and eyes

Several case-control studies of melanoma published subsequent to these reviews have confirmed the strong consistent associations between adult melanoma and intensity of recreational sun exposure and frequency of sunburns during childhood and youth (see, e.g., Pfahlberg et al., 2001). The number of skin nevi is a strong predictor of the adult melanoma risk. Ultraviolet B greatly increases the risk of melanoma in experimental animals.

Overall melanoma incidence and mortality rates increased substantially from the mid-1950s to the late 1980s in several countries, with evidence of age-specific rates stabilizing or even decreasing among post–World War II birth cohorts in Sweden, Connecticut, Canada, New Zealand, and Australia but not among similar birth cohorts in France, Italy, and Czechoslovakia (see, e.g., Marrett et al., 2001). Observed mortality rate decreases may have been partially caused by earlier diagnosis and improved survival.

Nonmelanoma Skin Cancers
The main known risk factor for basal cell carcinoma of skin is intermittent recreational sun exposure during childhood and adolescence among persons who tend to burn rather than tan. The other main type of nonmelanoma skin cancer, squamous cell carcinoma, has generally been associated with lifelong sun exposure, but site-specific lesions have been linked to site-specific sunburn frequency during childhood. In Finland, one of the few countries having population-based incidence data for nonmelanoma skin cancer, basal cell and other nonmelanoma skin cancer incidence rates increased from about 1960 to 1995.

Other Health Effects

Although there is strong evidence that chronic exposure to sunlight and occupational exposure to UV light are risk factors for cortical cataracts of the eye, there appear to have been no epidemiologic studies of the role of sun exposure during childhood and adolescence. Within the UV spectrum, UVB at 297 nm is most efficient in causing human lens epithelial cell death in vitro and is much more potent than UVA in causing posterior cortical cataracts in mice. The potential impact of sun exposure on childhood immune function remains largely undefined. Exposure of human skin to UVA or UVB reduces T-cell-mediated contact hypersensitivity. Animal studies showed that UV-mediated suppression of contact hypersensitivity is reduced by broad-spectrum sunscreens, especially those containing high levels of a UVA filter (Fourtanier et al., 2000). Animals exposed to UVB have reduced immune responses including increased susceptibility to infection and tolerance of highly antigenic UV-induced skin tumors.

EXPOSURE

Incident UV light intensity at ground level depends on the solar zenith angle, stratospheric ozone, atmospheric pollutants, weather, and altitude. In a network of ground-level solar UV monitoring stations in Australia, the main factors influencing daily total ground-level UV intensity at a given site were cloud cover and stratospheric ozone levels (Roy et al., 1998). Chlorofluorocarbons and bromine compounds are the main anthropogenic contaminants that reduce stratospheric ozone levels; a decrease in stratospheric ozone of 50% at 60 degrees north (e.g., Scandinavia) would give such regions the effective UV dose of California or Mediterranean countries.

Surveys in several countries have shown a continuing high prevalence of sunburns among children, including infants as young as 6 months of age. Skin exposure varies by ground-level UV intensity, the presence of reflective surfaces (e.g., water, snow), body region, behavior, and clothing. Personal UV dosimetry of children in Japan showed that average daily exposures measured during different seasons were not directly correlated with outdoor UV intensity but were related to sporadic outdoor activities, suggesting the dominant role of behavioral factors.

RISK MANAGEMENT

Prevention of adult skin cancer must start in childhood and adolescence, when people receive a large fraction of their lifetime UV exposure. Downward trends of melanoma incidence rates among post–World War II birth cohorts in several countries (noted above) suggest that preventive programs may have already had a favorable impact. Recent surveys of preventive sun behaviors indicate that a third to a half of children used sunscreen and protective clothing while outdoors on the preceding weekend, with a tendency for favorable behaviors to decrease with age among adolescents.

There are uncertainties concerning the most important wavelengths of UV and near-UV visible radiation that may contribute to the risk of melanoma; the genotoxic portion of solar radiation may even extend to the near-visible light range. Although sunscreens are highly effective in blocking UVB and preventing skin erythema, not all products, especially older ones, adequately block UVA. Given that UVA comprises over 90% of the energy in ground-level UV radiation and is known to be genotoxic in human cells, the public should be advised to use broad-spectrum sunscreens that block both UVA and UVB. It appears, however, that no mandated regulation exists to specify testing of sunscreens for UVA efficacy. Testing showed that 6 of 11 products claiming to provide UVA protection had actual effectiveness levels of 6%–52% in the UVA range. There have been no randomized trials with long-term follow-up to assess sunscreen efficacy during childhood in the prevention of skin cancers, but available studies indicate the following:

- Nevi—a survey of Israeli children showed an increased risk of nevi among sunscreen users, but a randomized trial of sunscreen use among young children in Canada showed a significant reduction in the number of nevi in the intervention arm within 3 years
- Melanoma—there was a twofold increased risk of melanoma among Swedes who used sunscreens regularly; the increase was mainly on the trunk and was related to increased frequency of sunbathing.
- Nonmelanoma skin cancers and actinic keratoses—randomized trials have shown the efficacy of sunscreens in reducing sunburn, actinic keratoses, and squamous cell but not basal cell skin cancers in adults.

Sunscreens reduce epidermal damage and the frequency of cyclobutane pyrimidine dimers, pyrimidine-pyrimidone (6-4) photoproducts, and photooxidative lesions in human skin in vitro models. Despite evidence that older sunscreens prevented nonmelanoma but not melanoma skin cancers in UVR-exposed animals, new broad-spectrum sunscreens with higher sun protection factors (SPFs) may prove to be effective in reducing the risk of melanoma as well as other skin cancers. In any event, there is a need to improve the appropriate use of existing sunscreens, including the amount applied and the frequency of application. Controlled trials are also needed to assess the potential value of population screening for early detection of melanomas.

The IARC concluded that protection of skin from solar damage ideally involves several actions and has recommended public health guidelines including the following (International Agency for Research on Cancer, 2001):

- Adopt multiple measures, that is, wear tightly woven protective clothing that adequately covers the arms, trunk, and legs and a hat that shades the whole head, seek shade, avoid outdoor activities during peak midday sun intensity, and use sunscreens.
- Educate the public that sunscreen use should not be the first or the only choice for skin cancer prevention, as a means to prolong solar exposure, or as a substitute for clothing on usually unexposed sites such as the trunk and buttocks (and labeling of sunscreen products to inform consumers of this recommendation).
- Recognize that adequate solar protection during childhood is more important than at any other time in life and promote adoption of the above recommendations by parents and school managers.
- Residents of areas with high sun intensity who work outdoors or enjoy regular outdoor recreation should use sunscreens with high SPFs (>15) daily on usually exposed skin.
- Stringent evaluation of sunscreen safety should be performed using the same regulatory safety requirements as for pharmaceuticals, with a particular focus on potential long-term effects; data on the safety evaluation of sunscreens must be in the public domain so that they are available for independent scientific evaluation.
- Once the optimal method for specifying protection against broad-spectrum UVA has been agreed upon, a labeling method should be introduced that is internationally congruent and understandable to the public.
- Advertising for sunscreens should promote a global sun protection strategy, avoid promoting sunscreen use for intentional exposure to the sun, and avoid using messages likely to provide a false sense of security among users.
- Health promotion interventions should be designed to increase the appropriate and effective use of sunscreens by the general public and by subgroups at risk of skin cancer because of their phenotype or a predisposition to intentional solar exposure.

Whereas sunbeds probably cause skin cancer, public education should also address this issue on a precautionary basis. Finally, a broad strategy should include measures to avoid further reductions in the earth's stratospheric ozone layer. With a 10% loss of stratospheric ozone, skin cancer rates may rise by 30% for basal cell carcinoma and by 50% for squamous cell carcinoma, assuming no adaptive changes in human behavior (Jones, 1992).

CONCLUSIONS

Proven Health Outcomes of Intense Sun Exposure During Childhood

* Nevi (moles)
* Skin cancer (malignant melanoma, basal cell carcinoma) during adulthood

Unresolved Issues and Knowledge Gaps

* Cancer—limited evidence that intermittent intense sun exposure during childhood may increase the risk of squamous cell carcinoma during adulthood
* Cataracts—inadequate evidence to assess the role of sun exposure during childhood and the risk of cortical cataracts during adulthood
* Immune function—inadequate evidence to assess adverse effects of sun exposure on children's immune system
* Knowledge development—need epidemiologic studies to detect potential delayed health effects of UV exposure (immunologic, cataracts) and sunscreen use (protective and/or adverse effects)

Risk Management Issues

* Prevention—need to reduce exposure of children to intense sun exposure through several actions including adequate clothing, use of a hat that shades the whole head, seeking shade, avoiding outdoor activities during peak midday sun intensity, and use of broad-spectrum sunscreens
* Monitoring—need to measure ground-level and personal UV exposure and sun-protective behaviors of children and their guardians, that is, to measure progress in exposure reduction and to identify high-risk groups for targeted interventions

REFERENCES

Agency for Toxic Substances and Disease Registry. (1999). Toxicological profile for ionizing radiation. Atlanta: Agency for Toxic Substances and Disease Registry.

Ahlbom IC, Cardis E, Green A, Linet M, Savitz D, Swerdlow A. (2001). Review of the epidemiologic literature on EMF and Health. Environ Health Perspect 109 (Suppl 6):911–33.

Ahlbom A, Day N, Feychting M, Roman E, Skinner J, Dockerty J, Linet M, McBride M, Michaelis J, Olsen JH and others. (2000). A pooled analysis of magnetic fields and childhood leukaemia. Br J Cancer 83:692–8.

Angelillo IF, Villari P. (1999). Residential exposure to electromagnetic fields and childhood leukaemia: a meta-analysis. Bull WHO 77:906–15.

Astakhova LN, Anspaugh LR, Beebe GW, Bouville A, Drozdovitch VV, Garber V, Gavrilin YI, Khrouch VT, Kuvshinnikov AV, Kuzmenkov YN, Minenko VP, Moschik KV, and others. (1998). Chernobyl-related thyroid cancer in children of Belarus: a case-control study. Radiat Res 150:349–56.

Auvinen A, Hietanen M, Luukkonen R, Koskela RS. (2002). Brain tumors and salivary gland cancers among cellular telephone users. Epidemiology 13:356–9.

Axelson O, Fredrikson M, Akerblom G, Hardell L. (2002). Leukemia in childhood and adolescence and exposure to ionizing radiation in homes built from uranium-containing alum shale concrete. Epidemiology 13:146–50.

Boice JD, Miller RW. (1999). Childhood and adult cancer after intrauterine exposure to ionizing radiation. Teratology 59:227–33.

Brusick D, Albertini R, McRee D, Peterson D, Williams G, Hanawalt P, Preston J. (1998). Genotoxicity of radiofrequency radiation. DNA/Genetox Expert Panel. Environ Mol Mutagen 32:1–16.

Coghill RW, Steward J, Philips A. (1996). Extra low frequency electric and magnetic fields in the bedplace of children diagnosed with leukaemia: a case-control study. Eur J Cancer Prev 5:153–8.

Cooke MS, Evans MD, Burd RM, Patel K, Barnard A, Lunec J, Hutchinson PE. (2001). Induction and excretion of ultraviolet-induced 8-oxo-2'-deoxyguanosine and thymine dimers in vivo: implications for PUVA. J Invest Dermatol 116:281–5.

Correa-Villasenor A, Ferencz C, Loffredo C, Magee C. (1993). Paternal exposures and cardiovascular malformations. The Baltimore-Washington Infant Study Group. J Expo Anal Environ Epidemiol 3(Suppl 1):173–85.

De Roos AJ, Teschke K, Savitz DA, Poole C, Grufferman S, Pollock BH, Olshan AF. (2001). Parental occupational exposures to electromagnetic fields and radiation and the incidence of neuroblastoma in offspring. Epidemiology 12:508–17.

Department of Health UK. (2000). Mobile phones and health. Located at www.doh.gov.uk/mobile.htm.

Doll R, Wakeford R. (1997). Risk of childhood cancer from fetal irradiation. Br J Radiol 70:130–9.

Elwood JM. (1999). A critical review of epidemiologic studies of radiofrequency exposure and human cancers. Environ Health Perspect 107(Suppl 1):155–68.

Elwood JM, Jopson J. (1997). Melanoma and sun exposure: an overview of published studies. Int J Cancer 73:198–203.

Erdreich LS, Klauenberg BJ. (2001). Radio frequency radiation exposure standards: considerations for harmonization. Health Phys 80:430–9.

Expert panel on the potential health risks of radiofrequency fields from wireless telecommunication devices. (1999). A review of the potential health risks of radiofrequency fields from wireless telecommunication devices. Ottawa: The Royal Society of Canada/La Société royale du Canada.

Federal Communications Commission. (1999). Questions and answers about biological effects and potential hazards of radiofrequency electromagnetic fields. Located at http://www.fcc.gov/Bureaus/Engineering_Technology/Documents/bulletins/oet56/oet56e4.pdf.

Ferrini RL, Perlman M, Hill L. (1998). American College of Preventive Medicine practice policy statement: skin protection from ultraviolet light exposure. The American College of Preventive Medicine. Am J Prev Med 14:83–6.

Finkelstein MM, Kreiger N. (1996). Radium in drinking water and risk of bone cancer in Ontario youths: a second study and combined analysis. Occup Environ Med 53:305–11.

Fourtanier A, Gueniche A, Compan D, Walker SL, Young AR. (2000). Improved protection against solar-simulated radiation-induced immunosuppression by a sunscreen with enhanced ultraviolet A protection. J Invest Dermatol 114:620–7.

Graham C, Cook MR, Gerkovich MM, Sastre A. (2001). Examination of the melatonin hypothesis in women exposed at night to EMF or bright light. Environ Health Perspect 109:501–7.

Green LM, Miller AB, Agnew DA, Greenberg ML, Li J, Villeneuve PJ, Tibshirani R. (1999). Childhood leukemia and personal monitoring of residential exposures to electric and magnetic fields in Ontario, Canada. Cancer Causes Control 10:233–43.

Greenland S, Sheppard AR, Kaune WT, Poole C, Kelsh MA. (2000). A pooled analysis of magnetic fields, wire codes, and childhood leukemia. Childhood Leukemia-EMF Study Group. Epidemiology 11:624–34.

Infante-Rivard C, Mathonnet G, Sinnett D. (2000). Risk of childhood leukemia associated with diagnostic irradiation and polymorphisms in DNA repair genes. Environ Health Perspect 108:495–8.

International Agency for Research on Cancer. (1992). IARC monographs on the evaluation of carcinogenic risks to humans. Vol. 55. Solar and ultraviolet radiation. Lyon, France: International Agency for Research on Cancer.

International Agency for Research on Cancer. (2000). IARC monographs on the evaluation of carcinogenic risks to humans. Vol. 75. Ionizing radiation, Part 1: X- and gamma-radiation, and neutrons. Lyon, France: International Agency for Research on Cancer.

International Agency for Research on Cancer. (2001). Cancer-preventive effect of sunscreens. Lyon, France: International Agency for Research on Cancer.

International Agency for Research on Cancer. (2002). IARC monographs on the evaluation of carcinogenic risks to humans. Vol. 80. Non-ionizing radiation, Part 1: Static and extremely low frequency electric and magnetic fields. Lyon, France: International Agency for Research on Cancer.

International Commission on Radiological Protection. (1991). 1990 recommendations of the International Commission on Radiological Protection, ICRP Publication 60. Oxford: Pergamon Press.

International Commission on Non-Ionizing Radiation Protection. (1998). Guidelines for limiting exposure to time-varying electric, magnetic, and electromagnetic fields (up to 300 GHz). Health Phys 74:494–522.

Jones RR. (1992). Ozone depletion and its effects on human populations. Br J Dermatol 127(Suppl 41):2–6.

Kaletsch U, Kaatsch P, Meinert R, Schuz J, Czarwinski R, Michaelis J. (1999). Childhood cancer and residential radon exposure—results of a population-based case-control study in Lower Saxony (Germany). Radiat Environ Biophys 38: 211–5.

Kallen B, Karlsson P, Lundell M, Wallgren A, Holm LE. (1998). Outcome of reproduction in women irradiated for skin hemangioma in infancy. Radiat Res 149:202–8.

Kaune WT, Savitz DA. (1994). Simplification of the Wertheimer-Leeper wire code. Bioelectromagnetics 15:275–82.

Kavet R, Zaffanella LE, Daigle JP, Ebi KL. (2000). The possible role of contact current in cancer risk associated with residential magnetic fields. Bioelectromagnetics 21:538–53.

Kheifets LI, Sussman SS, Preston-Martin S. (1999). Childhood brain tumors and residential electromagnetic fields (EMF). Rev Environ Contam Toxicol 159:111–29.

Lee GM, Neutra RR, Hristova L, Yost M, Hiatt RA. (2002). A nested case-control study of residential and personal magnetic field measures and miscarriages. Epidemiology 13:21–31.

Li DK, Odouli R, Wi S, Janevic T, Golditch I, Bracken TD, Senior R, Rankin R, Iriye R. (2002). A population-based prospective cohort study of personal exposure to magnetic fields during pregnancy and the risk of miscarriage. Epidemiology 13:9–20.

Linet MS, Ries LA, Smith MA, Tarone RE, Devesa SS. (1999). Cancer surveillance series: recent trends in childhood cancer incidence and mortality in the United States. J Natl Cancer Inst 91:1051–8.

Loffredo CA, Hirata J, Wilson PD, Ferencz C, Lurie IW. (2001). Atrioventricular septal defects: possible etiologic differences between complete and partial defects. Teratology 63:87–93.

London SJ, Thomas DC, Bowman JD, Sobel E, Cheng TC, Peters JM. (1991). Exposure to residential electric and magnetic fields and risk of childhood leukemia. Am J Epidemiol 134:923–37.

MacMahon B. (1962). Prenatal X-ray exposure and childhood cancer. J Natl Cancer Inst 28:1173–91.

Marrett LD, Nguyen HL, Armstrong BK. (2001). Trends in the incidence of cutaneous malignant melanoma in New South Wales, 1983–1996. Int J Cancer 92: 457–62.

McBride ML, Gallagher RP, Theriault G, Armstrong BG, Tamaro S, Spinelli JJ, Deadman JE, Fincham S, Robson D, Choi W. (1999). Power-frequency electric and magnetic fields and risk of childhood leukemia in Canada. Am J Epidemiol 149:831–42.

Meinert R, Kaletsch U, Kaatsch P, Schuz J, Michaelis J. (1999). Associations between childhood cancer and ionizing radiation: results of a population-based case-control study in Germany. Cancer Epidemiol Biomarkers Prev 8:793–9.

Meinert R, Michaelis J. (1996). Meta-analyses of studies on the association between electromagnetic fields and childhood cancer. Radiat Environ Biophys 35:11–8.

Miller MA, Murphy JR, Miller TI, Ruttenber AJ. (1995). Variation in cancer risk estimates for exposure to powerline frequency electromagnetic fields: a meta-analysis comparing EMF measurement methods. Risk Anal 15:281–7.

National Academy of Sciences. (1990). Biological effects of ionizing radiation (BEIR) V report: Health effects of exposure to low levels of ionizing radiation. Washington, DC: National Academy Press.

National Academy of Sciences. (1997). Possible health effects of exposure to residential electric and magnetic fields. Washington, DC: National Academy Press.

National Academy of Sciences. (1999). Biological effects of ionizing radiation (BEIR) VI report: The health effects of exposure to Indoor radon. Washington, DC: National Academy Press.

National Institute of Environmental Health Sciences. (1998). Assessment of health effects from exposure to power-line frequency electric and magnetic fields. Working group report. (NIH Publication No. 98–3981). Research Triangle Park, NC: National Institute of Environmental Health Sciences.

National Institute of Environmental Health Sciences. (1999). Report on health effects from exposure to power-line frequency electric and magnetic fields. (NIH Publication No. 99-4493). Research Triangle Park, NC: National Institute of Environmental Health Sciences.

Naumburg E, Bellocco R, Cnattingius S, Hall P, Boice JD Jr, Ekbom A. (2001). Intrauterine exposure to diagnostic X rays and risk of childhood leukemia subtypes. Radiat Res 156:718–23.

Parazzini F, Luchini L, La Vecchia C, Crosignani PG. (1993). Video display terminal use during pregnancy and reproductive outcome—a meta-analysis. J Epidemiol Commun Health 47:265–8.

Parker L, Pearce MS, Dickinson HO, Aitkin M, Craft AW. (1999). Stillbirths among offspring of male radiation workers at Sellafield nuclear reprocessing plant. Lancet 354:1407–14.

Pfahlberg A, Kolmel KF, Gefeller for the Febim Study Group O. (2001). Timing of excessive ultraviolet radiation and melanoma: epidemiology does not support the existence of a critical period of high susceptibility to solar ultraviolet radiation-induced melanoma. Br J Dermatol 144:471–5.

Pierce DA, Shimizu Y, Preston DL, Vaeth M, Mabuchi K. (1996). Studies of the mortality of atomic bomb survivors. Report 12, part I. Cancer: 1950–1990. Radiat Res 146:1–27.

Repacholi MH. (2001). Health risks from the use of mobile phones. Toxicol Lett 120:323–31.

Ron E, Lubin JH, Shore RE, Mabuchi K, Modan B, Pottern LM, Schneider AB, Tucker MA, Boice JD. (1995). Thyroid cancer after exposure to external radiation: a pooled analysis of seven studies. Radiat Res 141:259–77.

Roy CR, Gies HP, Lugg DJ, Toomey S, Tomlinson DW. (1998). The measurement of solar ultraviolet radiation. Mutat Res 422:7–14.

Royal Society of Canada. (1999). A review of the potential health risks of radiofrequency fields from wireless telecommunication devices. Ottawa: Royal Society of Canada.

Rutledge JC. (1997). Developmental toxicity induced during early stages of mammalian embryogenesis. Mutat Res 396:113–27.

Savitz DA. (1995). Exposure assessment strategies in epidemiological studies of health effects of electric and magnetic fields. Sci Total Environ 168:143–53.

Savitz DA, Kaune WT. (1993). Childhood cancer in relation to a modified residential wire code. Environ Health Perspect 101:76–80.

Savitz DA, Poole C. (2001). Do studies of wire code and childhood leukemia point towards or away from magnetic fields as the causal agent? Bioelectromagnetics Suppl 5:S69–85.

Savitz DA, Whelan EA, Kleckner RC. (1989). Self-reported exposure to pesticides and radiation related to pregnancy outcome—results from National Natality and Fetal Mortality Surveys. Public Health Rep 104:473–7.

Schuz J, Grigat JP, Stormer B, Rippin G, Brinkmann K, Michaelis J. (2000). Extremely low frequency magnetic fields in residences in Germany. Distribution of measurements, comparison of two methods for assessing exposure, and predictors for the occurrence of magnetic fields above background level. Radiat Environ Biophys 39:233–40.

Sever LE, Gilbert ES, Hessol NA, McIntyre JM. (1988). A case-control study of congenital malformations and occupational exposure to low-level ionizing radiation. Am J Epidemiol 127:226–42.

Shaw GM. (2001). Adverse human reproductive outcomes and electromagnetic fields: a brief summary of the epidemiologic literature. Bioelectromagnetics Suppl 5:S5–18.

Shea KM, Little RE. (1997). Is there an association between preconception paternal X-ray exposure and birth outcome? The ALSPAC Study Team. Avon Longitudinal Study of Pregnancy and Childhood. Am J Epidemiol 145:546–51.

Shibata Y, Yamashita S, Masyakin VB, Panasyuk GD, Nagataki S. (2001). 15 years after Chernobyl: new evidence of thyroid cancer. Lancet 358:1965–6.

Shu XO, Potter JD, Linet MS, Severson RK, Han D, Kersey JH, Neglia JP, Trigg ME, Robison LL. (2002). Diagnostic X-rays and ultrasound exposure and risk of childhood acute lymphoblastic leukemia by immunophenotype. Cancer Epidemiol Biomarkers Prev 11:177–85.

Stang A, Anastassiou G, Ahrens W, Bromen K, Bornfeld N, Jockel KH. (2001). The possible role of radiofrequency radiation in the development of uveal melanoma. Epidemiology 12:7–12.

Stewart A, Webb J, Hewitt D. (1958). A survey of childhood malignancies. Br Med J 1:1495–1508.

United Nations Scientific Committee on the Effects of Atomic Radiation. (2000). UNSCEAR 2000 report. Sources and effects of ionizing radiation. UNSCEAR 2000 report to the General Assembly, with scientific annexes. Vienna: United Nations Scientific Committee on the Effects of Atomic Radiation.

U.S. Environmental Protection Agency. (1993). Protocols for radon and radon decay product measurements in homes (EPA 402-R-93-003). Located at http://www.epa.gov/RadonPubs/homprot1.html.

U.S. Environmental Protection Agency. (2001). Current drinking water standards. Located at http://www.epa.gov/safewater/mcl.html.

U.S. Environmental Protection Agency. (2002). Radon resistant new construction. Located at http://www.epa.gov/iaq/radon/index.html.

Wartenberg D. (2001). Residential EMF exposure and childhood leukemia: meta-analysis and population attributable risk. Bioelectromagnetics S5:S86–S104.

Washburn EP, Orza MJ, Berlin JA, Nicholson WJ, Todd AC, Frumkin H, Chalmers TC. (1994). Residential proximity to electricity transmission and distribution equipment and risk of childhood leukemia, childhood lymphoma, and childhood nervous system tumors: systematic review, evaluation, and meta-analysis. Cancer Causes Control 5:299–309.

Wertheimer N, Leeper E. (1979). Electrical wiring configurations and childhood cancer. Am J Epidemiol 109:273–84.

Whiteman DC, Valery P, McWhirter W, Green AC. (1997). Risk factors for childhood melanoma in Queensland, Australia. Int J Cancer 70:26–31.

Zanzonico PB, Becker DV. (2000). Effects of time of administration and dietary iodine levels on potassium iodide (KI) blockade of thyroid irradiation by ^{131}I from radioactive fallout. Health Phys 78:660–7.

Zhang J, Cai WW, Lee DJ. (1992). Occupational hazards and pregnancy outcomes. Am J Ind Med 21:397–408.

Zheng T, Holford TR, Chen Y, Ma JZ, Flannery J, Liu W, Russi M, Boyle P. (1996). Time trend and age-period-cohort effect on incidence of thyroid cancer in Connecticut, 1935–1992. Int J Cancer 67:504–9.

10
Indoor Air

Young children in developed countries spend over 90% of their time in homes, day-care centers, schools, motor vehicles, and other indoor environments. The EPA's Science Advisory Board over the past several years has consistently ranked indoor air pollution among the top five risks to public health in the United States. Sources of indoor air contaminants include occupant behaviors (especially smoking), water, building materials, consumer products, pets, insects, fungi, inadequately ventilated cooking and heating devices, and influx of outdoor air pollutants. Children inhale relatively high amounts of air per unit body weight per day and play at floor level, where concentrations of airborne contaminants may be relatively high. Airborne contaminants can disrupt lung growth and function during early childhood, causing persistent functional deficits and respiratory diseases.

The major categories of indoor air contaminants are gases/vapors and particulate matter, ranging from small, respirable particles to large, transiently suspended particles including house dust (Table 10–1). Smoking is the main source of airborne fine particulate matter ($PM_{2.5}$) in homes with smokers; other sources include other indoor combustion processes and infiltration of outdoor air. Larger particles can originate from indoor materials (e.g., textiles, clothing), biologic sources (pets, insects, fungi),

TABLE 10–1. Types of Indoor Air Contaminants

Category	Examples	Sources
Gases and vapors	Carbon monoxide, nitrogen dioxide, formaldehyde, radon, volatile organic chemicals, pesticides	Influx of outdoor air, fuel combustion (cooking, heating), building materials, geologic formations (radon), solvents, cleaning agents, chlorinated water
Particulate matter	Toxicants—ETS, particulate matter from other combustion processes, asbestos	Tobacco smoking, fuel combustion (cooking, heating), influx of outdoor air, building materials, furnishings
	Biologics—animal dander, fungal spores, bacteria, viruses, pollens, arthropod antigens	Pets, molds (closely linked to dampness), insects, humans
Dust[a]	Pesticides, heavy metals	Interior use of pesticides, influx of outdoor air, tracking in of contaminated soil/dust

[a] Included because airborne contaminants often deposit and accumulate in house dust and carpets, on furnishings, and on other surfaces.

and soil tracked indoors from external sources. Economically disadvantaged children generally have higher exposures to indoor air hazards because of a higher prevalence of household smokers and microenvironmental conditions such as dampness, inadequate ventilation, and building deterioration that favor proliferation of molds, house-dust mites, and cockroaches.

The purpose of this chapter is to describe the known and suspected health impacts of indoor air contaminants, with a major focus on environmental tobacco smoke (ETS), biologic agents, and volatile organic chemicals (VOCs). Topics include known and suspected links between indoor air pollutants and fetal development, sudden infant death syndrome (SIDS), respiratory diseases, and cancer. Available data on exposure levels for ETS and major VOCs document high-risk groups. The section on risk management notes the important role of children's parents and caregivers to provide a safe indoor environment but also points to the need for regulatory measures. See Chapters 4, 5, 7, 9, 11, and 12 for discussion of other potential indoor air contaminants including heavy metals, pesticides, radon, ambient air pollutants, and volatile disinfection by-products.

ASTHMA

This section describes the general characteristics of asthma, the most common chronic disease among children in developed countries, to facilitate subsequent discussion of various airborne agents in this important childhood condition. Asthma has two main characteristics: chronic inflammation of the airways and recurrent episodes of wheezing and coughing. The etiology of asthma appears to involve the interaction of multiple genes, environmental allergens, and chemical toxicants. Genes possibly important in the onset of this disease include those for cytokine/chemokine and IgE regulation, glutathione-S-transferase, and 5-lipoxygenase (see, e.g., Ober and Moffatt, 2000). Asthma prevalence rates among children have increased substantially during recent decades; in Canada, for instance, the prevalence of physician-diagnosed childhood asthma increased from 2.5% to 11.2% during 1978–1995 (Millar and Hill, 1998). Although the presence and degree of airway inflammation determine the severity of asthma, the causes of airway inflammation remain uncertain (National Academy of Sciences, 2000).

The main types of childhood airway obstruction involve episodic wheezing (1) after bronchiolitis during infancy, often associated with maternal smoking and low birth weight, or (2) after sensitization to allergens, the dominant type among children aged 5–18 years. About 20% of children diagnosed with asthma before age 5 years may be asymptomatic by age 10 years, but many still have significant airway hyperreactivity. Diagnosis is facilitated by the use of standard criteria such as the CDC case definition for asthma.[1] Symptom questionnaires appear to best balance sensitivity and specificity for asthma prevalence studies, while highly specific diagnostic criteria are better suited for etiologic studies (Pekkanen and Pearce, 1999).

Asthma risk factors include those that cause the development of asthma (i.e., incident asthma) and those that exacerbate established asthma. Epidemiologists have studied prevalent asthma much more frequently than incident disease. The U.S. National Academy of Sciences (NAS) reviewed indoor air contaminants and assigned levels of evidence for their roles as causes of asthma development or as triggers of episodes in known asthmatics (Table 10–2). The NAS concluded that (1) house-dust mite antigen is the only known cause of asthma development, (2) ETS is associated with asthma development but causality remains uncertain, and (3) cat, cockroach, and house-dust mite antigens and ETS trigger episodes in known asthmatics.

Analysis of NHANES III showed that the risk of physician-diagnosed asthma in young children was approximately doubled for those with a family history of allergic disease, ETS exposure, home use of a gas stove or oven for heat, or the presence of a dog in the household; the population attributable risk for children with one or more risk factors was 39% (Lanphear et al., 2001). Recent evidence indicates that early childhood infections do not protect against asthma, arguing against the hypothesis that a reduced risk of such infections may have contributed to increased asthma prevalence rates (McKeever et al., 2002). Nonenvironmental risk factors (e.g., obesity) may also contribute to asthma (von Mutius et al., 2001). Asthma is discussed further below and in Chapter 11 (Outdoor Air); readers may consult other sources for more detailed information on asthma (National Academy of Sciences, 2000; Pearce et al., 1998).

---

[1] (1) The presence of wheezing lasting for 2 or more consecutive days that responds to bronchodilators, or a chronic cough that persists for 3–6 weeks in the absence of allergic rhinitis or sinusitis, or nocturnal awakening with dyspnea, cough, and/or wheezing in the absence of other medical conditions known to cause these symptoms and (2) a 12% increment in FEV_1 and/or FVC (See Lung Function later in Chapter for explanation of these terms) after inhaling a short-acting bronchodilator, or a 20% decrement in FEV_1 after a challenge by histamine, methacholine, exercise, or cold air, or a 20% diurnal variation in peak expiratory flow over 1 to 2 weeks. A confirmed case is a person who has had any of the clinical symptoms at least three times during the past year and had at least one of the laboratory criteria.

TABLE 10–2. Summary of Indoor Environmental Risk Factors for Asthma

Level of Evidence	Factors That Cause Development of Asthma	Factors That Precipitate Episodes in Known Asthmatics
Sufficient evidence of a causal relationship	House-dust mite antigens	Cat, cockroach, and house-dust mite antigens in specifically sensitized persons, ETS (preschool-age children)
Sufficient evidence of an association	ETS (preschool-age children)	Dog, rodent, and fungal antigens in specifically sensitized persons, rhinovirus, nitrogen dioxide from indoor sources
Limited or suggestive evidence of an association	Cockroach antigen (preschool-age children), respiratory syncytial virus	Domestic birds, C. pneumoniae, M. pneumoniae, respiratory syncytial virus, formaldehyde, fragrances, ETS (school-age children)
Inadequate or insufficient evidence to determine whether or not an association exists	Cat, cow, horse, dog, domestic bird, fungal, and rodent antigens, endotoxins, molds, rhinovirus (infants), Chlamydia pneumoniae, C. trachomatis, Mycoplasma pneumoniae, houseplants, indoor pollens, nitrogen dioxide (from indoor sources), pesticides, plasticizers, VOCs, formaldehyde, fragrances, ETS (school-age children)	Cow and horse antigens, down pillows, C. trachomatis, endotoxins, houseplants, indoor pollens, insects other than cockroaches or house-dust mites, pesticides, plasticizers, VOCs
Limited or suggestive evidence of no association	Rhinovirus (school-age children)	No agents

Source: National Academy of Sciences (2000).

Environmental Tobacco Smoke

Health Effects

Environmental tobacco smoke is a common indoor air contaminant and an important preventable cause of childhood illnesses and deaths (Table 10–3). The EPA concluded that ETS

- Causes lung function deficits, respiratory tract irritation (cough, sputum production, wheezing), lower respiratory tract infections, middle ear infections, and increased frequency and severity of asthmatic episodes
- Likely causes 8000–26,000 new asthma cases annually and a substantial fraction of SIDS deaths

Reviews since the 1992 EPA report was published support these conclusions and indicate that ETS likely increases the risk of childhood meningococcal infections (see, e.g., California Environmental Protection Agency, 1997). The estimated annual direct and indirect costs of the health effects of parental smoking in the United States were $13 billion in 1993 dollars.

TABLE 10–3. Child Health Impacts of Parental Smoking in the United States

Category	Attributable Events (per year)
Low birth weight (<2500 g)	46,000 cases 2,800 perinatal deaths
SIDS	2,000 deaths
Bronchiolitis (age <2 yr)	22,000 hospitalizations 1,100 deaths
Middle ear infections (age <15 yr)	3.4 million outpatient visits
Tympanostomies (age <15 yr)	110,000
Asthma (age <18 yr)	1.8 million outpatient visits 28,000 hospitalizations 14 deaths
Burns[a]	10,000 outpatient visits 590 hospitalizations 250 deaths

Source: Aligne and Stoddard (1997).

[a]Fires initiated by smoking materials.

Mechanisms of Toxicity

Particle deposition. Inhaled particles may be deposited in the (1) mouth, nose, and larynx, (2) tracheobronchial airways, and (3) terminal bronchioles and alveoli of the lungs. The first two regions have high flow rates, and large and some very small particles are deposited there by impaction; fine particles are deposited mainly by diffusion and sedimentation in regions with low airflow rates, that is, the terminal bronchioles and alveoli. Deposited particles may dissolve in body fluids, may be cleared by the mucociliary system, or may be transported to lymph nodes.

Genotoxicity. Tobacco smoke contains over 40 known carcinogens. Environmental tobacco smoke originates mainly from sidestream smoke; the lower temperatures of idling cigarettes cause less complete combustion and higher concentrations of most carcinogens in sidestream smoke compared to mainstream smoke (Table 10–4). In the absence of smoking, indoor air particulate matter has little detectable mutagenic activity; after smoking, however, genotoxic activity (mutagenicity and sister chromatid exchange) increases markedly. Levels of blood cotinine (a nicotine metabolite) and ETS-related adducts (4-aminobiphenyl-hemoglobin and PAH-albumin) in young children are associated with ETS exposure. Cord blood lymphocytes from infants prenatally exposed to maternal smoking had hypoxanthine-guanine phosphoribosyltransferase (HPRT) gene dele-

TABLE 10–4. Ratios of Sidestream to Mainstream Concentrations of Known and Probable Human Carcinogens in Tobacco Smoke

	SS/MS Ratio
Vapor phase	
Benzene	5–10
Hydrazine	3
Formaldehyde	0.1–50
N-nitrosodimethylamine	20–100
Particulate phase	
Total particulate phase	1.3–1.9
Benzo(a)pyrene	2.5–3.5
2-naphthylamine	30
4-aminodiphenyl	31
Cadmium	7.2
Nickel	13–30
Polonium-210	1–4

Source: Wigle et al. (1987).

tions similar to those associated with childhood acute lymphatic leuke-mia (e.g., the t(4;11) translocation) (Finette et al., 1998).

Developmental Effects

Maternal ETS exposure has been linked to an increased risk of sponta-neous abortion, particularly late events (see, e.g., Windham et al., 1992). Two recent reviews concluded that maternal ETS exposure is associated with average birth weight reductions of 25–90 g (adjusted for gestation length) and a pooled odds ratio for IUGR of 1.2 (CI 1.1–1.3) (Misra and Nguyen, 1999; Windham et al., 1999). Several studies published since these reviews showed links between maternal ETS exposure and preterm birth (see, e.g., Dejmek et al., 2002). Only a few of the studies reporting links between prenatal ETS exposure among nonsmoking women and adverse pregnancy outcomes (spontaneous abortions, low birth weight, preterm delivery) have used biomarkers of exposure (e.g., cotinine) during early or late pregnancy. Polymorphisms in *CYP1A1* and *GSTT1* have been linked to marked birth weight deficits among women who smoked dur-ing pregnancy (Wang et al., 2002); the potential role of such polymor-phisms in the risk of low birth weight among ETS-exposed nonsmoking women is not known. Height at age 5 years was not related to prenatal ETS exposure status among children of nonsmoking mothers (Eskenazi and Bergmann, 1995).

Lung Function

Spirometry. Depending on host characteristics and exposure intensity and duration, air pollutants may cause acute and reversible or chronic and persistent reductions in lung volumes and flow rates measured by spirometric tests including FEV_1 (forced expiratory volume 1, the volume in liters of air that is forcefully exhaled in 1 second), FVC (forced vital ca-pacity, the maximum volume of air that can be exhaled after full inspira-tion), FEV_1/FVC (ratio of FEV_1 to FVC, expressed as a percentage), MMEF (also referred to as FEF_{25-75}, the maximum midexpiratory flow rate in mil-liliters per second during the middle half of a FVC test), FEF_{75} (forced ex-piratory flow rate in milliliters per second at 75% of FVC), and PEF (peak expiratory flow rate, the peak flow rate in milliliters per second during expiration).

Deficits of 20% or more in FEV_1 and MMEF, respectively, indicate large or small airway obstruction. Measured flow rates may be compared to population norms for children of the same age, sex, and height. As-sessment may also include measurement of FEV_1 before and after inha-lation of a β-agonist bronchodilator; an increase of 0.2 L (or 15% of base-line FEV_1) after the use of a bronchodilator indicates the presence of reversible airflow obstruction characteristic of asthma.

Lung function deficits. Disruption of the signaling systems that control normal lung morphogenesis and growth during critical prenatal and childhood time periods can cause irreversible structural and/or functional deficits (Pinkerton and Joad, 2000). Lung volumes and flow rates grow until about age 25 years, plateau for several years, and then gradually decline. Although small lung function deficits generally do not cause symptoms or clinically obvious disability, they provide objective measures of preclinical respiratory tract damage. A meta-analysis of 22 surveys of school-age children exposed to parental smoking concluded that ETS exposure is associated with lung function deficits among asthmatic and healthy children, with evidence of exposure-risk relations (Table 10–5) (Cook et al., 1998). Longitudinal studies and investigations using biomarkers of ETS exposure have confirmed links between childhood ETS exposure and lung function deficits (see, e.g., Li et al., 2000; Mannino et al., 2001). A meta-analysis of 10 epidemiologic studies showed a significant association between maternal smoking and bronchial hyperreactivity (pooled $OR = 1.3$, CI 1.1–1.5) (Cook and Strachan, 1998). The biologic plausibility of these findings is shown by similar findings in experimental animal studies (Witschi et al., 1997).

Asthma

A meta-analysis of six longitudinal studies concluded that incident asthma development, especially before age 7 years, and asthma severity were associated with maternal smoking (Strachan and Cook, 1998b). It appears that prenatal maternal smoking and childhood ETS exposure are independently related to the risk of childhood asthma (Infante-Rivard et al., 1999; McGready et al., 2001). The NAS concluded that ETS: (*1*) causes exacerbations of asthma in preschool-age children, (*2*) is associated with new-onset asthma in young children, and (*3*) is a possible cause of asthma exacerbations in older children (National Academy of Sciences, 2000). The

TABLE 10–5. Meta-Analysis of
Parental Smoking and Children's
Lung Function

Parameter	Average Deficit[a]
FEV_1	1.4% (1.0–1.9)
FEF_{25-75}	5.0% (3.3–6.6)
FEF_{75}	4.3% (3.1–5.5)

Source: Cook et al. (1998).

[a]Reduction for children exposed to parental smoking compared to unexposed children.

Academy stated that there is inadequate evidence to determine if ETS is associated with new-onset asthma in school-age children.

Other Respiratory Diseases
In a pooled analysis of lower respiratory illness before age 3 years, all but one of 38 epidemiologic studies showed significant associations with smoking by either parent (pooled $OR = 1.6$, CI 1.4–1.7), and most studies showed exposure–risk relationships (Strachan and Cook, 1997). An independent meta-analysis indicated that ETS exposure during early childhood approximately doubled the risk of lower respiratory infections requiring hospitalization (Li et al., 1999). Environmental tobacco smoke exposure alone (from fathers and/or other household members) is a risk factor for respiratory illness among infants whose mothers never smoked. The frequency and duration of otitis media among young children are also strongly associated with ETS exposure; a meta-analysis of 42 epidemiologic studies yielded pooled odds ratios of 1.5 (CI 1.1–2.0) for recurrent middle ear infection and 1.4 (CI 1.2–1.6) for middle ear effusion among children exposed to parental smoking (Strachan and Cook, 1998a).

Cancer
Based mainly on studies of lung cancer among adults exposed to ETS for many years, the EPA determined that there is sufficient evidence that ETS causes cancer in humans (U.S. Environmental Protection Agency, 1992). Some 50 epidemiologic investigations of childhood cancer have shown that maternal smoking during pregnancy and postnatal ETS exposure are weakly associated with brain tumors, leukemia, and lymphomas (Sasco and Vainio, 1999). A meta-analysis showed moderately strong associations between paternal but not maternal smoking and non-Hodgkin's lymphoma, acute lymphatic leukemia, and brain tumors (Boffetta et al., 2000). The association with paternal smoking does not necessarily indicate a link to direct ETS exposure; the mechanism could involve paternal germ cell mutations. There is inadequate evidence to assess reported links between ETS exposure during childhood and breast cancer and nasopharyngeal cancer in adults. Although paternal smoking was associated with childhood cancers, no tobacco smoke carcinogen has been tested in animals with preconceptual exposure of male parents (Anderson et al., 2000).

Sudden Infant Death Syndrome
Sudden infant death syndrome is a diagnosis of exclusion based on the sudden unexpected death of an infant usually aged 2–5 months with no adequate cause of death identified at autopsy; SIDS likely includes deaths that have heterogeneous etiologies. A meta-analysis of 39 studies of SIDS yielded pooled, adjusted odds ratios of 2.1 (CI 1.8–2.4) for prenatal ma-

ternal smoking and 1.9 (CI 1.6–2.4) for postnatal maternal smoking (Anderson and Cook, 1997). Evidence includes the following: (1) consistent, strong, dose-related associations with maternal smoking during pregnancy were found, (2) infants of women who smoked prenatally and postnatally had the greatest risk of SIDS, and (3) maternal and household smoking intensity were independently associated with SIDS. Evidence on SIDS and prenatal maternal smoking meets these criteria for causality: strength of association, exposure–risk relationship, consistency across studies and study designs, biologic plausibility, and appropriate time relationship.

Exposures

Self-reported information, indoor air monitoring (air nicotine and fine particulate levels), and biomonitoring are useful for estimating ETS exposure. In homes and public buildings where smoking takes place, ETS is the main source of indoor fine particulate matter, with 24-hour average $PM_{2.5}$ levels increasing by about 1 $\mu g/m^3$ per cigarette smoked per day. During recent years, about 30% of nonsmoking Canadian children have experienced ETS exposure, primarily at home. Nicotine is almost specific to tobacco, and its major proximate metabolite, cotinine, is a very specific and sensitive biomarker of recent ETS exposures, having a half-life of 7–40 hours in urine, saliva, and blood. Cord serum cotinine, the most useful biomarker of fetal exposure during late pregnancy, distinguishes between mothers who smoked, who were passively exposed to ETS, and who had neither exposure. Maternal smoking is the major determinant of urinary and salivary cotinine and hair nicotine levels among young children. Hair nicotine level reflects adsorption of ETS onto hair but is rarely used in epidemiologic studies. During the period 1990–1999, the median plasma cotinine level among nonsmokers in the United States decreased fourfold (from 0.20 to 0.05 $\mu g/L$) (Centers for Disease Control and Prevention, 2001). Despite this progress, more than half of American youth are still exposed and have higher plasma cotinine levels than older persons. A known human carcinogen in ETS, 4-aminobiphenyl, forms adducts with hemoglobin, with a half-life of about 4 months.

Most epidemiologic studies of particulate matter have used measures of particle size and concentration, not toxicity. Although there are no calibration standards for measurement of the suspended particle mass, existing methods identify relative exposure levels and time trends. Indoor $PM_{0.1}$ and $PM_{2.5-10}$ concentrations vary substantially with brief peaks related to indoor activities. Peak indoor air and personal PM exposure levels are associated with ETS, influx of outdoor air, cooking, vacuuming, movement (resuspended particles), wood smoke, and motor vehicle travel. Freestanding kerosene heaters add about 40 $\mu g/m^3$ of $PM_{2.5}$ to background residential levels. Ambient $PM_{2.5}$ from motor vehicles, fuel combustion, incineration, and industries can permeate homes, school buses, and other indoor environments frequented by children, resulting in indoor/outdoor $PM_{2.5}$ ratios of 0.4 to 0.8, depending on particle size and density, the air exchange rate, and the surface-to-volume ratio of the indoor environment.

Asbestos fibers have been detected in air and dust in homes, schools, and other public buildings built approximately during the period 1920–1977 [the Consumer Product Safey Commission (CPSC) and the EPA started to restrict asbestos use during the 1970s]. Parents occupationally exposed to asbestos can carry fibers home on their clothing. Although the cancer risks associated with such exposures during childhood have not been assessed systematically, there have been sporadic reports of childhood mesothelioma linked to parental occupational exposure, presumably caused by asbestos contamination of residential indoor air.

Risk Management

Children are more likely than adults to develop health effects from ETS exposure, and the home is their most important exposure source. Although measures have variably been adopted to control ETS exposure in public places, transportation, schools, day-care centers, and workplaces, the protection of children from exposure at home has received relatively little attention. Only California meets the nation's Healthy People 2010 objective of eliminating exposure to ETS by either banning indoor smoking or limiting it to separately ventilated areas. Community programs and clinical interventions can reduce children's exposures to ETS at home; for instance, ETS exposure of adolescents living with adult smokers was reduced in homes with parent-imposed smoking restrictions (Biener et al., 1997).

BIOLOGIC AGENTS

Health Effects

Immunologic Sensitization and Inflammation
In sensitized persons, IgE is the main mediator of allergic responses to inhaled allergens, and serum IgE levels are associated with the development and severity of asthma. Allergen–IgE complexes bind to immune

system cells, triggering release of proinflammatory agents that cause early (airway constriction, mucus production, and airway edema) and delayed effects (prolonged bronchoconstriction) (National Academy of Sciences, 2000). Allergen priming of T_h cells begins prenatally because of transplacental transport of very small amounts of antigens. By age 5 years, most children convert to the normal adult T_{h1} cytokine pattern and respond to allergen exposure with moderate IgG and IgA production and no symptoms. If the dominant T_h cells produce the T_{h2} cytokine pattern, especially interleukin-4 (IL-4) and IL-5, antigen exposure will trigger IgE production, eosinophilia, and allergic symptoms.

Asthma

This section focuses on biologic agents in the home environment that are potential causes of asthma development or triggers of episodes in known asthmatics. Rhinovirus infection appears to trigger episodes among known asthmatics, and there is limited evidence for associations between respiratory syncytial virus, *Chlamydia pneumoniae*, and *Mycoplasma pneumoniae* infections and exacerbation of childhood asthma (Table 10–2). There is limited evidence for respiratory syncytial virus and inadequate evidence for other infectious agents to assess their role in asthma development.

Animal and insect aeroallergens. Important findings of the National Institute of Medicine and other studies include the following (see also Table 10–2):

Pets
• Sensitization—cat allergen *Fel d* 1 can sensitize children at very low levels (nanograms per cubic meter) and trigger severe asthma attacks in sensitized persons.
• Asthma development—the strongest risk factor for recent-onset, physician-diagnosed asthma among young children in NHANES III was allergy to a pet (Lanphear et al., 2001); a longitudinal cohort study of incident asthma in southern California also showed an association with pets in the home (McConnell et al., 2002).
• Asthma episodes—there is sufficient evidence that cat and dog allergens can cause episodes in sensitized asthmatics.

House-dust mites
• Sensitization—African American and Mexican American children in NHANES III had relatively high house-dust mite sensitization rates.
• Asthma development—there is sufficient evidence that house-dust mite antigens can cause asthma development.

- Asthma episodes—there is sufficient evidence that house-dust mite antigens can trigger episodes in sensitized asthmatics.

Cockroaches
- Sensitization—African American and Mexican American children in NHANES III had relatively high cockroach antigen sensitization rates; there was a dose–response relationship between cockroach allergen exposure and sensitization.
- Asthma development—there is suggestive evidence that cockroach antigens can cause asthma development in preschool children.
- Asthma episodes—there is sufficient evidence that cockroach antigens can trigger episodes in sensitized asthmatics.

Fungi
Measurement of fungal exposure is complicated by large numbers of fungi and fungal products. Many fungal products are potential allergens, and some have been characterized; the amounts and profiles produced depend on environmental factors and the type of substrate. Fungal mycotoxins comprise some 400 entities including aflatoxins, trichothecenes, fumonisins, and ochratoxin, with toxic activities including cytotoxicity, immunotoxicity, carcinogenicity, estrogenic activity, and inflammation. Few epidemiologic studies have directly measured indoor air fungal allergen levels, resorting instead to indirect indicators such as the presence of visible mold or dampness.

Approximately 6%–10% of the general population and 15%–50% of persons with allergic conditions are sensitized to fungal allergens. Dampness and other indicators of fungal allergens have been associated with asthma in several studies. A review of epidemiologic studies of indoor dampness and respiratory symptoms, asthma, and allergy concluded that dampness increases the risk of cough, wheezing, and asthma by up to twofold; the mechanism is unknown but may include house-dust mites or molds (Bornehag et al., 2001). The IOM concluded that there was sufficient evidence of an association between molds and triggering of asthma episodes but inadequate evidence of an association between molds and development of asthma (Table 10–2). See also Chapter 11 (Outdoor Air) for discussion of ambient molds and other aeroallergens in childhood respiratory disease.

Endotoxin. Endotoxin is a component of the outer membrane of gram-negative bacteria that is a potent toxin, activating human airway macrophages to release proinflammatory cytokines and other substances at levels as low as 1 ng/mL in vitro. Exposure to elevated endotoxin levels in house dust has been linked to airway inflammation when inhaled by adult volunteers, wheezing episodes before age 1 year, and asthma severity among adults. At present there is inadequate evidence to assess its role in asthma development or triggering of asthma episodes (Table 10–2).

Multiple exposures. Among asthmatic children, the likelihood of sensitization to house-dust mite or cockroach antigens is associated with their concentration in house dust. Deficits in FEV_1 among asthmatic children in NHANES II were greater among those sensitized to any indoor allergen than for those reactive to any outdoor allergen tested (Schwartz and Weiss, 1995). A recent review concluded that existing evidence does not prove a causal relationship between allergen exposure level and asthma development, noting that no published studies had linked allergen exposure during infancy to the risk of asthma after age 6 years in a random population sample (Pearce et al., 2000).

Other Diseases

An outbreak of idiopathic pulmonary hemosiderosis among 37 infants in Cleveland included 12 deaths; investigation showed strong associations with residence in households with major water damage, increased air levels of *Stachybotrys chartarum* fungal spores, and combined exposure to *S. chartarum* and ETS (Dearborn et al., 1999). Over 100 additional similar cases have since been reported in the United States. It is thought that trichothecene mycotoxins produced by *S. chartarum* inhibit protein synthesis in the rapidly growing infant lung, causing capillary fragility and hemorrhage.

Exposures

Comparison of results from health studies of indoor aeroallergens has been constrained by inconsistent use of the sampling sites, measurement devices, and sampling schedules needed to measure children's exposures during activities in different household areas; most studies have measured aeroallergen levels in reservoir dust, but air levels may better reflect respiratory tract exposures. But airborne particle levels from resuspended house dust vary substantially throughout the day and across seasons, making adequately integrated exposure measures difficult and expensive. The correlation between cat, dust mite, and cockroach antigen concentrations in floor dust and serum allergen-specific IgE levels appears to vary by type of dust sampler (Mansour et al., 2001). The first National Survey of Lead and Allergens in Housing in United States (1998–1999) measured cockroach allergen *Bla g* 1, the dust mite allergens *Der f* 1 and

Der p 1, the cat allergen *Fel d* 1, the dog allergen *Can f* 1, the rodent allergens *Rat n* 1 and mouse urinary protein, allergens of the fungus *Alternaria alternata,* and endotoxin in dust samples from a bed, the bedroom floor, a sofa or chair, the living room floor, the kitchen floor, and the basement floor (Vojta et al., 2002) (results to be published soon).

Animal and Insect Aeroallergens

Pets. About 30% of households in the United States keep cats or dogs as pets. The main cat allergen, *Fel d* I, occurs in settled dust and in fine airborne particles ($PM_{2.5}$) that remain airborne for prolonged times, are very adherent, spread throughout the house, and are ubiquitous even in households without cats. The main dog allergens, *Can f* I and *Can f* II, are also widely distributed in fine airborne particles and in settled dust. Most homes with dogs or cats and substantial proportions of pet-free homes have high levels of their specific antigens in dust and detectable levels in airborne fine particulate matter; curtains, desks, and chairs in school classrooms act as reservoirs for cat and dog allergens apparently transported to school on clothing.

House-dust mites. The house-dust mite (*Dermatophagoides pteronyssinus*) is a tiny insect that scavenges materials including human skin scales, pollen grains, insect scales, house dust, and plant fibers. Antigens from mite feces and dead body parts (*Der p* I and II) occur mainly as large particles (>10 μm) that accumulate in settled dust and remain airborne for short periods if disturbed; antigen concentrations in house dust are highest in geographic regions with persistent high humidity during several months annually. Within homes, concentrations (micrograms per gram of dust) are highest in mattresses, carpets, quilts, and sofas. Floor and mattress dust antigen levels vary by factors including type of ventilation (higher in the absence of forced air), season, type and age of home, age of mattress, and number of occupants. Young children spend a great deal of time on or near the floor, where allergens are concentrated in dust, and can be sensitized to house-dust mite antigens at very low levels.

Cockroaches. Blattella germanica and *Periplaneta americana* are the two most common cockroaches in the United States; high levels of their antigens (*Bla g* 1, 2, and 4) are linked to warm, humid climates, lower socioeconomic status, living in apartments, and availability of water and food (particularly in kitchens). Cockroach antigens are associated with large particles that accumulate in settled dust and remain airborne for short periods if disturbed. There is a strong association between poverty and high house dust cockroach antigen levels and skin sensitization.

Fungi

There are at least 1 million species of fungi including 200 to which humans are commonly exposed. The most prevalent mold genera in homes are *Alternaria, Cladosporium,* and *Penicillium*. Fungal spores are ubiquitous in the outdoor environment and indoor dust, and can readily grow indoors under conditions of persistent high humidity and in homes with a dirt floor or crawl space type of basement. Compared to white children, African American children are twice as likely to be sensitized to *A. alternata* ($OR = 2.1$, CI 1.5–2.8) (Stevenson et al., 2001). Indoor storage of organic wastes (for composting) for a week or longer is associated with a five- to eightfold increase in levels of fungal extracellular polysaccharides and β-glucans on living room and kitchen floors. Other factors contributing to mold growth include carpeted floors, dampness, past flooding, indoor storage of firewood, and unvented dryers.

Fungal exposure has often been assessed by crude indicators such as the presence of visible mold or dampness. Quantitative indices include spore counts, culturable fungi, ergosterol (a fungal cell membrane sterol), β(1-3)-glucans, extracellular polysaccharides, fungal volatile organic compounds (3-methylfuran, 1-octene-3-ol, geosmin), mycotoxins, specific DNA sequences, and fungal-specific lipids (Dillon et al., 1999). β(1-3)-Glucans are potent inflammatory agents that occur in cell walls of fungi, yeasts, some bacteria, and many plants. Concentrations of β(1-3)-glucans per unit area in settled house dust are associated with carpets, the presence of a dog, more than four persons, infrequent cleaning, and the presence of visible mold. Settled dust concentrations of β(1-3)-glucans are highly correlated with those of endotoxin, house-dust mite and cat allergens, and mold spores.

Endotoxin

High endotoxin levels in settled dust are associated with the presence of a dog or cat in the home, indoor storage of organic wastes (for composting), and farm environments where livestock and poultry are kept. Mattress dust endotoxin levels may better reflect exposure than floor dust or air levels (Park et al., 2000).

Risk Management

Animal and Insect Aeroallergens

   Pets. Removal of pets from the home is the most effective way to reduce cat or dog allergens but is often avoided; keeping pets out of bedrooms and regular cleaning reduce exposure levels somewhat. After removal of cats from homes, *Fel d* I levels fall but may remain elevated for several months unless carpets and upholstery are removed and mattresses and pillows are encased. Intervention using a high-efficiency particulate air cleaner (HEPA filter) over a 3-month period significantly reduced airborne but not settled dust cat allergen levels, and there was no significant improvement in cat-induced asthma or rhinitis symptom scores, sleep disturbance, medication use, or PEFs (Wood et al., 1998). Removal of dogs from homes appears to reduce dog allergen levels, but there is inadequate evidence to assess the impact of dog or cat removal or related interventions on symptoms of sensitized asthmatics (National Academy of Sciences, 2000).

House-dust mites. A review of 23 intervention trials that used chemical and physical methods to control house-dust mite antigen levels in homes of asthmatics concluded that there was negligible impact on symptom scores, medication use, and lung function (Gotzsche et al., 1998). Nevertheless, some randomized intervention trials have succeeded in reducing bedroom mite allergen levels, bronchial hyperreactivity, and bronchodilator use and in improving symptoms and FEV_1 levels (Carswell et al., 1996; Shapiro et al., 1999). Possible reasons for lack of efficacy include failure to reduce antigen levels adequately and sensitization to other allergens persistent in the home environment (atopic persons are usually sensitized to multiple indoor allergens). Aeroallergen levels can also be reduced to some degree by eliminating carpets and upholstered furniture (especially from bedrooms), vacuuming with a central vacuum or one with a HEPA filter, damp mopping floors, washing bedding weekly in hot water (at least 55°C), increasing ventilation, and keeping relative humidity below 50% and temperatures below 25°C.

Cockroaches. Insecticides are often used for cockroach control, especially in inner-city housing and apartments. This measure, however, introduces children to the risk of pesticide toxicity. Other measures include general cleanliness (especially removal of food debris), control of dampness, and caulking of crevices. A randomized intervention trial that recruited asthmatic children sensitized to cockroach antigen showed only a minor, transitory benefit of cockroach extermination and house cleaning education on house-dust antigen levels (Gergen et al., 1999). There is sufficient evidence that intensive cockroach exposure interventions can cause transiently reduced allergen levels, but there is inadequate evidence to assess its efficacy in improving symptoms or lung function in sensitized asthmatics (National Academy of Sciences, 2000).

Fungi and Endotoxins
Mold control depends mainly on maintenance of low humidity levels and avoidance of water damage. There are no recognized guidelines or stan-

dards for concentrations of fungi or fungal products in indoor air or house dust (Dillon et al., 1999). A review of the recent epidemiologic literature concluded that the use of cross-sectional study designs and inadequate validation of exposure measures precluded a quantitative risk assessment and an air standard for fungi (Verhoeff and Burge, 1997). Finland, apparently the only country that has done so, declared indoor visible mold growth to be a health hazard and legislated public health measures to control indoor dampness and molds (Husman, 1999). Some countries have developed guidelines for relative humidity and ventilation rates. There is suggestive evidence that interventions can reduce fungal allergen levels indoors but inadequate evidence to determine if such interventions improve asthma symptoms or lung function in sensitized asthmatics; there is inadequate evidence to determine if interventions reduce endotoxin levels in homes (National Academy of Sciences, 2000).

Mixed Exposures
The European Environment and Health Committee recommended that European Union member states take actions on asthma including (1) development of guidelines for house dust, humidity, molds, cockroaches, and pets, (2) promotion of improved ventilation, (3) communication of the dangers of ETS and smoking during pregnancy, and (4) strict enforcement of smoking prohibitions in areas frequented by children (European Centre for Environment and Health, 1999). There is sufficient evidence that intervention (ventilation, mattress and pillow encasement, regular hot washing of bedding, etc.) can reduce multiple house-dust allergen levels and cause an improvement in asthma symptoms but inadequate evidence to determine if mitigation can reduce asthma development (National Academy of Sciences, 2000).

VOLATILE ORGANIC CHEMICALS AND GASES

This section briefly addresses indoor volatile organic chemicals (VOCs) and gases (carbon monoxide and nitrogen dioxide) as potential threats to child health. See also Chapter 11 (Outdoor Air) for discussion of outdoor sources of VOCs and other toxic gases and their potential health effects.

Health Effects

Volatile Organic Chemicals
Among the over 300 chemicals that have been detected in indoor air, about 30 have been linked to asthma in occupational or animal studies; among

these, children may be exposed to several in their homes, such as, acrolein (ETS), formaldehyde (ETS, synthetic materials), and chlorine (chlorinated water, household bleach). There is limited evidence that exposure to mixed indoor air contaminants may be a factor in childhood asthma and other allergic diseases in children. Limited evidence links formaldehyde to wheezing and other respiratory symptoms, but there is inadequate evidence to determine if it can cause asthma development (National Academy of Sciences, 2000). The ability of relatively low-level formaldehyde to cause eye irritation among youth and young adults was shown in a controlled exposure study (Yang et al., 2001). Experimental animal evidence indicates that inhaled formaldehyde exposure increases sensitization to aeroallergens.

Home use of organic solvents for model building and artwork, and maternal prenatal exposure to extensive indoor painting, were associated with a two- to fourfold increased risk of childhood leukemia (Freedman et al., 2001). Benzene is a frequent contaminant of indoor air and a known cause of aplastic anemia and acute myeloid leukemia in persons with prolonged high occupational exposures. Sequential metabolism of benzene in liver and bone marrow generates semiquinone radicals that react covalently with tubulin, chromosomal proteins, and topoisomerase II and induce oxidative DNA damage. When attacked by free radicals, topoisomerase II can break DNA strands and cause the 11q23 chromosomal band abnormalities commonly seen in childhood leukemia. At high concentrations in air, formaldehyde is a known animal (nasal sinus cancer) and a probable human carcinogen, but the potential role of it and other VOCs in childhood cancer is unknown.

Carbon Monoxide and Nitrogen Dioxide
Carbon monoxide (CO) is a colorless, odorless gas produced by incomplete combustion of carbonaceous fuels and materials. The most serious health effect in children is acute, high-dose CO poisoning that can cause symptoms ranging from headache and dizziness to nausea, vomiting, loss of consciousness, and death. Inhaled CO is rapidly absorbed into the bloodstream, where it binds to hemoglobin with an affinity about 240 times that of oxygen. Carbon monoxide also binds to cytochrome aa3, blocking mitochondrial energy production, and to myoglobin, interfering with oxygen storage in skeletal and heart muscle. Children are at increased risk of CO poisoning because of their relatively high metabolic rates; the fetus is also susceptible because fetal hemoglobin has a higher affinity for CO than adult hemoglobin. Because of their high oxygen needs, the central nervous and cardiovascular systems are most adversely affected by CO poisoning. The American Association of Poison Control

Centers Toxic Exposure Surveillance System (TESS) received 1787 reports of moderate, severe, or fatal CO poisonings among children aged 0–5 years during 2000 (Litovitz et al., 2001). Potential health effects of low-level ambient CO levels are discussed in Chapter 11 (Outdoor Air).

There is limited but inconsistent evidence of associations between indoor nitrogen dioxide (NO_2) exposure and respiratory disease in children. The best evidence comes from studies that had reasonable sample sizes and direct measures of NO_2 exposure, such as, the Harvard Six Cities Study (Neas et al., 1991) and a large case-control study of incident asthma in Montreal (Infante-Rivard, 1993). Acute high-level NO_2 exposure in hockey arenas employing propane-powered ice resurfacers has caused high rates of acute respiratory symptoms (in 57% of adolescent players in one outbreak).

Exposures

Volatile Organic Chemicals

Exposure to VOCs can be estimated from their levels in indoor, ambient, and personal air and water, and VOC uptake can be assessed from urine and alveolar breath samples. Personal VOC exposures are dominated by indoor sources, with ambient outdoor exposures contributing only about 2%–25% of personal exposures for most toxic and carcinogenic VOCs (Wallace, 1993). Detailed monitoring of adult volunteers showed that most of 25 commonly performed activities increase personal exposure to one or more target VOCs, often by a factor of 10. Activities causing high VOC exposures included use of deodorizers (p-dichlorobenzene), washing clothes and dishes (chloroform), visiting a dry cleaner (1,1,1-trichloroethane, tetrachloroethylene), smoking (benzene, styrene), and painting and paint stripping (n-decane, n-undecane). Specific findings from studies of VOC exposures include the following:

- All VOCs—based on measured personal exposures and estimated upper-bound lifetime cancer risks, the most important indoor VOCs were benzene, vinylidene chloride, chloroform, and p-dichlorobenzene; airborne sources accounted for 80%–100% of the exposure to each of these VOCs (Wallace, 1991).
- Benzene
  - Children—personal air benzene levels of urban children are higher than those of suburban children; levels of urinary trans-muconic acid (a benzene metabolite) among inner-city children are associated with time spent playing near the street (note: motor vehicles emit benzene).

o Adults—the main sources are active and passive smoking, auto exhaust, and driving or riding in automobiles; built-in garages are a major source for nonsmokers

Indoor air formaldehyde levels may be elevated in homes, especially mobile homes, containing large amounts of particleboard and other building materials that release formaldehyde and have low air exchange rates. An indoor air quality survey of homes in southern Louisiana showed indoor air formaldehyde levels of up to 6.6 mg/m^3, with 60% of homes exceeding the ASHRAE guideline (123 μg/m^3) (Lemus et al., 1998). See Chapter 12 (Water) for discussion of exposure to chloroform and other VOCs while showering or swimming in indoor chlorinated pools.

Carbon Monoxide and Nitrogen Dioxide

Carbon monoxide binds tightly to hemoglobin, forming carboxyhemoglobin with a half-life of 2–6 hours. Carboxyhemoglobin blood levels reflect the concentration and duration of CO exposure, exercise, and other factors and can be estimated by direct blood analysis or by measuring CO in exhaled breath. Ambient NO$_2$ monitoring does not adequately reflect children's personal exposures because they spend over 90% of their time indoors, where NO$_2$ levels reflect sources such as gas stoves and smokers. Homes with inadequately ventilated gas stoves generally have markedly higher NO$_2$ levels than those with electric stoves, particularly in winter.

Risk Management

Volatile Organic Chemicals

Indoor sources of VOCs include built-in garages, smoking, building materials and furnishings, chlorinated water, dry-cleaned clothes, cleaning solutions, solvents, paint, and other consumer products (Table 10–6). Potential control measures for indoor air contaminants include ventilation, source removal or substitution, source modification, air cleaning, and behavioral change (Moeller, 1997). Parents and other child-care providers can reduce children's exposures to certain VOCs by, for example, not using moth balls or bathroom deodorizers containing *p*-dichlorobenzene, avoiding dry-cleaning (or at least storing dry-cleaned materials outdoors for 24 hours), and not storing volatile solvents, gasoline, or gasoline-containing machines in attached garages.

Major indoor sources of formaldehyde include products containing formaldehyde-based resins such as finishes, plywood, paneling, fiberboard, particleboard, permanent press fabric, draperies, and urea formaldehyde foam. Given the ubiquitous and largely unavoidable exposure to such prod-

TABLE 10–6. VOCs: Sources and Levels in Indoor Air, Exhaled Breath, and Blood

VOC	Main Indoor Sources	Indoor air levels ($\mu g/m^3$)[a]	Exhaled breath levels ($\mu g/m^3$)[b]	Blood levels (ng/L)[c]
Formaldehyde	Building materials, furniture, cabinets, acid-cured floor finishes	50	NA	NA
Chloroform	Chlorinated water (drinking, showering/bathing, washing dishes or clothes, indoor swimming pools)	1	ND–2.3	NA
Carbon tetrachloride	Past uses—aerosol cans, cleaning fluids, degreasing agents, fire extinguishers, spot removers	<5	ND–0.7	NA
Benzene	Gasoline or motor vehicle in built-in garage, smoking	5	0.9–12	460
Ethylbenzene	Gasoline or motor vehicle in built-in garage, smoking	5	0.2–2.9	225
1,1,1-Trichloroethane	Past uses—glues, paints, aerosol sprays	NA	0.1–6.6	340
Trichloroethylene	Adhesives, paint removers, and spot removers	5	ND–0.9	NA
Tetrachloroethane	Past uses—paints	NA	NA	580
Tetrachloroethylene	Dry-cleaned fabrics, ingredient in some consumer products	5	1.8–6.8	NA
p-Dichlorobenzene	Mothballs, toilet deodorizers	1	ND–1.3	2050
Styrene	Smoking	2	ND–0.8	190
Toluene	Gasoline or motor vehicle in built-in garage, smoking, paints, paint thinners, fingernail polish, lacquers, adhesives	20	NA	1460
Xylenes (o,m,p)	Gasoline or motor vehicle in built-in garage, smoking, cleaning agent, thinner for paint, paints, varnishes	15	0.6–8.6	1040

[a]U.S. Environmental Protection Agency (1998).

[b]Exhaled breath median concentrations (Wallace et al., 1996).

[c]95th percentiles (estimated from graph) (Needham et al., 1995).

ND = not detectable.

ucts at present, improved ventilation is one of the few potential interventions in the short term; even this measure is complicated by the associated energy cost. Longer term, there is the potential for introduction of safer products.

The European Environment and Health Committee recommended that European Union member states take actions on VOCs and other indoor air toxicants by (1) establishment of pollution-free schools by limiting access of vehicles, especially diesel-powered vehicles, and by restricting the siting of pollution-emitting sources around schools, (2) elimination of wall-to-wall carpets and irritant chemical cleaning products in schools, (3) establishment of guidelines for the quality of the home environment to minimize risk factors including gas stoves, and (4) promotion of improved home ventilation (European Centre for Environment and Health, 1999).

Carbon Monoxide and Nitrogen Dioxide
Potential sources of CO in indoor air include inadequately ventilated non-electric space heaters and stoves, leaking furnaces or chimneys, back-drafting from furnaces, gas water heaters, wood stoves, and fireplaces, running cars in attached closed garages, indoor use of barbeques, and smoking. The main indoor sources of NO_2 are inadequately ventilated gas appliances for cooking and heating. Preventive measures for both CO and NO_2 include proper installation, maintenance, and use of fuel-burning appliances, adequate ventilation, avoidance of unventilated space heaters (or at least avoiding prolonged use), and use of CO detectors.

CONCLUSION

Proven Child Health Outcomes

- Environmental tobacco smoke
  - Prenatal maternal smoking increases the risk of SIDS
  - Childhood ETS exposure increases the risk of bronchiolitis, pneumonia, and middle ear infections, the number and severity of asthma episodes in preschool-age children, bronchial hyperreactivity, lung function deficits, and reduced lung function growth rates during childhood.
- Biologic agents
  - House-dust mite antigen exposure can cause new-onset (incident) asthma.
  - Cat, cockroach, and house-dust mite antigen exposure can precipitate episodes in sensitized asthmatics.

- Volatile chemicals and gases
  - Carbon monoxide from combustion sources can cumulate indoors to levels capable of causing acute toxicity and death.
  - Acute exposure to formaldehyde or high-level NO_2, respectively, can cause acute eye irritation or respiratory symptoms.

Unresolved Issues and Knowledge Gaps

- Environmental tobacco smoke
  - There is limited evidence that prenatal maternal ETS exposure can cause spontaneous abortions, birth weight deficits, and preterm birth.
  - There is limited evidence that postnatal ETS exposure can cause SIDS, independent of prenatal maternal smoking.
  - There is limited evidence that prenatal and postnatal maternal smoking can cause new-onset, persistent asthma in preschool-age children, independent of other risk factors.
  - There is limited evidence that ETS causes asthma exacerbations in school-age children but inadequate evidence to determine if ETS can cause new-onset asthma in this age group.
  - There is limited evidence that paternal smoking is associated with childhood brain tumors, acute lymphatic leukemia, and non-Hodgkin's lymphoma.
  - There is inadequate evidence that childhood ETS exposure is linked to adult breast and nasopharyngeal cancers.
- Biologic agents
  - Dog antigens, molds, and rhinovirus are associated with episodes in known asthmatics but causality is uncertain.
  - There is limited evidence that cockroach antigen can cause new-onset asthma in preschool-age children.
  - There is limited evidence that dog, rodent, and fungal antigens can exacerbate asthma among preschool-age children.
  - There is limited evidence that the fungus *Stachybotrys chartarum* can cause idiopathic pulmonary hemosiderosis in infants, especially those also exposed to ETS.
- Volatile chemicals and gases
  - There is limited evidence that personal air or indoor NO_2 levels are associated with lung function deficits, respiratory symptoms, and early-onset asthma.
  - Children have low-level exposures to several VOCs in indoor air that are known human or animal carcinogens, but their potential role in childhood or adult cancer remains undefined (occupational exposure to benzene, however, can cause adult leukemia).

Risk Management

- Prevention
  - It appears that no country has comprehensive programs to address indoor air health hazards and to evaluate progress in reducing children's exposures.
  - Although paternal smoking is linked to childhood cancer, no tobacco smoke carcinogen has been tested for intergenerational carcinogenicity in animals.
- Monitoring
  - Biomonitoring—periodic population-based measurement of indicators of internal dose of ETS and selected VOCs is needed.
  - Indoor environment surveys—periodic population-based measurement of the prevalence of key indoor air hazards (e.g., aeroallergens, dampness/molds, VOCs, CO, NO_2) is needed.

See Chapter 11 (Outdoor Air) for further discussion of CO, NO_2, and certain VOCs and other chapters for other indoor pollutants (e.g., radon, pesticides, metals, volatile drinking water disinfection by-products).

REFERENCES

Aligne CA, Stoddard JJ. (1997). Tobacco and children. An economic evaluation of the medical effects of parental smoking . Arch Pediatr Adolesc Med 151:648–53.

Anderson HR, Cook DG. (1997). Passive smoking and sudden infant death syndrome: review of the epidemiological evidence. Thorax 52:1003–9.

Anderson LM, Diwan BA, Fear NT, Roman E. (2000). Critical windows of exposure for children's health: cancer in human epidemiological studies and neoplasms in experimental animal models. Environ Health Perspect 108(Suppl 3):573–94.

Biener L, Cullen D, Di ZX, Hammond SK. (1997). Household smoking restrictions and adolescents' exposure to environmental tobacco smoke. Prev Med 26: 358–63.

Boffetta P, Tredaniel J, Greco A. (2000). Risk of childhood cancer and adult lung cancer after childhood exposure to passive smoke: a meta-analysis. Environ Health Perspect 108:73–82.

Bornehag CG, Blomquist G, Gyntelberg F, Jarvholm B, Malmberg P, Nordvall L, Nielsen A, Pershagen G, Sundell J. (2001). Dampness in buildings and health. Nordic interdisciplinary review of the scientific evidence on associations between exposure to "dampness" in buildings and health effects (NORDDAMP). Indoor Air 11:72–86.

California Environmental Protection Agency. (1997). Health effects of exposure to environmental tobacco smoke. Sacramento: Office of Environmental Health Hazard Assessment.

Carswell F, Birmingham K, Oliver J, Crewes A, Weeks J. (1996). The respiratory effects of reduction of mite allergen in the bedrooms of asthmatic children—a double-blind controlled trial. Clin Exp Allergy 26:386–96.

Centers for Disease Control and Prevention. (2001). National report on human exposure to environmental chemicals. Cotinine. Atlanta: Centers for Disease Control and Prevention.

Cook DG, Strachan DP. (1998). Parental smoking, bronchial reactivity and peak flow variability in children. Thorax 53:295–301.

Cook DG, Strachan DP, Carey IM. (1998). Parental smoking and spirometric indices in children. Thorax 53:884–93.

Dearborn DG, Yike I, Sorenson WG, Miller MJ, Etzel RA. (1999). Overview of investigations into pulmonary hemorrhage among infants in Cleveland, Ohio. Environ Health Perspect 107:495–9.

Dejmek J, Solansky I, Podrazilova K, Sram RJ. (2002). The exposure of nonsmoking and smoking mothers to environmental tobacco smoke during different gestational phases and fetal growth. Environ Health Perspect 110:601–6.

Dillon HK, Miller JD, Sorenson WG, Douwes J, Jacobs RR. (1999). Review of methods applicable to the assessment of mold exposure to children. Environ Health Perspect 107(Suppl 3):473–80.

Eskenazi B, Bergmann JJ. (1995). Passive and active maternal smoking during pregnancy, as measured by serum cotinine, and postnatal smoke exposure. I. Effects on physical growth at age 5 years. Am J Epidemiol 142:S10–8.

European Centre for Environment and Health WHO. (1999). Children's health and the environment (EUR/ICP/EHCO 02 02 05/16). Rome: European Centre for Environment and Health.

Finette BA, O'Neill JP, Vacek PM, Albertini RJ. (1998). Gene mutations with characteristic deletions in cord blood T lymphocytes associated with passive maternal exposure to tobacco smoke. Nat Med 4:1144–51.

Freedman DM, Stewart P, Kleinerman RA, Wacholder S, Hatch EE, Tarone RE, Robison LL, Linet MS. (2001). Household solvent exposures and childhood acute lymphoblastic leukemia. Am J Public Health 91:564–7.

Gergen PJ, Mortimer KM, Eggleston PA, Rosenstreich D, Mitchell H, Ownby D, Kattan M, Baker D, Wright EC, Slavin R, and others. (1999). Results of the national cooperative inner-city asthma study (NCICAS) environmental intervention to reduce cockroach allergen exposure in inner-city homes. J Allergy Clin Immunol 103:501–6.

Gotzsche PC, Hammarquist C, Burr M. (1998). House dust mite control measures in the management of asthma: meta-analysis. BMJ 317:1105–10.

Husman TM. (1999). The Health Protection Act, national guidelines for indoor air quality and development of the national indoor air programs in Finland. Environ Health Perspect 107(Suppl 3):515–7.

Infante-Rivard C. (1993). Childhood asthma and indoor environmental risk factors. Am J Epidemiol 137:834–44.

Infante-Rivard C, Gautrin D, Malo JL, Suissa S. (1999). Maternal smoking and childhood asthma. Am J Epidemiol 150:528–31.

Lanphear BP, Aligne CA, Auinger P, Weitzman M, Byrd RS. (2001). Residential exposures associated with asthma in U.S. children. Pediatrics 107:505–11.

Lemus R, Abdelghani AA, Akers TG, Horner WE. (1998). Potential health risks from exposure to indoor formaldehyde. Rev Environ Health 13:91–8.

Li JS, Peat JK, Xuan W, Berry G. (1999). Meta-analysis on the association between environmental tobacco smoke (ETS) exposure and the prevalence of lower respiratory tract infection in early childhood. Pediatr Pulmonol 27:5–13.

Li YF, Gilliland FD, Berhane K, McConnell R, Gauderman WJ, Rappaport EB, Peters JM. (2000). Effects of in utero and environmental tobacco smoke exposure on lung function in boys and girls with and without asthma. Am J Respir Crit Care Med 162:2097–2104.

Litovitz TL, Klein-Schwartz W, White S, Cobaugh DJ, Youniss J, Omslaer JC, Drab A, Benson BE. (2001). 2000 Annual report of the American Association of Poison Control Centers Toxic Exposure Surveillance System. Am J Emerg Med 19:337–95.

Mannino DM, Moorman JE, Kingsley B, Rose D, Repace J. (2001). Health effects related to environmental tobacco smoke exposure in children in the United States: data from the Third National Health and Nutrition Examination Survey. Arch Pediatr Adolesc Med 155:36–41.

Mansour M, Lanphear BP, Hornung R, Khoury J, Bernstein DI, Menrath W, Decolongon J. (2001). A side-by-side comparison of sampling methods for settled, indoor allergens. Environ Res 87:37–46.

McConnell R, Berhane K, Gilliland F, Islam T, Gauderman WJ, London SJ, Avol E, Rappaport EB, Margolis HG, Peters JM. (2002). Indoor risk factors for asthma in a prospective study of adolescents. Epidemiology 13:288–95.

McGready R, Hamilton KA, Simpson JA, Cho T, Luxemburger C, Edwards R, Looareesuwan S, White NJ, Nosten F, Lindsay SW. (2001). Safety of the insect repellent *N,N*-diethyl-*M*-toluamide (DEET) in pregnancy. Am J Trop Med Hyg 65:285–9.

McKeever TM, Lewis SA, Smith C, Collins J, Heatlie H, Frischer M, Hubbard R. (2002). Early exposure to infections and antibiotics and the incidence of allergic disease: a birth cohort study with the West Midlands General Practice Research Database. J Allergy Clin Immunol 109:43–50.

Millar WJ, Hill GB. (1998). Childhood asthma. Health Rep 10:9–21.

Misra DP, Nguyen RH. (1999). Environmental tobacco smoke and low birth weight: a hazard in the workplace? Environ Health Perspect 107:879–904.

Moeller DW. (1997). Environmental health. Cambridge, MA: Harvard University Press.

National Academy of Sciences. (2000). Clearing the air. Asthma and indoor air exposures. Washington, DC: National Academy Press.

Neas LM, Dockery DW, Ware JH, Spengler JD, Speizer FE, Ferris BG Jr. (1991). Association of indoor nitrogen dioxide with respiratory symptoms and pulmonary function in children. Am J Epidemiol 134:204–19.

Needham LL, Hill RH, Ashley DL, Pirkle JL, Sampson EJ. (1995). The priority toxicant reference range study: interim report. Environ Health Perspect 103 (Suppl 3):89–94.

Ober C, Moffatt MF. (2000). Contributing factors to the pathobiology. The genetics of asthma. Clin Chest Med 21:245–61.

Park JH, Spiegelman DL, Burge HA, Gold DR, Chew GL, Milton DK. (2000). Longitudinal study of dust and airborne endotoxin in the home. Environ Health Perspect 108:1023–8.

Pearce N, Beasley R, Burgess C, Crane J. (1998). Asthma epidemiology. principles and methods. New York: Oxford University Press.

Pearce N, Douwes J, Beasley R. (2000). Is allergen exposure the major primary cause of asthma? Thorax 55:424–31.

Pekkanen J, Pearce N. (1999). Defining asthma in epidemiological studies. Eur Respir J 14:951–7.

Pinkerton KE, Joad JP. (2000). The mammalian respiratory system and critical windows of exposure for children's health. Environ Health Perspect 108(Suppl 3): 457–62.

Sasco AJ, Vainio H. (1999). From in utero and childhood exposure to parental smoking to childhood cancer: a possible link and the need for action. Hum Exp Toxicol 18:192–201.

Schwartz J, Weiss ST. (1995). Relationship of skin test reactivity to decrements in pulmonary function in children with asthma or frequent wheezing. Am J Respir Crit Care Med 152:2176–80.

Shapiro GG, Wighton TG, Chinn T, Zuckrman J, Eliassen AH, Picciano JF, Platts-Mills TA. (1999). House dust mite avoidance for children with asthma in homes of low-income families. J Allergy Clin Immunol 103:1069–74.

Stevenson LA, Gergen PJ, Hoover DR, Rosenstreich D, Mannino DM, Matte TD. (2001). Sociodemographic correlates of indoor allergen sensitivity among United States children. J Allergy Clin Immunol 108:747–52.

Strachan DP, Cook DG. (1997). Parental smoking and lower respiratory illness in infancy and early childhood. Thorax 52:905–14.

Strachan DP, Cook DG. (1998a). Parental smoking, middle ear disease and adenotonsillectomy in children. Thorax 53:50–6.

Strachan DP, Cook DG. (1998b). Parental smoking and childhood asthma: longitudinal and case-control studies. Thorax 53:204–12.

U.S. Environmental Protection Agency. (1992). Respiratory health effects of passive smoking: lung cancer and other disorders (EPA/600/9-90/006F). Washington, DC: U.S. Environmental Protection Agency.

U.S. Environmental Protection Agency. (1998). Inside IAQ (EPA/600/N-98/002). Research Triangle Park, NC: U.S. Environmental Protection Agency.

Verhoeff AP, Burge HA. (1997). Health risk assessment of fungi in home environments. Ann Allergy Asthma Immunol 78:544–54.

Vojta PJ, Friedman W, Marker DA, Clickner R, Rogers JW, Viet SM, Muilenberg ML, Thorne PS, Arbes SJ Jr, Zeldin DC. (2002). First national survey of lead and allergens in housing: survey design and methods for the allergen and endotoxin components. Environ Health Perspect 110:527–32.

von Mutius E, Schwartz J, Neas LM, Dockery D, Weiss ST. (2001). Relation of body mass index to asthma and atopy in children: the National Health and Nutrition Examination Study III. Thorax 56:835–8.

Wallace L. (1993). A decade of studies of human exposure: what have we learned? Risk Anal 13:135–9.

Wallace L, Buckley T, Pellizzari E, Gordon S. (1996). Breath measurements as volatile organic compound biomarkers. Environ Health Perspect 104(Suppl 5): 861–9.

Wallace LA. (1991). Comparison of risks from outdoor and indoor exposure to toxic chemicals. Environ Health Perspect 95:7–13.

Wang X, Zuckerman B, Pearson C, Kaufman G, Chen C, Wang G, Niu T, Wise PH, Bauchner H, Xu X. (2002). Maternal cigarette smoking, metabolic gene polymorphism, and infant birth weight. JAMA 287:195–202.

Wigle DT, Collishaw NE, Kirkbride J. (1987). Exposure of involuntary smokers to toxic components of tobacco smoke. Can J Public Health 78:151–4.

Windham GC, Eaton A, Hopkins B. (1999). Evidence for an association between environmental tobacco smoke exposure and birthweight: a meta-analysis and new data. Paediatr Perinat Epidemiol 13:35–57.

Windham GC, Swan SH, Fenster L. (1992). Parental cigarette smoking and the risk of spontaneous abortion. Am J Epidemiol 135:1394–1403.

Witschi H, Joad JP, Pinkerton KE. (1997). The toxicology of environmental tobacco smoke. Annu Rev Pharmacol Toxicol 37:29–52.

Wood RA, Johnson EF, Van Natta ML, Chen PH, Eggleston PA. (1998). A placebo-controlled trial of a HEPA air cleaner in the treatment of cat allergy. Am J Respir Crit Care Med 158:115–20.

Yang X, Zhang YP, Chen D, Chen WG, Wang R. (2001). Eye irritation caused by formaldehyde as an indoor air pollution—a controlled human exposure experiment. Biomed Environ Sci 14:229–36.

11
Outdoor Air

About 1.5 billion people in developed countries live in urban areas and are chronically exposed to outdoor air pollution, mainly from vehicular and industrial emissions. The WHO forecasts that urban populations will grow fastest in economically disadvantaged countries, comprise 62% of the world's population by the year 2025, and live in increasingly dense centers of anthropogenic emissions. Over 150 million tons of air pollutants are emitted annually in United States alone. Closely related to population growth and urbanization are the uncertain potential impacts of global climatic change on local, regional, and global air quality.

A severe air pollution episode in a river valley in Belgium during 1930 caused several thousand acute respiratory illnesses and about 60 deaths. A similar air pollution episode was associated with several thousand respiratory illness cases and 19 deaths in Donora, Pennsylvania, in 1948 when industrial emissions were trapped in a river valley by a temperature inversion. The severe London smog episode of December 1952 caused about 4000 excess deaths over a 5-day period during which visibility was reduced to as little as 1–5 m. Although most of the excess deaths were from cardiorespiratory diseases among the elderly, death rates doubled among young children. The smog was caused by a persistent temperature inversion combined with extensive use of coal by industry and for home heating; estimated particulate matter (PM) and sulfur dioxide (SO$_2$) levels were greatly elevated. A similar episode in London during 1956 lasted for only 18 hours but was associated with about 1000 excess deaths. These incidents showed that severe air pollution can cause substantial excess mortality and led to the U.K. 1956 Clean Air Act.

The EPA has defined two major air pollutant categories: (*1*) criteria air pollutants—CO, NO$_2$, SO$_2$, PM, lead, and ozone are clearly recognized human health threats and are regulated under national ambient air quality standards (NAAQS) and (*2*) hazardous air pollutants (HAPs)—this group comprises 189 substances reasonably expected to cause serious health effects and under review for establishment of emission standards. Motor vehicles produce most of the CO, NO$_2$, and VOCs in ambient urban air. Fossil fuels combusted by industry (especially coal) and motor vehicles (especially diesel fuel) are the major sources of ambient air PM$_{2.5}$ and SO$_2$. Photochemical smog was first recognized in California during the 1940s and 1950s when greatly increased motor vehicle emissions and secondary pollutants from photochemical reactions were trapped in the Los Angeles basin; about 75% of southern urban Californians reported eye irritation during peak smog periods in 1960.

Although concentrations of individual toxic chemicals in ambient air are highly correlated, substantial evidence links each of the criteria air pollutants to respiratory and other health effects in children. Children may be more exposed than adults to outdoor air pollutants because they breathe more air per unit body weight at rest, spend more time outdoors, and have higher activity levels. Asthmatic children are generally more susceptible than healthy children to respiratory impacts of outdoor air pollution.

The objective of this chapter is to describe the major known and probable effects of outdoor air pollution, with a focus on children living in modern urban environments. The discussion includes the relationships between major categories of outdoor air toxics and potential developmental and respiratory effects. The chapter closes with a discussion of major sources of outdoor air toxics and interventions aimed at reducing their health effects. Chapters 4 and 5 (Metals), Chapter 7 (Pesticides), Chapter 9 (Radiation), and Chapter 10 (Indoor Air) address other indoor and outdoor air contaminants.

HEALTH EFFECTS

Many studies have shown consistent associations between daily ambient PM levels and daily cardiovascular, respiratory, and total deaths involving mainly older persons; associations have generally been stronger after applying lag periods of up to a few days. The estimated average increases in daily total, cardiovascular, and respiratory disease mortality, respectively, are about 1%, 1.4%, and 3.4% per 10 $\mu g/m^3$ increment in PM_{10} levels (Dockery and Pope, 1994). Elevations of PM_{10} have also been accompanied by increased hospitalizations and emergency room and physician visits of children for asthma and other respiratory diseases.

Mechanisms of Toxicity

Particulate Matter

Particulate matter comprises solid, liquid, or mixed particles suspended in air with variable size, composition, and origins (Table 11–1). Because the health effects of PM are strongly related to particle size, PM size categories have been defined for regulatory purposes. Primary PM is emitted directly into the atmosphere and occurs in ultrafine, fine, and coarse size ranges. Older studies measured total suspended particles (TSP), a fraction including particles up to 40 μm in diameter. Whereas fine ($PM_{1.0-2.5}$) particles can remain in the atmosphere for days to weeks and may travel through the atmosphere hundreds to thousands of kilometers from sources, coarse particles ($PM_{2.5-10}$) usually settle to earth within minutes to hours and within tens of kilometers from sources. Coarse particles often originate from the earth's crust and usually contain oxides of iron, calcium, silicon, and aluminum.

Secondary PM is formed in the atmosphere through chemical and physical transformations of ultrafine particles ($PM_{1.0}$) and gases that coalesce to form $PM_{2.5}$; the latter contains sulfates, nitrates, ammonium ion, elemental carbon, PAHs, other toxic organic carbon compounds, and metals. Particle size is influenced by humidity; uptake of water by airborne particles increases their size and contributes to visible haze during summer smog episodes.

Toxicity of inhaled particles depends on their physical and chemical properties, particularly the size, solubility, and content of toxic substances including organic chemicals and metals. Health concerns about PM have increasingly focused on fine and ultrafine particles because they are deposited in peripheral airways and alveoli and contain higher concentrations of toxic chemicals than larger particles. Fine particles are highly respirable and have very large surface areas, making excellent carriers for adsorbed inorganic and organic toxics, particularly PAHs, nitro-PAHs, and oxidized PAH derivatives. Coarse particles are deposited mainly in the upper airways or larger bronchi and larger particles (≥ 10 μm) in the nasopharynx.

TABLE 11–1. Criteria Air Pollutants

Contaminant	Characteristics	Sources
PM		
1. Coarse particles (PM$_{2.5-10}$)	2.5 μm $\leq$ diameter < 10 μm	Mechanical processes, such as crushing or grinding activities, construction, farming, and mining activities, paved and unpaved roadways; fuel combustion; biologic sources—grass, tree, and other plant pollens, mold spores
2. Fine particles (PM$_{1.0-2.5}$)	1.0 μm $\leq$ diameter < 2.5 μm	Direct emissions from motor vehicles, industries, wood burning, construction, tilled fields, unpaved roads, stone crushing; secondary formation in atmosphere from gases emitted by motor vehicles and industry (SO$_2$, NO$_x$, ammonia, and VOCs)
3. Ultrafine particles (PM$_{1.0}$)	Diameter < 1.0 μm	Condensation of hot vapors formed during high-temperature combustion, such as in motor vehicle catalytic converters
NO$_x$	Odorless, highly reactive gases; NO$_2$ contributes to reddish-brown color of urban smog	Fuel combustion at high temperature, such as in internal combustion engines, electric utilities
SO$_2$	Colorless gas with a choking odor	Combustion of fossil fuels such as diesel fuel, high-sulfur gasoline, coal
CO	Colorless, odorless gas	Incomplete combustion, such as in internal combustion engines, industries, wood burning
Ozone	Pale blue gas with strong odor; potent oxidizing agent and respiratory tract irritant	Photochemical reactions of NO$_x$ and VOCs mainly from motor vehicle emissions in the presence of sunlight under summer conditions
Lead[a]	Metal	Leaded gasoline, lead smelters

[a]See Chapter 4 for further discussion of lead.

Deposited PM is cleared from the larger ciliated airways by the mucociliary ladder to the pharynx and swallowed or expectorated; impaired clearance at high exposure levels appears to be greater among children than adults. Fine particles deposited in peripheral airways and alveoli are phagocytosed by lung macrophages that migrate via the mucociliary ladder or enter the lymphatic system and migrate to regional lymph nodes. In human volunteers, inhaled ultrafine carbon particles labeled with technetium-99 were rapidly absorbed into the bloodstream and distributed to the liver and other tissues, showing the potential for inhaled particles to cause toxic effects in extrapulmonary tissues (Nemmar et al., 2002). Some particles are retained in the lungs; a comparison of autopsy lung tissue from never-smoking women in Mexico City and Vancouver, Canada, showed that the Mexican women had sevenfold higher geometric mean particles per gram of lung tissue, a finding consistent with the higher PM levels in Mexico City (Brauer et al., 2001).

Diesel particles have a mass median aerodynamic diameter of 0.2 μm and comprise a carbonaceous core (about 80% of the particle mass) and organic chemicals (about 20% of the mass). Based on human lung models, about 10% of inhaled diesel exhaust particles are deposited in alveoli; the modeled particle mass deposited per unit alveolar surface area per minute peaked at age 2 years at levels twice those of adults. Diesel exhaust PM promotes release of cytokines, chemokines, immunoglobulins, and oxidants that can cause respiratory tract inflammation (Pandya et al., 2002). In adult volunteers exposed to diesel exhaust, there were increased neutrophils and myeloperoxidase in sputum and increased expression of inflammatory response genes (IL-5, IL-8, and growth-regulated oncogene-α) in bronchial tissue and bronchial wash cells. Diesel exhaust PM contains several known carcinogens including polycyclic mononitroarenes; exposure is widespread, as shown by the presence of mononitroarene-hemoglobin adducts in blood samples from most persons, with levels being higher among urban compared to rural residents. Among toxic chemicals in diesel exhaust, 3-nitrobenzanthrone is a particularly powerful mutagen.

Gases
Ozone reacts with polyunsaturated fatty acids and with sulfhydryl, amino, and other tissue compounds and generates free radicals that cause further oxidative tissue damage. Ozone exposure of healthy and atopic children is associated with nasal lavage inflammatory reaction biomarkers (increased leukocyte counts, eosinophilic cationic protein, and myeloperoxidase activity) and urinary eosinophil protein X levels (a marker of

eosinophil activation). Controlled exposure of human volunteers to ozone, NO_2, or diesel exhaust causes an acute inflammatory response in airways (Krishna et al., 1998). Acute effects in animals exposed to ozone at near-ambient levels or to NO_2 at levels far above ambient concentrations include lipid peroxidation, inflammation and increased permeability of airways, bronchial hyperreactivity to inhaled aeroallergens and broncho-constrictive agents, lung function deficits, and reduced mucociliary clearance. Monkeys exposed to high-level ozone for 90 days develop a dose-related bronchiolar inflammatory response with thicker walls and increased nonciliated bronchiolar epithelial cells, interstitial smooth muscle cells, macrophages, mast cells, and neutrophils; monkeys exposed for a year develop persistent pulmonary fibrosis.

Acute exposure to high SO_2 levels in controlled exposure studies also causes an inflammatory response indicated by neutrophilia in broncho-alveolar lavage fluid. Ozone appears to be much potent than NO_2 in triggering airway inflammation in healthy persons. But NO_2 is a precursor of photochemically produced stronger oxidants including ozone, nitric oxide (NO), peroxyacetyl nitrate (PAN), and peroxypropionyl nitrate. Exposure of human nasal or bronchial epithelial cells in vitro to NO_2, ozone, and diesel exhaust PM causes release of proinflammatory mediators; the latter increase eosinophil chemotaxis and adherence to endothelial cells, possibly offering a mechanism for pollution-induced airway inflammation.

Carbon monoxide binds with high affinity to the iron present in heme-proteins, that is, hemoglobin, myoglobin, and cytochromes. At low CO levels, toxicity is mainly caused by tissue hypoxia due to conversion of hemoglobin to carboxyhemoglobin, a relatively stable complex incapable of transporting oxygen to tissues. Secondary toxic mechanisms include binding of CO to myoglobin in heart and skeletal muscle and to cytochromes in various tissues, thereby interfering with oxygen storage and mitochondrial energy generation.

Volatile Organic Carbons
Emissions by motor vehicles of incompletely combusted hydrocarbons and evaporative fuel losses are the major sources of ambient urban VOCs. There are over 600 VOCs having three main types of toxicity: (1) participation in atmospheric photochemical reactions that increase ground-level ozone levels, (2) genotoxicity, and (3) carcinogenicity. In the absence of anthropogenic air pollution, ozone levels remain relatively low because ozone reacts with NO to produce NO_2 and oxygen, reactions that equilibrate in the absence of VOCs. By reacting with NO, VOCs cause a net increase in ozone levels. Photochemically driven oxidation of VOCs pro-

duces highly reactive hydrocarbon radicals that react with other smog components to form PAN and aldehydes, reactive chemicals that contribute to eye and respiratory tract irritation.

Volatile organic chemicals include benzene, a known human carcinogen that causes acute myeloid leukemia after prolonged occupational exposure at relatively high levels. It is not known if lifelong low-level exposure to benzene in ambient air increases the risk of cancer (see also Chapter 10, Indoor Air, for further discussion of benzene).

Developmental Effects

Birth Weight

Several epidemiologic studies have demonstrated fairly consistent associations between low birth weight, preterm birth, IUGR, and forms of ambient air pollution including CO, SO_2, and PM during pregnancy, particularly during the first trimester (Bobak, 2000; Bobak and Leon, 1999; Ha et al., 2001; Maisonet et al., 2001; Ritz and Yu, 1999; Ritz et al., 2000; Wang et al., 1997). There is some indication that IUGR is associated with ambient air PAHs, independent of PM_{10} levels (Dejmek et al., 2000). Sensitivity of the fetus during organogenesis to mutagens such as PAHs may relate in part to their ability to inhibit trophoblast invasion of the endometrium and impair placental function. Ambient CO levels routinely exceeded 300 ppm in the Los Angeles basin during the early 1970s, levels that could produce maternal blood carboxyhemoglobin levels equivalent to those due to smoking 20 cigarettes per day (6%–10% of total hemoglobin), thereby reducing the fetal oxygen supply. Ambient CO levels also increase fetal blood carboxyhemoglobin levels, further reducing the oxygen supply to rapidly growing fetal tissues. Animal models have shown that low-level CO (75–150 ppm) caused reduced birth weight and postnatal weight gain in rats.

Stillbirths and Early Childhood Deaths

There is some epidemiologic evidence, mainly from time series ecologic studies, of associations between multiple ambient air pollutants and stillbirths (Pereira et al., 1998), PM and SIDS (Woodruff et al., 1997), and multiple pollutants and early childhood respiratory deaths (Conceicao et al., 2001).

Birth Defects

The first large, population-based study of outdoor air pollution and birth defects was a record-based case-control study of orofacial clefts and cardiac defects in the Los Angeles region (Ritz et al., 2002). There were exposure–risk relationships between average ambient CO levels near the mother's residence during the second month of gestation and the risk of cardiac ventricular septal defects ($OR = 3.0$, CI 1.4–6.1, for the fourth versus the first CO quartiles) and aortic/pulmonary artery valve defects. No clear relationships between these birth defects and other air pollutants were apparent.

Respiratory Function and Diseases

Respiratory health effects from exposure to ambient air pollution during childhood range from subtle transient lung function deficits to coughing, asthma episodes, and irreversible lung function deficits. Supporting evidence for health effects of individual major air pollutants comes from controlled exposure, epidemiologic, and animal studies. Controlled exposure studies have generally involved acute exposures of volunteers in test chambers or through mouthpieces to air/contaminant mixtures over periods ranging from less than an hour to a few hours, small sample sizes (often fewer than 20 subjects), intermittent exercise (to increase ventilation rates and contaminant doses), and spirometry to measure changes in lung function indicators (see Chapter 10, Indoor Air, for a description of spirometry tests).

Observational epidemiologic studies of ambient air quality enable assessment of the mixed, variable, and chronic exposures common in the general population over periods of days to years, for example, major air pollution episodes lasting a few days, intermittent exposure to summertime smog episodes, or average air quality during pregnancy or childhood. Commonly used variations of general epidemiologic study designs in this field include (1) panel studies involving small cohorts (often fewer than 100 subjects) that are intensively studied for a limited time (weeks to months), for example, through daily symptom diaries, daily self-administered peak expiratory flow (PEF) tests, frequent ambient air monitoring, and, sometimes, personal air monitoring, (2) ecologic time-trend analytic studies of daily respiratory health events (e.g., emergency room visits or physician contacts) and daily ambient air quality data, and (3) hybrid studies—many cohort and cross-sectional studies have collected certain exposure and health outcome data for individual subjects and regional ambient air quality data. Only a few epidemiologic studies have used personal air sampling (and these were small, short-term studies) or repeated standardized respiratory function tests (instead of self-administered PEF tests).

Lung function deficits after brief exposure to ambient air pollutants or intense air pollution episodes are generally reversible within hours or days but may cause clinically significant effects in sensitive groups including children (especially asthmatics) and the elderly. Although small lung function deficits are not clinically obvious, some children experience relatively large effects and chronic exposure to intermittently high air pollution levels is associated with lung function growth deficits in preadolescent children, that is, reduced growth rates of lung capacity. Epidemiologic studies have not shown clear evidence of a threshold for the inverse relationships between ozone or PM and lung function deficits in children. The majority of studies have focused on the relation between ambient air pollution and exacerbation of existing asthma rather than incident disease. Bronchial hyperreactivity is a major feature of asthma and appears to predispose children to larger decrements of lung function during air pollution episodes. See Chapter 10 (Indoor Air) for further discussion of childhood asthma.

Particulate Matter
Ambient air PM, acid, and NO_2 levels are highly correlated, precluding conclusive attribution of health effects to any one pollutant. Reviews by the California Environmental Protection Agency and the EPA concluded that PM_{10} is associated with exacerbation of asthma and increased respiratory illness in children, with no evidence of a threshold (California Environmental Protection Agency, 2000; U.S. Environmental Protection Agency, 2001a). Specific findings from these reviews and individual studies include

- Acute exposure—elevated daily PM levels appear to cause PEF deficits, cough, asthma exacerbation, and acute respiratory illness in healthy and/or asthmatic children.
- Chronic exposure—average PM (or acid aerosol) levels are associated with lung function deficits, lung function growth deficits, respiratory symptoms, acute respiratory illness, and school absenteeism in healthy and/or asthmatic children.

Ozone
Ozone is a powerful oxidant and a pulmonary irritant that causes average FEV_1 deficits of 5%–10% after controlled exposure (up to 3 hours) of adolescents or young adults to levels as low as 80–120 ppb while exercising intermittently (see, e.g., McDonnell et al., 1999). After such exposure, some sensitive subjects develop much higher FEV_1 deficits. Chronic ambient ozone exposure appears to cause persistent lung function deficits, but the exposure–risk relationship between average daily exposures and

chronic effects remains poorly defined (California Environmental Protection Agency, 2000). Associations between ozone and respiratory effects are stronger during the summer because of the higher ambient ozone levels (Burnett et al., 2001; Kopp et al., 2000). Asthmatics are more susceptible than nonasthmatics to lung function deficits, airway inflammation, and bronchial hyperreactivity after ozone exposure.

Personal air ozone levels are generally much lower than ambient levels except during outdoor activities (Suh et al., 2000); thus, ambient levels tend to misclassify individual ozone exposures, a factor that may explain some inconsistencies in observational epidemiologic studies. Ozone appears to produce stronger effects among active children in field settings than in controlled exposure studies, possibly because of (1) longer exposures, (2) potentiation by other ambient air pollutants, (3) persistence of effects from exposures on previous days, and (4) persistence of a transient response associated with the daily peak of exposure. Findings concerning respiratory effects of ozone include the following:

- Acute exposure
  - Daily ozone levels while exercising outdoors during summer are associated with lung function deficits among healthy and asthmatic children, with exposure–risk relationships extending to levels below the current ozone 1-hour NAAQS (120 ppb); a pooled analysis of six summer camp panel studies of nonasthmatic children yielded a slope of -0.50 ml FEV_1/ppb ozone ($p < .0001$) based on the average ozone level during the hour before lung function measurements (Kinney et al., 1996).
  - Asthma exacerbations severe enough to require medical care and school absenteeism are linked to ozone, especially after prolonged episodes (see, e.g., Burnett et al., 2001; Gilliland et al., 2001).
- Chronic exposure
  - Recent studies produced conflicting evidence of lung function growth deficits among preadolescent children living in areas subject to high summertime ozone levels (Frischer et al., 1999; Gauderman et al., 2000).
  - Average lifetime ozone exposure appeared to cause persistent lung function deficits among nonsmoking, nonasthmatic college freshmen (Kunzli et al., 1997).
  - Asthma—incident asthma was strongly associated with involvement in three or more sports in high-ozone areas in southern California (McConnell et al., 2002); asthma symptom scores were much more closely associated with personal air than ambient ozone levels (Delfino et al., 1996).

Sulfur Dioxide and Related Pollutants

Sulfur dioxide and sulfuric acid are strong irritants that appear to cause transient lung function deficits, reduced bronchial mucociliary clearance, respiratory symptoms, asthma exacerbation, and respiratory illness (California Environmental Protection Agency, 2000). Sulfur dioxide is very soluble in water and tends to be absorbed in the upper airways by subjects at rest, but some of it reaches peripheral lung airways at higher ventilation rates. In air, SO_2 is converted to sulfuric acid and sulfate, substances associated with the fine PM fraction; the health effects attributed to fine PM may, therefore, be partially caused by the sulfate component. Health effects attributable to SO_2 and derivatives include the following (see "Particulate Matter" above for effects of chronic exposure to acid aerosols):

- Lung function deficits—adolescent asthmatics are more sensitive than nonasthmatics to lung function deficits after exposure to SO_2 or sulfuric acid aerosol during controlled studies or intense air pollution episodes; the exposure–risk relationship between controlled SO_2 concentration and FEV_1 deficits appears to be continuous, with no evidence of a threshold (World Health Organization, 2000).
- Respiratory symptoms—many asthmatics and some nonasthmatics with allergies develop respiratory symptoms after brief exposure to SO_2 in controlled exposure studies; such effects are found consistently in exercising asthmatics at SO_2 levels of 400 ppb or greater (California Environmental Protection Agency, 2000).

Nitrogen Dioxide

Nitrogen dioxide is a much weaker oxidant than ozone and appears to be much less potent in causing airway inflammation in healthy persons. A meta-analysis of controlled NO_2 exposure studies of adults indicated a trend for airflow rates to decrease among healthy persons at levels above 1 ppm and among asthmatics at lower levels. Exposure to NO_2 at levels as low as 260 ppb for 30 minutes increased the bronchial responsiveness of asthmatics to subsequent challenge with common aeroallergens (California Environmental Protection Agency, 2000). Relatively high personal air NO_2 levels were associated with incident asthma in Montreal (Infante-Rivard, 1993) and asthma exacerbation (Linaker et al., 2000). Prevalent and recent-onset asthma among children in Austria were associated with ambient NO_2 levels in communities where children had lived for at least 2 years (Studnicka et al., 1997). Firm conclusions are not possible, however, because ambient NO_2 is correlated with PM and other emissions from high-temperature combustion processes (California Environmental Protection Agency, 2000).

Mixed Pollutants

There is limited evidence of lung function deficits after controlled exposure of asthmatic children to mixed air pollutants, possibly because of the small sample sizes and short duration of exposure and observation. For instance, controlled exposure of young adult asthmatics to NO_2 and ozone or to NO_2 and SO_2 increased bronchoconstriction after challenge with house-dust mite antigen. Several cross-sectional and longitudinal studies showed associations between prolonged exposure to multiple ambient air pollutants and lung function deficits and lung function growth deficits (see, e.g., Gauderman et al., 2000; Schwartz, 1989). Asthma exacerabation and respiratory symptoms have been associated with long-term exposure to multiple air pollutants and traffic density indices (see, e.g., Boezen et al., 1999; McConnell et al., 1999). Daily asthma events severe enough to require medical care have been associated with exposure to two or more major ambient air pollutants (see, e.g., Hajat et al., 1999).

Aeroallergens

Aeroallergens are usually proteins carried on inhalable particles, the major outdoor sources being plant pollens and mold spores. Approximately 80% of asthmatic children are skin-prick positive to one or more aeroallergens (see Chapter 10, Indoor Air, for discussion of indoor aeroallergens). Increased daily ambient air spore counts for specific fungi or total spore counts have been linked to respiratory symptoms, asthma exacerbation, and daily asthma deaths. Other findings include

- Acute exposure—daily ambient air fungal spore counts and soybean allergen concentrations have been associated with asthma exacerbation severe enough to require medical care and asthma deaths among children and young adults (see, e.g., Dales et al., 2000; Downs et al., 2001).
- Chronic exposure—skin prick sensitization to *Alternaria* has been linked to incident and prevalent asthma among children and young adults (Gergen and Turkeltaub, 1992; Halonen et al., 1997).

Cancer

Diesel exhaust is a major source of fine and ultrafine particles in urban ambient air and has been identified as a probable human carcinogen by the IARC, the U.S. National Toxicology Program, and the EPA (International Agency for Research on Cancer, 1989; National Institute for Environmental Health Sciences, 2001; U.S. Environmental Protection Agency, 2000b). A cohort study of 1.2 million U.S. adults showed that each $PM_{2.5}$ increment of 10 $\mu g/m^3$ was associated with an 8% increased risk of lung cancer mortality, independent of smoking, occupation, and other risk factors (Pope et al., 2002). The role of childhood ambient air exposures in adult lung cancer is unknown.

The few epidemiologic studies of childhood cancer in relation to ambient air pollution were relatively small and used relatively crude exposure measures such as neighborhood traffic density or parent's occupation. There is limited evidence of associations between childhood leukemia and prenatal parental occupational exposure to benzene or gasoline or childhood exposure to high-density traffic (Fig. 11–1). A large Danish case-control study showed no association between maternal occupational benzene exposure or residential NO_2 exposure and childhood leukemia or CNS cancers but did show associations with childhood Hodgkin's disease (Raaschou-Nielsen et al., 2001). Two ecologic studies showed generally negative results but used very crude exposure indicators.

EXPOSURES

Under the Clean Air Act, the EPA was required to set NAAQS, to ensure that NAAQS are met through source control, and to monitor the effectiveness of the program. The act also required each state to establish a network of air monitoring stations for criteria air pollutants (CO, NO_2, ozone, PM_{10}, $PM_{2.5}$, SO_2, lead). The State and Local Monitoring Network (SLAMS) is a network of about 4000 monitoring stations sited and designed to meet the needs of state and local air pollution control agencies to support air program activities. The National Air Monitoring Network (NAMS) is a subset of about 1000 stations in SLAMS sited and designed to monitor the highest contaminant levels in areas of greatest population density. A separate network of stations monitors ozone precursors (about 60 VOCs and carbonyl) in 24 large population areas with extremely high ozone levels with two to five sites per area, depending on the population. Ideally, air-monitoring stations would provide accurate indices relevant to the occurrence of health effects in populations exposed to air pollutants. Obstacles to achieving this goal include the limited number of stations, sampling infrequency (e.g., 24-hour averages obscure short-term peaks), small-area variations in air contaminants (e.g., CO levels may vary substantially over short distances, depending on traffic density and other factors), and the dependence of personal exposure levels on behavioral factors.

The concentrations of pollutants in ambient air depend on the rate of emissions and the efficiency of dispersion; daily variations in pollutant levels depend more on meteorological conditions than on changes in

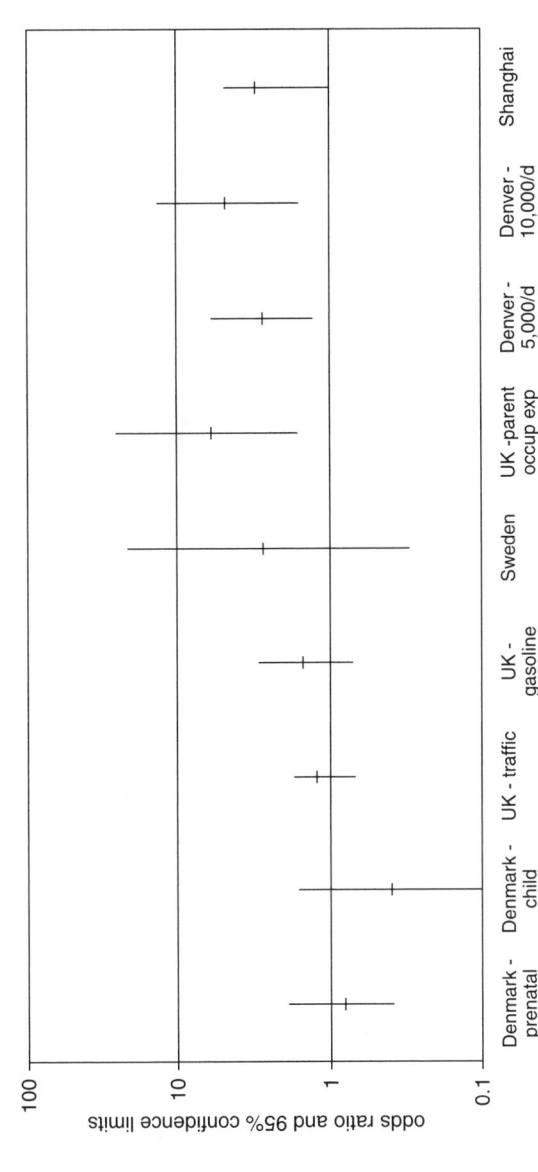

FIGURE 11–1. Epidemiologic studies of childhood leukemia and indicators of exposure to benzene and other motor vehicle emissions in outdoor air. Shanghai (Shu et al., 1988), Denver traffic density (Savitz and Feingold, 1989), U.K. parent occupational exposure (McKinley et al., 1991), Sweden NO$_2$ levels (Feychting et al., 1998), U.K. proximity to gasoline stations and main roads (Harrison et al., 1999), Denmark prenatal maternal and childhood residential exposure (Raaschou-Nielsen et al., 2001).

emission rates. Wind speed is the major factor influencing efficiency of dispersion; other factors depend on local conditions and include the effective trapping of atmospheric pollutants in valleys or basins by wind or atmospheric thermal inversions. Trends in ambient air levels of major air pollutants in the United States are shown in Table 11–2. Annual average ambient air levels decreased by 36% for CO and SO_2, 18% for PM_{10}, and 10% for NO_x (NO and NO_2) but by only 4% for ozone during the 1990s.

Particulate Matter

Early epidemiologic studies measured (TSP), that is particles up to about 40 μm in diameter. The TSP values include nonrespirable particles and are subject to measurement artifacts; since the late 1970s, most studies have measured PM_{10}, $PM_{2.5}$, and, occasionally, $PM_{1.0}$. Polycyclic aromatic hydrocarbons, other toxic organic carbon compounds, and sulfate occur mainly in $PM_{2.5}$. Ambient air $PM_{2.5}$ concentrations tend to be relatively uniform across large cities in eastern United States during the summer months, unlike PM_{10} levels, which show more spatial variation. The dependence of $PM_{2.5}$ levels on traffic volume is reflected in peak hourly levels during morning and evening rush hours and peak 24-hour averages during midweek, particularly at roadway monitoring sites. Both $PM_{2.5}$ and PM_{10} particles penetrate buildings, with indoor to outdoor concentration ratios approaching unity at high air exchange rates. Levels of PM vary by microenvironment; for example, geometric mean PM_{10} levels in subways and buses may be two to four times those in ambient outdoor air.

TABLE 11–2. Percent Change in Annual Average Emission and Ambient Air Pollutant Levels, United States, 1991–2000

Pollutant	Percent Change	
	Emissions	Ambient Air Levels
CO	−5	−41
NO_x	+3	−11
Ozone (1-hr)	na	−10
VOCs	−16	na
PM_{10}	−6[a]	−19
SO_2	−24	−37

Source: U.S. Environmental Protection Agency (2001b).
[a]Direct PM_{10} emissions.

Ozone

Elevated ambient ozone levels arise mainly from photochemical reactions of air pollutants under summer conditions. Indoor ozone levels are usually much lower than ambient levels because ozone is highly reactive and the indoor environment is rich in substances that react with ozone. Children are at risk of ozone exposure because they are often outdoors and physically active during summer, when ozone levels are highest; for example, children in summer camps may inhale ozone doses close to those that produce lung function deficits and respiratory symptoms in adults during controlled exposure studies. Annual average ozone levels in 24 communities in Canada and the United States varied from 16 to 35 ppb; 1-hour ozone levels exceeded the Canadian guideline (100 ppb) in 18 communities and the U.S. NAAQS (120 ppb) in 10 communities (Spengler et al., 1996). Monitoring of children in southern California during the summer ozone season showed that average personal summer ozone exposures were three to four times winter levels.

Sulfur Dioxide and Strong Acidity

Sulfurous and sulfuric acids, partially neutralized ammonium bisulfate salts, and fine PM are formed in atmospheric reactions between SO_2 and other fossil fuel emissions. Ambient air concentrations of these pollutants are highly correlated; for example, sulfates may comprise 20% or more of the $PM_{2.5}$ mass in regions such as the northeastern United States subject to air pollution from combustion of high-sulfur fuels, especially coal-burning electric power utility and diesel engine emissions. Total airborne acidic species are higher in summer because of atmospheric conversion of SO_2 and NO_2, respectively, to sulfuric acid (H_2SO_4) and nitric acid (HNO_3) through photochemical processes. The main vapor phase strong acids in the southwestern United States are HNO_3 and hydrochloric acid (HCl). Annual average particle strong acidity levels in 24 Canadian and U.S. communities ranged from below detection limits to about 50 nM/m^3, but single-day levels often exceeded 150 nM/m^3 during the summer in the "sulfate belt" comprising major portions of Tennessee, Kentucky, Ohio, Virginia, Pennsylvania, New York, and West Virginia (Spengler et al., 1996).

Nitrogen Dioxide

The annual average ambient NO_2 level in U.S. cities in 1998 was 18 ppb (U.S. Environmental Protection Agency, 2000d). Urban outdoor NO_x levels display diurnal variation related to morning and late afternoon rush hour traffic but little seasonal variation. In cities with high traffic density,

1-hour outdoor NO_2 levels reach about 100 ppb and occasionally reach 400 ppb during urban air pollution episodes.

Volatile Organic Chemicals

Modeled estimates of long-term outdoor air levels of 148 VOCs in the United States indicated an average of 14 VOCs in each census tract for which concentrations exceeded health-based benchmarks for cancer or noncancer outcomes (Woodruff et al., 1998). Formaldehyde, benzene, and 1,3-butadiene levels exceeded cancer benchmark levels in over 90% of all census tracts (Table 11–3). About 10% of census tracts had one or more VOCs at levels conferring a cancer risk of at least 10^{-4}.

Personal Air

Individual exposure to air pollutants varies with ambient and indoor air pollutant concentrations in the microenvironments that a person moves through during daily activities, the time spent and activities undertaken in each microenvironment, and ventilation rates. Personal air $PM_{2.5}$ levels among nonsmoking children and adults living in nonsmoking homes were correlated with ambient $PM_{2.5}$ but not with personal gaseous pollutant levels (Sarnat et al., 2001). Personal exposures to reactive gaseous pollutants are driven more by time spent outdoors than by ambient air levels, suggesting that they should not be confounders of ambient $PM_{2.5}$ and health effects. A person may be exposed to more ozone during an

TABLE 11–3. Hazardous Air Pollutants with Ambient Concentrations Above Cancer Benchmark Levels

HAP	Average Level ($\mu g/m^3$)	Cancer Benchmark ($\mu g/m^3$)	Ratio	% of Census Tracts Above Level
Formaldehyde	0.25	0.077	3.2	94
Benzene	0.48	0.12	4.0	92
Ethylene dichloride	0.061	0.038	1.6	21
Chloroform	0.083	0.043	1.9	8
Carbon tetrachloride	0.88	0.067	13	3
Ethylene dibromide	0.0077	0.0045	1.7	1
Bis(2-ethylhexyl) phthalate	1.6	0.25	6.4	<1
Methyl chloride	1.2	0.56	2.2	<1

Source: Woodruff et al. (1998).

hour of vigorous exercise outdoors than while spending several hours indoors with low average physical activity.

Findings from monitoring of children's personal air contaminant levels include:

- Particulate matter—personal air $PM_{2.5}$ levels among children without ETS exposure were strongly correlated with but higher than ambient levels.
- Ozone—in southern California, average personal air ozone exposure levels were about 22 ppb during summer months and 6 ppb during winter months.
- Nitrogen dioxide—personal air exposures among children tend to be more closely related to indoor sources (gas appliances, smokers) than to ambient NO_2 levels.
- Volatile organic chemicals—personal air benzene levels were associated with front-door ambient levels, riding in cars, moped driving, and refueling of cars (Raaschou-Nielsen et al., 1997).

Biomarkers

There are relatively few biomarkers of ambient air pollution uptake. Hemoglobin adducts of 1-nitropyrene and 2-nitrofluorene and urinary 1-hydroxypyrene are non-specific biomarkers of exposure to diesel PM (other sources include mainstream tobacco smoke and cooked animal fats). Urinary 1-hydroxypyrene was detected in the majority of Harlem seventh-grade students, including nonsmokers (Northridge et al., 1999). Urinary levels of trans-muconic acid (a metabolite of benzene) among inner-city children were associated with time spent playing near the street but not with ETS exposure or urinary cotinine (Weaver et al., 1996). Carbon monoxide binds tightly to hemoglobin, forming carboxyhemoglobin (half-life of 2–6 hours); carboxyhemoglobin blood levels reflect the concentration and duration of CO exposure, exercise, and other factors and can be estimated by direct blood analysis or by measuring CO in exhaled breath.

RISK MANAGEMENT

Sources

The major sources of ambient air pollutants in the United States are motor vehicles (53% of NO_x, 79% of CO, 44% of VOCs) and electricity generation (67% of SO_2) (Table 11–4). Emissions from these sources are ex-

TABLE 11–4. Major Sources of Ambient Air Pollutant Emissions, United States, 1998 (Percent by Source)

Source	$PM_{2.5}$[a]	SO_2	NO_2	CO	VOCs
Electricity generation	2.0	67.3	25.8	0.5	0.3
Motor vehicles	7.3	7.2	53.3	78.6	43.5
Industries	11.7	25.3	19.9	9.6	12.6
Solvent use	<0.1	<0.1	<0.1	<0.1	29.5
Biogenic sources	9.5	<0.1	<0.1	<0.1	<0.1
Other	69.4[b]	0.3	1.8	11.4[c]	14.1[c]
Total (percent)	100.0	100.0	100.0	100.0	100.0
Total (thousands of tons)	8,379	19,647	24,454	89,454	17,917

Source: U.S. Environmental Protection Agency (2000c).

[a]Directly emitted particles; secondary fine particles also formed from SO_2, NO_x, NH_s, and VOCs in the atmosphere.

[b]Includes agriculture, forestry, fugitive dust (roads, construction), and other combustion.

[c]Includes domestic gasoline-powered devices, recreational marine vessels, aircraft, and other sources.

tremely complex, with hundreds of identified compounds, including PM, gases, VOCs, and metals. See Chapters 4 and 5 (Metals) for further discussion of selected metals.

Particulate Matter

Exhaust emissions from gasoline and diesel engines of similar power contain similar types of toxic chemicals, but diesel engines are more important sources of NO_2, PM, and certain PAH carcinogens (e.g., nitroarenes) than gasoline engines with catalytic converters. Diesel engines produce 69% of the PM_{10} emissions from motor vehicles in the United States (U.S. Environmental Protection Agency, 2000c). Catalytic converters of the type used with gasoline vehicles substantially reduce total PM and VOC emissions but increase emissions of ultrafine particles. In many rural temperate and northern regions, wood burning for heat and cooking and forest fires, respectively, are major sources of ambient PM during winter and summer months.

Ozone

Ground-level ozone has two main origins: downward transport of ozone from the stratosphere and photochemical reactions near the earth's surface driven by anthropogenic emissions. The former contributes about 5–15 ppb to background terrestrial ozone levels. The major reactions driving the formation of ground-level ozone are illustrated in Figure 11–2; the

Motor vehicles emit NO_2 and VOCs

NO_2 + solar energy $\longrightarrow$ NO + O (ground state oxygen)

$O + O_2 \longrightarrow O_3$ (ozone)

$NO + O_3 \longrightarrow NO_2 + O_2$

O_3 + solar energy $\longrightarrow O_2 + O^c$ (charged oxygen)

$O^c + H_2O \longrightarrow 2\ OH^*$ (hydroxyl radicals)

$CO + OH^* \longrightarrow CO_2 + HO_2^*$ (hydroperoxy radical)

$HO_2^* + NO \longrightarrow NO_2 + OH^*$

$O_3 + NO_2 \longrightarrow O_2 + NO_3^*$ (nitrate radical – forms mainly at night)

$2\ NO_3^* + H_2O \longrightarrow 2HNO_2 + O_3$

$HNO_2 + hv \longrightarrow OH^* + NO$

$R + OH^* \longrightarrow R^* + H_2O$ (R = a volatile organic carbon)

$R^* + O_2 \longrightarrow ROO^*$ (peroxy radical)

$ROO^* + NO \longrightarrow RO + NO_2$

$NO_2 + OH^* \longrightarrow HNO_3$ (nitric acid – forms inorganic vapor acid)

$SO_2 + 2\ OH^* \longrightarrow H_2SO_4$

FIGURE 11–2. Formation of ground-level ozone and related photochemical oxidative reactions.

net result is to produce peak ground-level NO_2 levels by midmorning and maximum ozone levels by midday or early afternoon. Ozone from urban sources is transported over considerable distances to rural downwind locations and is relatively persistent there because of lower NO levels (NO reacts with and depletes ozone).

Sulfur Dioxide
Coal contains about 4% sulfur by weight and was the first fossil fuel to be extensively exploited during the nineteenth-century Industrial Revolution. Initially, coal was used primarily in industrial boilers to create steam to power machinery. The 1952 London smog incident was caused by the combination of a prolonged inversion and widespread use of low-grade coal for home heating; at its peak, smog extended for 30 km around London and reduced visibility to 1–5 m. During recent decades, coal has been widely used in electricity-generating utilities and releases more SO_2 than either oil or gas. A 1000 MW plant burns about 700 tons of coal per

hour and emits about a half million tons of SO_2 annually; similar amounts are generated by utilities burning high-sulfur oil. Other sources of SO_2 include pulp and paper mills, oil refineries, and smelters.

Levels of SO_2 vary by season, with generally higher levels during winter months. Total airborne acidic species, however, are higher in summer months because of atmospheric conversion of SO_2 and NO_2, respectively, to H_2SO_4 and HNO_3 through photochemical processes (Figure 11.2). The oxidation of SO_2 by molecular oxygen occurs very slowly in clean, dry air but much faster in air containing particulates and moisture. Sulfuric acid reacts with atmospheric ammonia (from animal, human, and other sources), forming ammonium sulfate and bisulfate salts that accumulate in the $PM_{2.5}$ fraction.

Nitrogen Oxides
Nitric oxide and NO_2 are formed at high combustion temperatures from nitrogen and oxygen in air, electric utilities and motor vehicles being the two main sources. Diesel engines produce 50% of the NO_2 emissions from motor vehicles. Emissions of NO_x increased 17% in the United States between 1970 and 1999, mainly from heavy-duty diesel vehicles and coal-fired electric generation plants. Natural NO_x sources include stratospheric intrusion, oceans, lightning, soil, and wildfires. In the United States, natural and anthropogenic NO_x emissions, respectively, are about 2.2 and 21.4 Tg annually.

Carbon Monoxide
Motor vehicle interiors have the highest average CO levels (10–29 mg/m^3 or 9–25 ppm) of all microenvironments; commuting exposures are highly variable, with some commuters breathing CO in excess of 40 mg/m^3 (35 ppm). Important sources of CO exposure for children include living in homes with elevated levels (related to cigarette smoking, inadequately ventilated nonelectric cooking and heating appliances, vehicle start-up and idling in attached garages), commuting in cars or buses, and engaging in physical activity (e.g., playing, running, bicycling) adjacent to high-traffic roadways.

Volatile Organic Carbons
Leading sources of VOC emissions are vegetation, motor vehicles, consumer and commercial solvent use, open burning and forest fires, dry cleaning, and pulp and paper production. The VOCs emitted by vegetation are mainly monoterpenes and isoprene, which are widely dispersed, while anthropogenic VOCs are concentrated in population centers. Older, poorly maintained vehicles have far higher VOC emissions than newer models. Benzene and MTBE were added to gasoline at low levels in the

late 1970s during the phase-out of tetraethyl lead to enhance fuel combustion. Children may be exposed to MTBE in air (from incomplete fuel combustion and other emissions into ambient air) or water (groundwater contaminated by leaking underground storage tanks or surface water contaminated by recreational water crafts). See also Chapter 5 (Metals—Mercury, Arsenic, Cadmium, and Manganese) for discussion of manganese exposure from emissions of motor vehicles using gasoline containing MTBE. Monitoring of ambient air and personal exposures to toxic VOCs in the United States showed that the major sources were motor vehicle exhaust, gasoline vapors, or ETS for personal exposures and motor vehicle exhaust or gasoline vapors for ambient air levels (Anderson et al., 2001; Wallace, 1996).

Over the period 1900–1998, PM_{10} emissions increased until about 1950 and then decreased by about 50% by 1998, while emissions of other pollutants generally increased until about 1970 (Fig. 11–3); total emissions of the six principal air pollutants decreased 31% between 1970 and 1999, mainly due to reduced SO_2 and VOC emissions. During 1990–1999, emissions of PM_{10}, $PM_{2.5}$, SO_2, CO, and VOCs decreased by 9%–17% but NO_x emissions increased slightly (2%) (Table 11–2). The observed emission trends are likely related to several factors including:

- Coal consumption by electric utilities and their PM_{10} and SO_2 emissions approximately doubled every decade from 1940 to 1970; subsequent regulation led to reduced SO_2 and PM_{10} emissions by electric utilities.

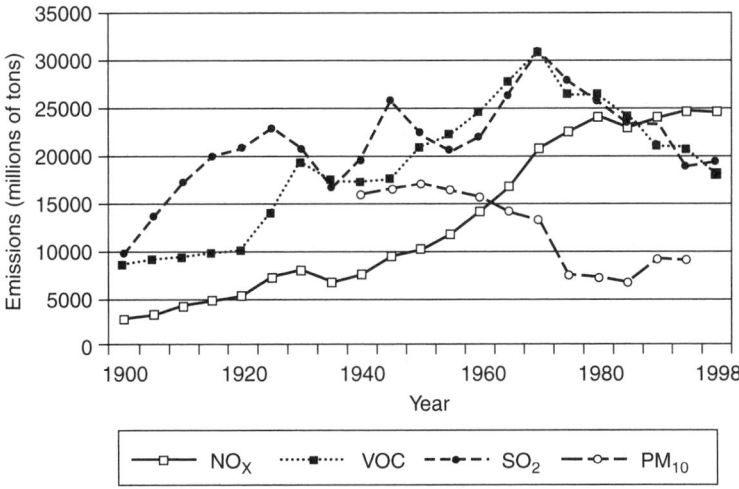

FIGURE 11–3. Trends in national emissions of major air pollutants, United States, 1900–1998. PM_{10} represents directly emitted PM from sources other than fugitive dust, agriculture, or forestry (U.S. Environmental Protection Agency, 2000c).

- Fossil fuel combustion increased during periods of strong economic growth and decreased during recessions; for example, emissions of SO_2 and VOCs declined during the 1930s and after the 1974 energy crisis (Figure 11–3).
- Emission reductions per motor vehicle (related to the introduction of catalytic converters in 1975, improved fuels, and new engine technologies) have been offset by greatly increased numbers of motor vehicles and greater fuel consumption.
- Ground-level ozone levels have remained fairly constant since the 1970s in parallel with levels of their precursors, that is, VOCs and NO_x.
- Decreased use of wood for residential heating and cooking has contributed to the long-term decline in PM_{10}.

Limited data on emissions of hazardous air pollutants by the EPA indicate decreases of 23% in total HAPs, 66% in tetrachloroethylene, and 39% in benzene during the mid-1990s. Ambient air benzene levels in Canadian urban areas decreased by about 25% during 1990–1997.

Intervention

Air Quality Guidelines and Standards

Air quality standards legally define clean air by specifying maximum concentrations and durations of pollutants that pose a threat to public health. The WHO developed air quality guidelines for Europe in 1987 to help countries develop their own national air quality standards and broadened the guidelines in 2000 to address air quality issues in developing countries (World Health Organization, 2000). The WHO air quality guidelines, the EPA NAAQS, and the California ambient air quality standards (AAQS) are shown in Table 11–5. The main differences are the higher values in the United States for annual NO_2 (100 vs. 40 $\mu g/m^3$) and 24-hour SO_2 (365 vs. 125 $\mu g/m^3$), but the WHO values are proposed guidelines and the EPA NAAQS are legally binding standards. The number of persons living in U.S. counties where 1-hour or 8-hour average ambient levels of any criteria air pollutant exceeded NAAQS in 1999 were, respectively, 62 million and 125 million.

The EPA is required by the Clean Air Act to review NAAQSs every 5 years to identify any revisions needed to adequately protect public health with an adequate margin of safety. The EPA NAAQS review process is very lengthy and can substantially delay needed revisions. For instance, the EPA introduced revised ozone and PM standards in 1997, but they have not been implemented because of a legal challenge initiated by the American Trucking Association. The EPA planned to (1) phase out

TABLE 11–5. Guidelines for Major Air Pollutants

Pollutant	Type of Average	Units	EPA NAAQS[a]	California AAQS[b]	WHO Guideline[c]
Ozone	1-hour	$\mu g/m^3$ (ppb)	235 (120)	180 (90)	NA
	8-hour[d]	$\mu g/m^3$ (ppb)	157 (80)	NA	120 (61)
PM_{10}	24-hour	$\mu g/m^3$	150	50	NA
	Annual	$\mu g/m^3$	50	30[e]	NA
$PM_{2.5}$	24-hour[d]	$\mu g/m^3$	65	NA	NA
	Annual[d]	$\mu g/m^3$	15	NA	NA
SO_4	24-hour	$\mu g/m^3$	NA	25	NA
SO_2	1-hour	$\mu g/m^3$ (ppb)	NA	655 (250)	NA
	3-hour	$\mu g/m^3$ (ppb)	1300 (500)	NA	NA
	24-hour	$\mu g/m^3$ (ppb)	365 (140)	105 (40)	125 (48)
	Annual	$\mu g/m^3$ (ppb)	80 (30)	NA	50 (19)
CO	1-hour	mg/m^3 (ppm)	40 (35)	23 (20)	30 (26)
	8-hour	mg/m^3 (ppm)	10 (9)	10 (9)	10 (9)
NO_2	1-hour	$\mu g/m^3$ (ppb)	NA	470 (250)	200 (106)
	Annual	$\mu g/m^3$ (ppb)	100 (53)	NA	40 (21)

[a]*Source:* U.S. Environmental Protection Agency (2001c).

[b]*Source:* California Environmental Protection Agency (2000).

[c]*Source:* World Health Organization (2000).

[d]A 1999 federal court ruling blocked implementation of these standards, proposed by the EPA in 1997; the EPA has appealed this decision to the U.S. Supreme Court (U.S. Environmental Protection Agency, 2001c).

[e]Geometric mean.

the 1-hour primary ozone standard with an 8-hour standard of 80 ppb based on the 3-year average of the annual fourth highest daily maximum 8-hour ozone concentrations and (2) add new $PM_{2.5}$ standards for annual (15 $\mu g/m^3$) and 24-hour (65 $\mu g/m^3$) averages and retain existing PM_{10} standards (Table 11–5). As of early 2002, the EPA had still not implemented these proposals. About 121 million persons in the United States lived in counties that exceeded the NAAQS for 8-hour ozone in 2000 (Table 11–6).

TABLE 11–6. Population in Counties that
Exceeded NAAQS, United States, 2000

Pollutant	Number of People (millions)
CO	9.7
NO_2	0
Ozone[a]	
8-hour	81.5
1-hour	34.7
PM_{10}	8.3
$PM_{2.5}$	75.0
SO_2	0
Any NAAQS	121.4

Source: U.S. Environmental Protection Agency
(2001b).

[a] A 1999 federal court ruling blocked implementation of these standards, proposed by the EPA in
1997; the EPA has appealed this decision to the
U.S. Supreme Court (U.S. Environmental Protection Agency, 2001c).

Under the Children's Environmental Health Protection Act, California has reviewed state AAQSs to assess whether they adequately protect
infants and children (California Environmental Protection Agency, 2000).
The California Environmental Protection Agency conducted critical reviews of potential health effects of eight major air pollutants and concluded that health effects may occur in infants, children, and other potentially susceptible subgroups at or near the maximum levels specified
by California AAQSs. The Agency concluded that PM_{10}, ozone, and NO_2
posed the greatest public health threats at current AAQS levels and should
be included in the first tier of pollutants for review and potential changes
in air quality standards; the review of PM_{10} included sulfates because they
occur in this component. Pollutants in the second tier included lead, CO,
hydrogen sulfide, and SO_2. The review of tier one pollutants concluded
that

- PM_{10}—has the potential to produce health effects in infants and children including reduced birth weight, premature birth, asthma exacerbation, acute respiratory infections, and death; most Californians are
  exposed to levels above the state standard during parts of the year.
- Ozone—has adverse effects on lung function and exacerbates asthma
  and other respiratory illnesses; many Californians are exposed to ozone
  levels above the state standard during the day in summer months.

- Nitrogen dioxide—may enhance the response of asthmatics to aeroallergens at NO_2 levels close to the standard; NO_2 levels in California are occasionally close to the state standard.
- Carbon monoxide and SO_2—SO_2 levels are very low relative to the standard throughout the state, and ambient CO levels are only weakly related to personal air levels; existing AAQSs are reasonably protective of public health, including that of infants and children.

Motor Vehicles

Motor vehicle emissions can be reduced by three main means: engine modifications, exhaust system technologies, and fuel reformulation. Introduction of catalytic converters and lead-free gasoline beginning in the United States in 1976 (in response to regulations under the 1970 Clean Air Act) substantially reduced emissions of VOCs per car, but total motor vehicle VOC emissions have declined only slowly during recent years because of the greatly increased number of vehicles. During smog episodes, some European cities limit car use to alternate days based on odd/even vehicle registration numbers. The Ontario (Canada) Medical Association has called for measures to reduce health impacts of air pollution on children and adults including California-level emission standards for light and heavy-duty vehicles, expanded vehicle inspection and maintenance programs, and tougher standards for sulfur levels in gasoline.

Fuels

The 1990 amendments to the U.S. Clean Air Act required the use of oxygenated gasoline in areas that did not meet the federal ambient air standard for CO, a problem most frequent during winter months. To meet the requirement for 2.7% oxygen content in gasoline, gasoline producers may add 15% MTBE, 7.5% ethanol, or other oxygenates. Oxygenates reduce total VOC emissions, but alcohol increases emissions of formaldehyde. Use of oxygenated gasoline appears to reduce CO levels when ambient temperatures are above 50°F but has little benefit at lower temperatures. Quantification of the public health benefits of fuel oxygenates is problematic because exposure–response relationships for ozone and respiratory health are not well understood for the population subgroups most likely to be affected.

Leaking underground gasoline storage tanks have produced high concentrations of benzene, MTBE, and other VOCs in groundwater. The first publicized incident (1996) involved MTBE contamination of two well fields supplying 50% of the drinking water to Santa Monica, California. Air emissions of MTBE from motor vehicle exhaust and evaporation from gasoline partition into water and enter the hydrologic cycle, for example, via storm drain runoff. Given the low biodegradability of MTBE and its low affinity for soil particles, it can remain free in water (especially groundwater) for extended times and quickly migrate long distances. California has served notice of its intent to phase out MTBE by the end of 2002, and an expert group advised the EPA to remove the requirement for oxygenates from the Clean Air Act because they provide less benefit in modern motor vehicles. In Canada, federal regulations in 1997 limited the gasoline benzene content to an annual average of 1% and to 1.5% at any one time.

Industry
In response to the London smog episode, the U.K. government introduced its first Clean Air Act in 1956 to control domestic sources of air pollution. The introduction of cleaner coals and the increased use of North Sea gas helped reduce SO_2 emissions; also, some electric power stations were relocated from urban to more rural areas. The U.K. Clean Air Act of 1968 required the use of tall chimneys for industries burning fossil fuels, but increased stack height has increased residence time in air and promoted conversion of atmospheric SO_2 to sulfate compounds including acids. After the U.S. EPA was formed in 1970, it was immediately engaged in meeting requirements under the Clean Air Act to establish national air quality and emission standards. This led to the NAAQS for six criteria pollutants (CO, NO_2, PM, lead, SO_2, and ozone) that are proven human health threats. In 1995, the EPA finalized a rule aimed at reducing NO_x emissions from coal-fired power plants by over 400,000 tons per year during 1996–1999 and by over 2 million tons per year beginning in 2000.

The EPA has developed objectives to reduce potential health risks of HAPs including cancer, birth defects, and reproductive effects related to emissions from stationary and mobile sources (U.S. Environmental Protection Agency, 2000e). To achieve these objectives, the EPA plans to (1) develop standards to address sources of 33 HAPs that present the greatest threats to public health, (2) ensure that sources accounting for 90% of area-source emissions are subject to standards, with specific priorities to reduce benzene and formaldehyde emissions from motor vehicles, (3) conduct air toxics assessments to identify areas of concern and priorities, (4) track progress through emission inventories and monitoring networks (there is no national ambient air quality monitoring network to measure ambient HAP levels), (5) initiate national and local initiatives focusing on multimedia and cumulative risks within urban areas, and (6) educate and engage state, local, and other stakeholders.

Public Education
The EPA has developed an air quality index (AQI) to communicate information on potential health risks of local air levels of the five criteria

TABLE 11-7. Air Quality Index

AQI	Air Quality Level	Color	Pollutant Concentration at Upper Limit of AQI Category							
			Ozone (8-hr) (ppb)	Ozone (1-hr) (ppb)	$PM_{2.5}$ (24-hr) ($\mu g/m^3$)	PM_{10} (24-hr) ($\mu g/m^3$)	CO (8-hr) (ppm)	SO_2 (8-hr) (ppb)	NO_2 (24-hr) (ppm)
0–50	Good	Green	0–64	—	0–15.4	0–54	0–4.4	0–34	—
51–100	Moderate	Yellow	65–84	—	15.5–40.4	55–154	4.5–9.4	35–144	—
101–150	Unhealthy for sensitive groups	Orange	85–104	125–164	40.5–65.4	155–254	9.5–12.4	145–224	—
151–200	Unhealthy	Red	105–124	165–204	65.5–150.4	255–354	12.5–15.4	225–304	—
201–300	Very unhealthy	Purple	125–374	205–504	150.5–350.4	355–524	15.5–40.4	305–804	0.65–1.64
301–500	Hazardous	Maroon	NA[a]	≥505	≥350.5	≥525	≥40.5	≥805	≥1.65

Source: U.S. Environmental Protection Agency (1999, 2000a).

[a]Not available (1-hr ozone levels are used to identify hazardous ozone levels).

air pollutants other than lead. The AQI is designed with a range of 0–500 for each criterion air pollutant and six color-coded health concern categories (Table 11–7). The AQI for a given day is the highest of the five individual pollutant AQIs. For large metropolitan areas (>350,000 people), state and local agencies are required to report AQIs to the public daily and, if two or more individual pollutant AQIs exceed 100, specify susceptible population groups such as children and people with asthma or heart disease. Cautionary statements to the public vary somewhat, depending on the pollution profile.

CONCLUSIONS

Proven health effects

- Acute exposure effects
  - Airway inflammation—controlled exposure of human volunteers to ozone, NO_2, or diesel exhaust causes an acute inflammatory response in airways
  - Transient lung function deficits
    After controlled exposure to individual air pollutants (ozone, SO_2), especially among asthmatics
    After same-day exposure to summer elevated ozone levels while engaged in outdoor activities or after moderately severe PM air pollution episodes among healthy and asthmatic children
  - Bronchial hyperreactivity—after brief controlled exposure to high levels of individual air pollutants (ozone, NO_2)
  - Exacerbation of asthma—after controlled exposure to SO_2 and after same-day exposure to increased ambient air pollution (ozone, PM_{10})
  - Acute respiratory disease—after ambient air pollution increases (PM_{10})

Unresolved Issues and Knowledge Gaps

- Acute exposure effects
  - Lung function deficits—limited evidence from controlled exposure to high NO_2 levels
  - Bronchial hyperreactivity—limited evidence from controlled exposure studies that moderately elevated ozone and high NO_2 or mixed pollutant exposure levels increase bronchial reactivity to aeroallergens
  - Asthma exacerbation—limited evidence of an association with ambient air fungal spore counts and soybean allergen
  - Acute childhood respiratory disease—limited evidence of an association between daily respiratory disease events serious enough to re-

quire medical care or to cause death and daily concentrations of individual and multiple outdoor air pollutants (SO_2, ozone, PM_{10})

- Prenatal maternal exposure effects
  - Preterm delivery or intrauterine growth retardation—limited evidence of associations with first trimester exposure (CO, SO_2, PM)
  - Stillbirths—inadequate evidence of an association with exposure to multiple outdoor air pollutants
  - Birth defects—suggestive evidence of an association between orofacial clefts and cardiac defects and first trimester CO exposure in one study
- Chronic exposure effects
  - Lung function deficits and respiratory symptoms—limited evidence of associations with residence in regions with intermittent exposure to elevated ozone, PM_{10}, particle strong acidity, multiple pollutants, or residence in areas of high traffic density (in both healthy and asthmatic children)
  - Lung function growth deficits—limited evidence of an association with residence for at least a few years in areas with high ambient pollution levels (PM_{10}, ozone, multiple pollutants)
  - Incident asthma—limited evidence of associations with outdoor activity in high-ozone regions and personal NO_2 exposure levels; inadequate evidence of association with the fungus *Alternaria.*
  - Childhood cancer—inadequate evidence of an association between leukemia or other childhood cancers and traffic density or ambient benzene levels
- Knowledge gaps—need epidemiologic studies with improved exposure assessment, statistical power, and biomarkers of susceptibility to assess the relative importance of ambient air pollutants and other risk factors for incident asthma, other respiratory diseases, and other potential health effects including developmental effects and childhood cancer

Risk Management Issues

- Prevention—need to prevent exposure of children and pregnant women to ambient air pollutant levels in excess of existing standards; interventions should target major sources including motor vehicles and industry
- Monitoring—need to monitor personal air exposure levels of children to ambient air pollutants, prevalence of lung function deficits and lung function growth deficits, and incidence of asthma and other respiratory diseases

REFERENCES

Anderson MJ, Miller SL, Milford JB. (2001). Source apportionment of exposure to toxic volatile organic compounds using positive matrix factorization. J Expo Anal Environ Epidemiol 11:295–307.

Bobak M. (2000). Outdoor air pollution, low birth weight, and prematurity. Environ Health Perspect 108:173–6.

Bobak M, Leon DA. (1999). Pregnancy outcomes and outdoor air pollution: an ecological study in districts of the Czech Republic 1986–8. Occup Environ Med 56:539–43.

Boezen HM, van der Zee SC, Postma DS, Vonk JM, Gerritsen J, Hoek G, Brunekreef B, Rijcken B, Schouten JP. (1999). Effects of ambient air pollution on upper and lower respiratory symptoms and peak expiratory flow in children. Lancet 353:874–8.

Brauer M, Avila-Casado C, Fortoul TI, Vedal S, Stevens B, Churg A. (2001). Air pollution and retained particles in the lung. Environ Health Perspect 109: 1039–43.

Burnett RT, Smith-Doiron M, Stieb D, Raizenne ME, Brook JR, Dales RE, Leech JA, Cakmak S, Krewski D. (2001). Association between ozone and hospitalization for acute respiratory diseases in children less than 2 years of age. Am J Epidemiol 153:444–52.

California Environmental Protection Agency. (2000). Adequacy of California ambient air quality standards: Children's Environmental Health Protection Act. Sacramento: Office of Environmental Health Hazard Assessment.

Conceicao GM, Miraglia SG, Kishi HS, Saldiva PH, Singer JM. (2001). Air pollution and child mortality: a time-series study in São Paulo, Brazil. Environ Health Perspect 109(Suppl 3):347–50.

Dales RE, Cakmak S, Burnett RT, Judek S, Coates F, Brook JR. (2000). Influence of ambient fungal spores on emergency visits for asthma to a regional children's hospital. Am J Respir Crit Care Med 162:2087–90.

Dejmek J, Solansky I, Benes I, Lenicek J, Sram RJ. (2000). The impact of polycyclic aromatic hydrocarbons and fine particles on pregnancy outcome. Environ Health Perspect 108:1159–64.

Delfino RJ, Coate BD, Zeiger RS, Seltzer JM, Street DH, Koutrakis P. (1996). Daily asthma severity in relation to personal ozone exposure and outdoor fungal spores. Am J Respir Crit Care Med 154:633–41.

Dockery DW, Pope CA III. (1994). Acute respiratory effects of particulate air pollution. Annu Rev Public Health 15:107–32.

Downs SH, Mitakakis TZ, Marks GB, Car NG, Belousova EG, Leuppi JD, Xuan W, Downie SR, Tobias A, Peat JK. (2001). Clinical importance of *Alternaria* exposure in children. Am J Respir Crit Care Med 164:455–9.

Feychting M, Svensson D, Ahlbom A. (1998). Exposure to motor vehicle exhaust and childhood cancer. Scand J Work Environ Health 24:8–11.

Frischer T, Studnicka M, Gartner C, Tauber E, Horak F, Veiter A, Spengler J, Kuhr J, Urbanek R. (1999). Lung function growth and ambient ozone: a three-year population study in school children. Am J Respir Crit Care Med 160:390–6.

Gauderman WJ, McConnell R, Gilliland F, London S, Thomas D, Avol E, Vora H, Berhane K, Rappaport EB, Lurmann F, Margolis HG, Peters J. (2000). Association between air pollution and lung function growth in southern California children. Am J Respir Crit Care Med 162:1383–90.

Gergen PJ, Turkeltaub PC. (1992). The association of individual allergen reactivity with respiratory disease in a national sample: data from the second National Health and Nutrition Examination Survey, 1976–80 (NHANES II). J Allergy Clin Immunol 90:579–88.

Gilliland FD, Berhane K, Rappaport EB, Thomas DC, Avol E, Gauderman WJ, London SJ, Margolis HG, McConnell R, Islam KT, Peters JM. (2001). The effects of ambient air pollution on school absenteeism due to respiratory illnesses. Epidemiology 12:43–54.

Ha EH, Hong YC, Lee BE, Woo BH, Schwartz J, Christiani da VC. (2001). Is air pollution a risk factor for low birth weight in Seoul? Epidemiology 12:643–8.

Hajat S, Haines A, Goubet SA, Atkinson RW, Anderson HR. (1999). Association of air pollution with daily GP consultations for asthma and other lower respiratory conditions in London. Thorax 54:597–605.

Halonen M, Stern DA, Wright AL, Taussig LM, Martinez FD. (1997). *Alternaria* as a major allergen for asthma in children raised in a desert environment. Am J Respir Crit Care Med 155:1356–61.

Harrison RM, Leung PL, Somervaille L, Smith R, Gilman E. (1999). Analysis of incidence of childhood cancer in the West Midlands of the United Kingdom in relation to proximity to main roads and petrol stations. Occup Environ Med 56:774–80.

Infante-Rivard C. (1993). Childhood asthma and indoor environmental risk factors. Am J Epidemiol 137:834–44.

International Agency for Research on Cancer. (1989). IARC monographs on the evaluation of carcinogenic risks to humans. Vol. 46. Diesel and gasoline engine exhausts and some nitroarenes. Lyon, France: International Agency for Research on Cancer.

Kinney PL, Thurston GD, Raizenne M. (1996). The effects of ambient ozone on lung function in children: a reanalysis of six summer camp studies. Environ Health Perspect 104:170–4.

Kopp MV, Bohnet W, Frischer T, Ulmer C, Studnicka M, Ihorst G, Gardner C, Forster J, Urbanek R, Kuehr J. (2000). Effects of ambient ozone on lung function in children over a two-summer period. Eur Respir J 16:893–900.

Krishna MT, Chauhan AJ, Frew AJ, Holgate ST. (1998). Toxicological mechanisms underlying oxidant pollutant-induced airway injury. Rev Environ Health 13:59–71.

Kunzli N, Lurmann F, Segal M, Ngo L, Balmes J, Tager IB. (1997). Association between lifetime ambient ozone exposure and pulmonary function in college freshmen—results of a pilot study. Environ Res 72:8–23.

Linaker CH, Coggon D, Holgate ST, Clough J, Josephs L, Chauhan AJ, Inskip HM. (2000). Personal exposure to nitrogen dioxide and risk of airflow obstruction in asthmatic children with upper respiratory infection. Thorax 55:930–3.

Maisonet M, Bush TJ, Correa A, Jaakkola JJ. (2001). Relation between ambient air pollution and low birth weight in the northeastern United States. Environ Health Perspect 109(Suppl 3):351–6.

McConnell R, Berhane K, Gilliland F, London SJ, Islam T, Gauderman WJ, Avol E, Margolis HG, Peters JM. (2002). Asthma in exercising children exposed to ozone: a cohort study. Lancet 359:386–91.

McConnell R, Berhane K, Gilliland F, London SJ, Vora H, Avol E, Gauderman WJ, Margolis HG, Lurmann F, Thomas DC, Peters JM. (1999). Air pollution and bronchitic symptoms in Southern California children with asthma. Environ Health Perspect 107:757–60.

McDonnell WF, Stewart PW, Smith MV, Pan WK, Pan J. (1999). Ozone-induced respiratory symptoms: exposure–response models and association with lung function. Eur Respir J 14:845–53.

McKinney PA, Alexander FE, Cartwright RA, Parker L. (1991). Parental occupations of children with leukaemia in west Cumbria, north Humberside, and Gateshead. BMJ 302:681–7.

National Institute of Environmental Health Sciences. (2001). Ninth report on carcinogens. Research Triangle Park, NC: National Toxicology Program.

Nemmar A, Hoet PH, Vanquickenborne B, Dinsdale D, Thomeer M, Hoylaerts MF, Vanbilloen H, Mortelmans L, Nemery B. (2002). Passage of inhaled particles into the blood circulation in humans. Circulation 105:411–4.

Northridge ME, Yankura J, Kinney PL, Santella RM, Shepard P, Riojas Y, Aggarwal M, Strickland P. (1999). Diesel exhaust exposure among adolescents in Harlem: a community-driven study. Am J Public Health 89:998–1002.

Pandya RJ, Solomon G, Kinner A, Balmes JR. (2002). Diesel exhaust and asthma: hypotheses and molecular mechanisms of action. Environ Health Perspect 110 (Suppl 1):103–12.

Pereira LA, Loomis D, Conceicao GM, Braga AL, Arcas RM, Kishi HS, Singer JM, Bohm GM, Saldiva PH. (1998). Association between air pollution and intrauterine mortality in São Paulo, Brazil. Environ Health Perspect 106:325–9.

Pope CA 3rd, Burnett RT, Thun MJ, Calle EE, Krewski D, Ito K, Thurston GD. (2002). Lung cancer, cardiopulmonary mortality, and long-term exposure to fine particulate air pollution. JAMA 287:1132–41.

Raaschou-Nielsen O, Hertel O, Thomsen BL, Olsen JH. (2001). Air pollution from traffic at the residence of children with cancer. Am J Epidemiol 153:433–43.

Raaschou-Nielsen O, Lohse C, Thomsen BL, Skov H, Olsen JH. (1997). Ambient air levels and the exposure of children to benzene, toluene, and xylenes in Denmark. Environ Res 75:149–59.

Ritz B, Yu F. (1999). The effect of ambient carbon monoxide on low birth weight among children born in southern California between 1989 and 1993. Environ Health Perspect 107:17–25.

Ritz B, Yu F, Chapa G, Fruin S. (2000). Effect of air pollution on preterm birth among children born in Southern California between 1989 and 1993. Epidemiology 11:502–11.

Ritz B, Yu F, Fruin S, Chapa G, Shaw GM, Harris JA. (2002). Ambient air pollution and risk of birth defects in Southern California. Am J Epidemiol 155:17–25.

Sarnat JA, Schwartz J, Catalano PJ, Suh HH. (2001). Gaseous pollutants in particulate matter epidemiology: confounders or surrogates? Environ Health Perspect 109:1053–61.

Savitz DZ, Feingold L. (1989). Association of childhood cancer with residential traffic density. Scand J Work Environ Health 15:360–3.

Schwartz J. (1989). Lung function and chronic exposure to air pollution: a cross-sectional analysis of NHANES II. Environ Res 50:309–21.

Shu XO, Gao YT, Brinton LA, Linet MS, Tu JT, Zheng W, Fraumeni JF. (1988). A population-based case-control study of childhood leukemia in Shanghai. Cancer 62:635–44.

Spengler JD, Koutrakis P, Dockery DW, Raizenne M, Speizer FE. (1996). Health effects of acid aerosols on North American children: air pollution exposures. Environ Health Perspect 104:492–9.

Studnicka M, Hackl E, Pischinger J, Fangmeyer C, Haschke N, Kuhr J, Urbanek R, Neumann M, Frischer T. (1997). Traffic-related NO_2 and the prevalence of asthma and respiratory symptoms in seven year olds. Eur Respir J 10:2275–8.

Suh HH, Bahadori T, Vallarino J, Spengler JD. (2000). Criteria air pollutants and toxic air pollutants. Environ Health Perspect 108(Suppl 4):625–33.

U.S. Environmental Protection Agency. (1999). Air quality index reporting; final rule (40 CFR Part 58). Fed Reg 64:42530–49.

U.S. Environmental Protection Agency. (2000a). Air quality index. A guide to air quality and your health (EPA-454/R-00-005). Research Triangle Park, NC: U.S. Environmental Protection Agency.

U.S. Environmental Protection Agency. (2000b). Health assessment document for diesel exhaust. Washington, DC: U.S. Environmental Protection Agency.

U.S. Environmental Protection Agency. (2001b). Latest findings on national air quality: 2000 status and trends. Research Triangle Park, NC: U.S. Environmental Protection Agency.

U.S. Environmental Protection Agency. (2000c). National air pollutant emission trends, 1900–1998. Research Triangle Park, NC: U.S. Environmental Protection Agency.

U.S. Environmental Protection Agency. (2000d). National air quality and emissions trends report, (1998). Research Triangle Park, NC: U.S. Environmental Protection Agency.

U.S. Environmental Protection Agency. (2000e). National air toxics program: the integrated urban strategy report to Congress. Research Triangle Park, NC: U.S. Environmental Protection Agency.

U.S. Environmental Protection Agency. (2001a). Air quality criteria for particulate matter (third external review draft). Located at http://cfpub.epa.gov/ncea/cfm/partmatt.cfm.

U.S. Environmental Protection Agency. (2001c). National ambient air quality standards (NAAQS). Located at http://www.epa.gov/airs/criteria.html.

Wallace L. (1996). Environmental exposure to benzene: an update. Environ Health Perspect 104(Suppl 6):1129–36.

Wang X, Ding H, Ryan L, Xu X. (1997). Association between air pollution and low birth weight: a community-based study. Environ Health Perspect 105:514–20.

Weaver VM, Davoli CT, Heller PJ, Fitzwilliam A, Peters HL, Sunyer J, Murphy SE, Goldstein GW, Groopman JD. (1996). Benzene exposure, assessed by urinary trans,trans-muconic acid, in urban children with elevated blood lead levels. Environ Health Perspect 104:318–23.

Woodruff TJ, Axelrad DA, Caldwell J, Morello-Frosch R, Rosenbaum A. (1998). Public health implications of 1990 air toxics concentrations across the United States. Environ Health Perspect 106:245–51.

Woodruff TJ, Grillo J, Schoendorf KC. (1997). The relationship between selected causes of postneonatal infant mortality and particulate air pollution in the United States. Environ Health Perspect 105:608–12.

World Health Organization. (2000). Guidelines for air quality. Geneva: World Health Organization.

12
Water

I. CHEMICAL CONTAMINANTS

The introduction of chlorinated drinking water during the early twentieth century virtually eliminated cholera, typhoid fever, and other waterborne infectious diseases in the regions served. Chlorine, a potent oxidizing agent, not only kills microbial agents but also reacts with natural organic material in raw water to produce hundreds of disinfection byproducts (DBPs). These DBPs include trihalomethanes (THMs), haloacetic acids, haloacetonitriles, haloketones, halophenols, halogenated furanones, and other halogenated hydrocarbons. There is limited epidemiologic evidence of associations between DBPs and adverse reproductive outcomes and certain cancers. Drinking water is also subject to contamination by natural sources (e.g., nitrate from agricultural operations), waste disposal (including leachates from hazardous waste disposal sites), and leakage from solvent storage containers. Trichloroethylene, for instance, is the most frequently reported organic contaminant in groundwater in the United States and is a probable human carcinogen; it has been used extensively as a degreaser in metal and automotive industries since the 1920s and was widely used in dry cleaning for several decades.

Part I of this chapter considers chemical contaminants from disinfection and hazardous waste disposal, and Part II focuses on certain childhood infectious diseases for which waterborne transmission is an important route of infection. The objective of Part I is to describe potential threats to child health from widespread drinking water chemical contaminants, with a major focus on risks of adverse developmental effects and cancer. The discussion includes recent developments in the epidemiology and risk management of DBPs. See other chapters for contaminants that may occur in water including lead and arsenic (Chapters 4 and 5, Metals), pesticides (Chapter 7, Pesticides), and radionuclides (Chapter 9, Radiation).

HEALTH EFFECTS

Genotoxicity

Formation of THMs (chloroform, dichlorobromomethane, dibromochloromethane, and bromoform) during chlorination of water was reported in 1974. Although only a fraction of chlorinated DBPs, THM concentrations have been widely used by regulators and researchers as a proxy for total DBPs. Organic extracts of chlorinated drinking water were later shown to be mutagenic in the Ames Salmonella assay, while extracts of raw water had little or no activity; most of the mutagenic activity in chlorinated water was associated with nonvolatile DBPs. The DBP 3-chloro-4-(dichloromethyl)-5-hydroxy-2[5H]-furanone (MX) and related chlorohydroxyfurnanones are potent mutagens; MX alone comprised about 30%–60% of the total mutagenic activity of chlorinated drinking water in Finland and Massachusetts (Wright et al., 2002).

Ozonation of raw water has been shown to produce considerably lower mutagenic activity than chlorination, and high ozone doses virtually eliminate mutagenicity. Other findings from studies of DBP mutagenicity include the following: (1) ingested chloroform and bromoform both cause chromosome abnormalities, and inhaled chloroform causes increased micronuclei in rats, (2) MX and three related chlorohydroxyfurnanones at low doses produce DNA strand breaks and complex chromatid rearrangements in human and rodent cells in vitro, (3) chlorinated and brominated acetonitriles produce DNA strand breaks in human cells in vitro, and (4) trichloroacetic acid, dichloroacetic acid, and chloral hydrate are all weakly mutagenic in mouse lymphoma cells in vitro.

Under the Comprehensive Environmental Response, Compensation, and Liability Act (CERCLA), the Agency for Toxic Substances and Disease Registry (ATSDR) and the EPA are responsible for identifying contaminants and groups of contaminants at hazardous waste sites that pose the greatest public health risks in the United States. The ATSDR is required to periodically prepare a list (known as the CERCLA list) of such substances in priority order based on frequency, known toxicity, and potential for human exposure. Most of the highest-ranked chemicals on the 2001 CERCLA list are genotoxic and probable or known human carcinogens (Table 12–1).

TABLE 12–1. Highest-Priority Contaminants at Hazardous Waste Sites in the United States, in Rank Order by Risk to Public Health[a]

Contaminant	Genotoxicity[b]	Carcinogenicity in humans[c]
Arsenic (inorganic) (highest ranked)	Clastogenic in vitro and in vivo; mutagenic in vitro	Known
Lead (inorganic)	Clastogenic in vitro and in vivo	Possible
Mercury—inorganic	Clastogenic in vitro and in vivo; mixed evidence of point mutations in vitro; inhibits mitotic spindle formation	Not classifiable
Mercury-elemental	Possibly clastogenic in occupationally exposed persons	Not classifiable
Vinyl chloride	Metabolites are mutagenic and clastogenic in vitro and in vivo	Known
PCBs	Most studies showed no mutagenicity; induces Phase I cytochrome enzymes that can activate procarcinogens and generate reactive oxygen species	Probable
Benzene	Metabolites appear to be clastogenic	Known
Cadmium	Mixed evidence of mutagenicity and clastogenicity; interferes with mitotic spindle in vitro and in vivo	Known
Benzo[a]pyrene, benzo[a]fluoranthene, other PAHs	Mutagenic and clastogenic in vitro	Probable
Chloroform	Not strongly mutagenic	Possible
p,p'-DDT	Mixed evidence of mutagenicity and clastogenicity	Possible
Trichloroethylene	EPA-not available; mixed evidence of mutagenicity in vitro noted in IARC review	Probable
Dieldrin	Clastogenic in vitro; mixed evidence of mutagenicity	Not classifiable
Chromium (hexavalent)	Mutagenic and clastogenic; causes oxidative DNA and chromosomal damage	Known

[a]Agency for Toxic Substances and Disease Registry (2001).

[b]U.S. Environmental Protection Agency (2001b).

[c]International Agency for Research on Cancer (2002).

Developmental Outcomes

Given the widespread exposure to DBPs and the evidence of reproductive toxicity in experimental animals, there have been surprisingly few epidemiologic studies incorporating strong statistical power and exposure assessment. Until recently, evidence of links between DBPs and adverse reproductive outcomes in humans came from a few epidemiologic studies involving diverse exposure assessments and health outcomes, precluding a meaningful synthesis (Reif et al., 1996). Subsequent epidemiologic studies have strengthened the case that DBPs may be reproductive toxicants in humans; recent reviews concluded that

- The weight of evidence from toxicologic and epidemiologic studies of DBPs was suggestive of associations between DBP exposure and IUGR and urinary tract birth defects, but the limited exposure data precluded definitive conclusions (Graves et al., 2001).
- Epidemiologic studies provide moderate evidence of associations between THMs and IUGR, neural tube defects, and spontaneous abortions; evidence of a role for other VOCs in drinking water is weaker because there have been fewer studies (Bove et al., 2002).

Fetal Deaths

Epidemiologic studies have yielded limited evidence of an association between spontaneous abortion and exposure to THMs during early pregnancy (Savitz et al., 1995; Waller et al., 1998). Important findings included a moderately strong association with a specific THM, bromodichloromethane (BDCM), independent of several potential confounders (Waller et al., 1998). The latter finding is consistent with evidence that BDCM causes fetal death in rodents. Drinking water may contain non-DBP VOCs such as tetrachloroethylene and trichloroethylene; there is fairly consistent evidence of associations between spontaneous abortion and occupational exposure to tetrachloroethylene, trichloroethylene, toluene, xylene, and chloroform.

There is also limited evidence of an association between stillbirths and THMs, particularly BDCM levels (Fig. 12–1). The subgroup of stillbirths caused by asphyxia was strongly associated with total THMs ($OR =$ 4.6, CI 1.9–11) in what appears to be the first epidemiologic study to assess this category of stillbirths in relation to environmental hazards (King et al., 2000). Asphyxia-related stillbirths include those related to placental vascular abnormalities (e.g., placental abruption). Trichloroacetic acid and other DBPs deplete folic acid in experimental animals (possibly through a free radical mechanism that induces vitamin B_{12} and folate deficiencies); folate deficiency increases the plasma homocysteine level, a

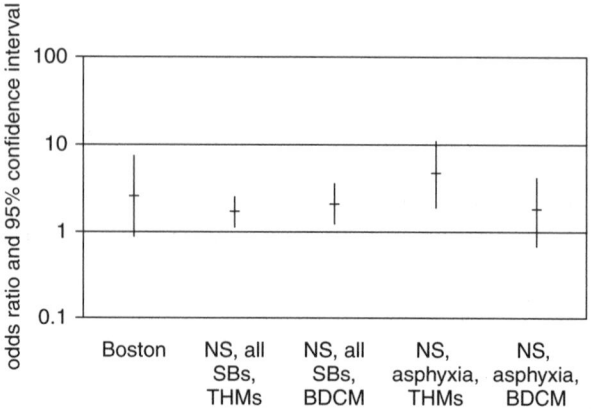

FIGURE 12–1. Associations between DBPs and stillbirths (SBs). Boston (Aschengrau et al., 1993), Nova Scotia (NS) (Dodds et al., 1999; King et al., 2000).

risk factor for neural tube defects and placental abruption (Dow and Green, 2000).

Birth Defects

The main findings from epidemiologic studies of DBPs and birth defects include

- Neural tube defects—fairly consistent associations with DBPs, the highest risks being those among women in the highest BDCM category and women in the highest tertile of THM levels who did not take multivitamin or folate supplements during the 3 months before pregnancy (Fig. 12–2)
- Urinary tract defects—limited evidence of an association with a chlorinated surface water source (Magnus et al., 1999)
- Oral clefts—inconsistent associations with DBPs
- Cardiac defects—generally no association with DBPs

There is inadequate evidence to assess the role of drinking water nitrate in neural tube defects; epidemiologic studies have shown associations with nitrate in well water but not in municipal water or diet (Arbuckle et al., 1988; Croen et al., 2001; Dorsch et al., 1984). Given that dietary nitrate intake is usually much greater than that from water, it is possible that nitrate is a marker for another toxicant(s) in water (especially groundwater). Animal studies have shown reproductive toxicity but not birth defects at high exposure levels to nitrate or nitrite.

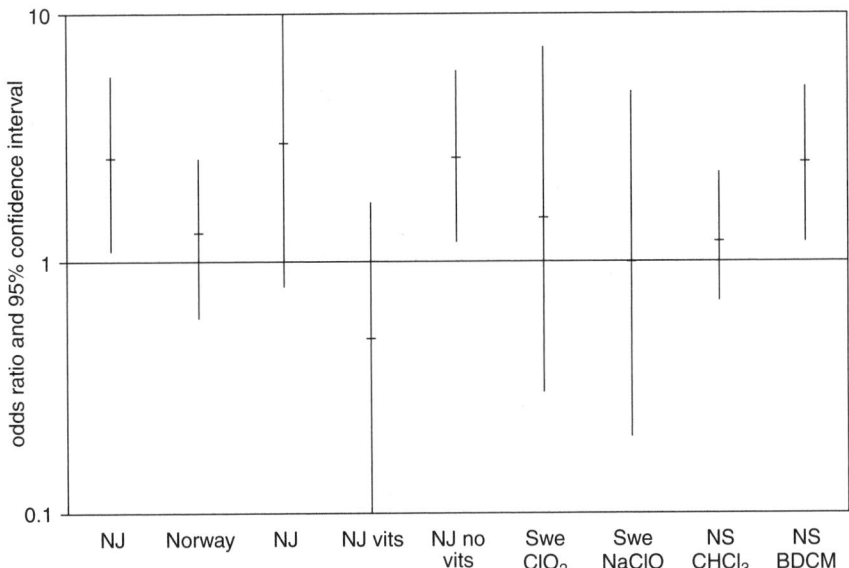

FIGURE 12–2. Associations between DBPs in drinking water and the risk of neural tube birth defects (Sweden restricted to spina bifida). Nova Scota (Dodds and King, 2001), Swe (Sweden) (Kallen and Robert, 2000), NJ (New Jersey: no vits, took vits, all subjects) (Klotz and Pyrch, 1999), Norway (Magnus et al., 1999), New Jersey (Bove et al., 1995).

Exposure to non-THM VOCs from contaminated wells or proximity to hazardous waste disposal sites has been linked to cardiac and neural tube defects (Croen et al., 1997; Dolk et al., 1998; Goldberg et al., 1990). Recent reviews of epidemiologic studies of pregnancy outcome and water contaminants or proximity to hazardous waste disposal sites concluded that (Bove et al., 2002; Vrijheid, 2000).

- There was limited and inconsistent evidence of associations between trichloroethylene or tetrachloroethylene in drinking water and cardiac, neural tube, and cleft defects.
- Some studies of individual and multiple hazardous waste disposal sites have shown associations with adverse health effects including low birth weight and birth defects; the potential for exposure to hazardous wastes through contaminated groundwater is real, but epidemiologic studies have generally lacked direct exposure measures, adequate statistical power, and control of potential confounders.

In summary, there is insufficient evidence to infer or reject a causal relationship between specific drinking water contaminants and birth defects.

In general, however, there is suggestive evidence of possible associations between neural tube and urinary tract defects and THMs. Importantly, an association between neural tube defects and THMs was restricted to women who did not take daily multivitamins or folate supplements during the 3 months before pregnancy (Klotz and Pyrch, 1999). Although based on small numbers, this finding is consistent with evidence that DBPs create folate deficiency, thereby increasing the plasma homocysteine level, a risk factor for neural tube defects (Dow and Green, 2000; Eskes, 2000).

Low Birth Weight

The most consistent findings in epidemiologic studies of DBPs and birth weight and gestation length were associations between THMs and IUGR (Fig. 12–3). Findings include evidence of exposure-risk relationships between IUGR and chloroform and BDCM (Kramer et al., 1992) and an association between third trimester THM exposure and IUGR (Gallagher et al., 1998). These findings are consistent with the observation of reduced birth weight among offspring of experimental animals that ingested chloroform at high doses during pregnancy (Thompson et al., 1974). Exposure to tetrachloroethylene-contaminated water was associated with re-

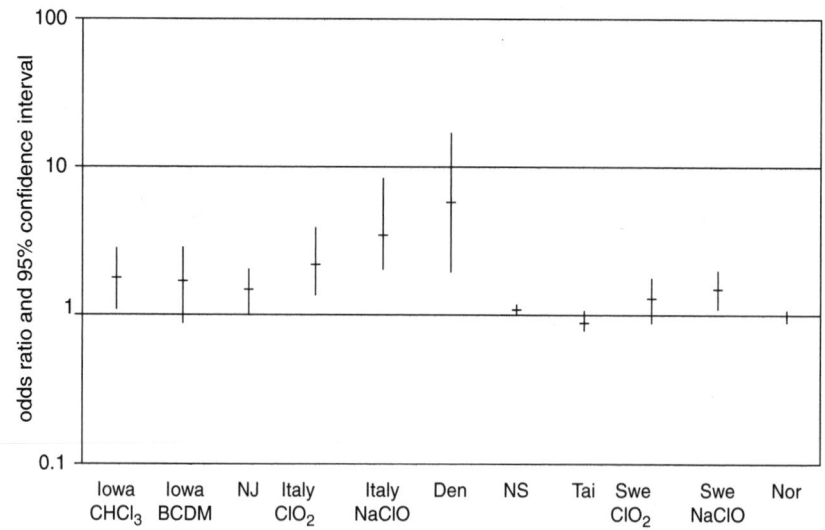

FIGURE 12–3. Associations between DBPs and the risk of IUGR (or small head circumference—Italy and Sweden); Nor (Norway) (Jaakkola et al., 2001), Sweden (Kallen and Robert, 2000), Tai (Taiwan) (Yang et al., 2000), Nova Scotia (Dodds et al., 1999), Den (Denver) (Gallagher et al., 1998), Italy (Kanitz et al., 1996), New Jersey (Bove et al., 1995), Iowa (Kramer et al., 1992).

duced birth weight and a twofold increased risk of IUGR among mothers aged 35 years or older but not among younger women (Sonnenfeld et al., 2001). There were significant exposure–risk relations between groundwater nitrate levels and IUGR and preterm birth in an agricultural region dependent on groundwater potentially contaminated by agricultural activities (Bukowski et al., 2001).

Cancer

Evidence from the few epidemiologic studies of childhood cancer and drinking water is inadequate to assess the potential etiologic roles of DBPs and other contaminants. There were weak or no associations between childhood cancer or childhood leukemia and DBP exposure in two studies (Infante-Rivard et al., 2001; Kallen and Robert, 2000). Further analysis of the leukemia study showed strong but imprecise associations with total THM exposure among children with polymorphisms involving a *CYP2E1* variant with increased transcriptional activity or a *GSTT1* null genotype, that is, variants that may increase generation or reduce detoxification of reactive THM metabolites (Infante-Rivard et al., 2002). Childhood leukemia was linked to drinking water containing trichloroethylene in women but not men in an ecologic study (Cohn et al., 1994). The THMs cause liver, kidney, and large intestinal tumors in rodents; BDCM and bromoform each caused substantially increased risks of large intestinal tumors. Rats of both sexes exposed to MX in drinking water had dose-related increases in thyroid and liver bile duct tumors, including increases at the lowest dose tested; the highest MX doses caused adrenal, lung, breast, and pancreatic tumors, lymphomas, and leukemias.

Investigation of a cluster of childhood leukemia in Woburn, Massachusetts, showed increased risk in an area served by water that may have been contaminated by trichloroethylene and other toxicants from a hazardous waste disposal site (Cutler et al., 1986); this incident led to legal actions popularized in the book and the motion picture *A Civil Action*. Childhood brain tumors were linked to maternal well water consumption in western Washington state (Mueller et al., 2001). Until studies with adequate statistical power and exposure assessment are conducted, assessment of the role of drinking water contaminants in childhood cancer will be problematic.

Epidemiologic studies have shown fairly consistent associations between THMs and adult bladder cancer and less consistent links to other adult cancers. Evidence from studies of persons occupationally exposed to trichloroethylene indicates increased risks of kidney cancer, liver cancer, non-Hodgkin's lymphoma, Hodgkin's disease, multiple myeloma, and cervical cancer (Wartenberg et al., 2000). Although most subjects had exposures to other solvents, it appears that trichloroethylene likely contributes to human cancers caused by solvent exposures. Biologic plausibility comes from evidence that trichloroethylene causes dose-related increased risks of liver and kidney cancers in experimental animals, with no evidence of a threshold within the observable dose range; the trichloroethylene metabolites trichloroacetic acid and dichloroacetic acid are also rodent carcinogens (liver cancer).

Other Health Effects

Infantile methemoglobinemia has been attributed to high water nitrate levels, particularly from farm wells. Compared to older persons, infants under age 6 months have lower levels of NADH-cytochrome b_5 reductase, an enzyme that converts methemoglobin to hemoglobin. Recent evidence suggests that infantile methemoglobinemia may be caused by gastrointestinal infection; NO is produced in gastrointestinal and other tissues in response to infection and inflammation and can oxidize hemoglobin to methemoglobin; thus water nitrate levels may be a proxy for waterborne enteric pathogens. There is inadequate evidence of an association between nitrate/nitrite in drinking water and the risk of childhood type I diabetes from ecologic studies; the only analytical study showed associations with prenatal maternal dietary nitrite intake and postnatal child dietary nitrite intake but not with drinking water nitrate or nitrite.

EXPOSURES

Chlorination Disinfection By-Products

Measurement of DBP exposure is complicated by variation in DBP concentrations in relation to

- Place—DBP formation increases with time after chlorination, and levels vary among sites including water treatment facilities, distribution systems, and homes.
- Time—DBP levels are generally higher during warmer months because of increased precursor levels in raw water (natural organic carbon from plant and other sources) and increased DBP formation rates.
- Raw water characteristics—DBP formation after chlorination varies by total organic carbon content, pH, ammonium and bromide ion concentrations, and temperature.

• Water treatment practices—filtration (if done before chlorination, especially for surface water, this substantially reduces the concentration of total organic carbon available to react with chlorine), choice of disinfection agent (e.g., chloramination produces lower DBP levels compared to chlorine or hypochlorite), and use of carbon filters to remove DBPs (either at the treatment facility or the point of use).

Epidemiologic studies of DBPs have usually collected self-reported information on residential history and water consumption habits but not on bathing/showering habits. The extent and quality of current and historic water quality data vary by jurisdiction, as do the frequency and number of specific DBP measurements. For monitoring DBPs in drinking water, the EPA requires individual and total THMs, dichloroacetic acid, trichloroacetic acid, total haloacetic acids, and bromate (U.S. Environmental Protection Agency, 1998). The infrequency of DBP measurements is a problem for epidemiologic studies of developmental outcomes; for example, the critical exposure period for birth defects is only a few weeks early in the first trimester. The limited ability of epidemiologic studies to accurately assess exposure to DBPs has likely caused some of the inconsistencies among studies (Arbuckle et al., 2002).

Exposure studies of human volunteers have shown that THM concentrations in water and exhaled alveolar breath or blood, collected after swimming in chlorinated pools or after showering, are strongly correlated. A 1-hour swim in water with a chloroform level of 160 μg/L produced an average chloroform uptake of about 65 μg/kg body weight (75% dermal, 25% inhalation); this is about thirtyfold higher than the dose from ingesting 2 L of water with a THM level of 80 μg/L (the current EPA maximum contaminant level [MCL]). Blood bromoform levels spiked sharply after showering in a region with high brominated THM levels (Lynberg et al., 2001). Such spikes could be etiologically significant if they occur during critical exposure periods for adverse developmental outcomes. Although THM levels in exhaled breath and blood and urinary haloacetic acid levels are promising biomarkers of recent exposure, technical and cost problems must be overcome before such biomarkers are widely used in epidemiologic studies (Arbuckle et al., 2002).

Most monitoring of DBP levels in chlorinated drinking water has been limited to total THMs, a fraction that contains only a small fraction of the mutagenic activity of chlorinated water. Only very limited or no data on MX or total mutagenicity levels in chlorinated drinking water are available in most countries. A tap water survey in Massachusetts surface water systems showed that the average MX concentration was 27.5 ng/L (range, 5–88 ng/L) and that MX comprised about half of the mutagenicity (Wright et al., 2002).

Other Toxics

The most frequently detected non-THM VOCs in Canadian and American drinking water supplies have been trichloroethylene, tetrachloroethylene, 1,2-dichloroethane, dichloromethane, benzene, toluene, ethylbenzene, xylenes, vinyl chloride, and 1,1,1-trichloroethane. For all regulated VOCs, 6% of groundwater and 8% of surface water supplies had one or more VOCs at levels exceeding the MCL (Table 12–2). Groundwater systems serving populations of over 10,000 experience relatively frequent VOC exceedances because of the shallow, unconfined groundwater supplies needed to sustain large flow rates but vulnerable to contamination. Solvents persist in groundwater because of relatively low biologic and chemical reactivity, low temperatures, absence of light, lack of contact with the atmosphere, and relatively low microbial concentrations. Rural groundwater supplies are vulnerable to nitrate contamination from animal and human feces, other organic waste, and chemical fertilizers; high drinking water nitrate levels are associated with shallow or dug wells and large farms.

Three to 4 million children in the United States live within 1.6 km of a major hazardous waste disposal site and are at risk of exposure to VOCs and other contaminants. Exposure pathways of VOCs for children include ingestion of contaminated soil and drinking water and inhalation of VOCs (e.g., volatilization during showers or from groundwater into basements). Contaminated groundwater was an exposure pathway at 91% of the 1300 sites on the National Priority List targeted for remediation because of public health threats and for several of the 20 priority contaminants on the

TABLE 12–2. Relative Frequency of Regulated VOC Occurrences in Exceedance of MCLs in Surface Water and Ground Water Supplies, United States

VOC	% of Surface Water Supplies	% of Ground-Water Supplies
Methylene chloride	4.7	2.3
Tetrachloroethylene	1.7	1.8
Trichloroethylene	1.2	1.5
Benzene	0.3	0.4
Vinyl chloride	0.3	0.2
All regulated VOCs[a]	8.2	6.1

Source: U.S. Environmental Protection Agency (1999).

Note: limited to those solvents for which at least 1% of water systems had MCL exceedances.

[a] There are 21 regulated VOCs including those shown above.

2001 CERCLA list, including arsenic, vinyl chloride, benzene, cadmium, chloroform, trichloroethylene, chromium VI, and hexachlorobutadiene (Table 12–1). The average drinking water trichloroethylene level in the United States during 1998 was 3.0 μg/L, with average daily intakes of about 11–33 μg by inhalation and 2–20 μg by ingestion; higher exposures may occur in homes with private wells located near waste disposal sites. Volatile organic chemicals are readily measured in exhaled breath and generally reflect recent exposures; exhaled breath tetrachloroethylene reflects exposures over somewhat longer periods because its half-life in vivo is much longer than that of most VOCs.

Risk Management

The provision of safe drinking water to a large population is a massive enterprise. There are about 170,000 public water systems in the United States alone, among which about 54,000 community water systems serve the majority of the population (U.S. Environmental Protection Agency, 2001c). The EPA regulates public water systems (publicly or privately owned water systems that serve at least 25 people or 15 service connections for at least 60 days annually) and has promulgated drinking water standards that address several hazard categories including microorganisms, disinfectant chemicals and DBPs, inorganic chemicals, organic chemicals, and radionuclides. This chapter addresses the first four categories to some degree; the reader should consult Chapter 9 for radionuclides, Chapter 7 for pesticides, and Chapters 4 and 5 for metals.

Disinfection By-Products

Trihalomethanes and other DBPs in drinking water originate mainly from the reaction of chlorine with humic and fulvic acids, natural organic substances arising from the decomposition of lignins and other phenolic compounds in vegetation. Levels of natural organics are generally higher in surface waters because of runoff from land, and thus chlorinated drinking surface water usually has higher average DBP levels than water from ground sources (Fig. 12–4). Most exposure to THMs comes from water and beverages. Trihalomethane levels in hot water are higher than those in cold water, tending to increase exposures through inhalation and bathing/showering. Chlorinated swimming pools are an important source of exposure, especially for children who swim frequently. Brominated DBPs tend to occur at higher levels in water from coastal areas and in sys-

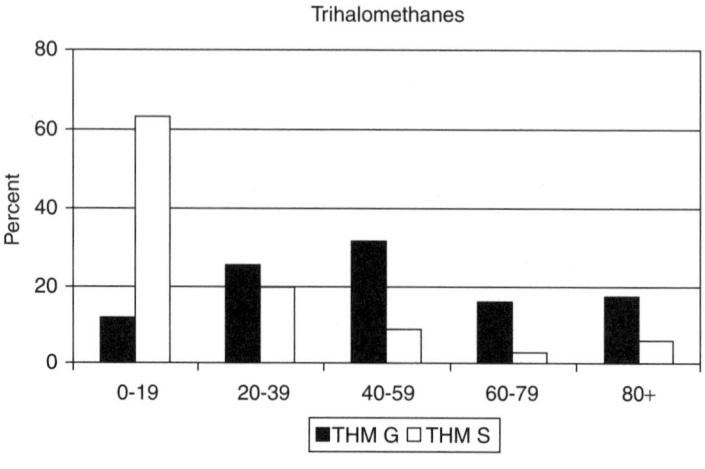

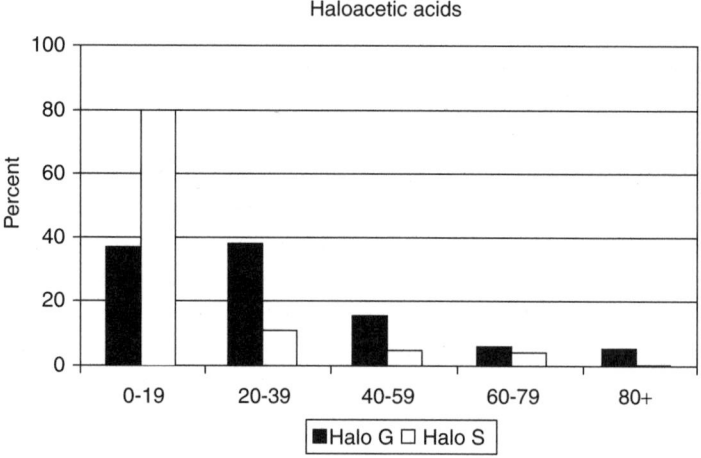

FIGURE 12–4. Distribution of total THM and haloacetic acid levels (μg/L) in U.S. ground and surface water supplies, 1998 (U.S. Environmental Protection Agency, 2000). G = ground water, S = surface water, Halo = haloacetic acids.

tems that use ozone. Reduction of DBP levels in drinking water, while preserving adequate disinfection, can be achieved through means such as

• Using raw water supplies low in natural organic material; this generally means groundwater or surface waters not prone to runoff with high organic content

- Protecting surface waters from contamination with natural organic material, for example, controlled disposal of animal manure and agricultural fertilizer runoff
- Filtration of raw water before disinfection, thereby reducing both the disinfectant dose needed and the microbial risks
- Using disinfection methods that reduce DBP formation (e.g., chloramination, ozonation, UV light)
- Removing DBPs from disinfected water with activated carbon filters (at the source or the point of use).

The main problem with many of these options relates to cost, particularly in older water systems that do not include filtration and serve relatively small populations. Although chlorination remains the dominant method in North America, ozonation is commonly used in several European countries; in such systems, some chlorinating agent is generally added to water before it enters the distribution system to maintain disinfection. Also, ozonation of water containing bromide increases production of bromate, a known animal carcinogen (kidney and thyroid tumors), and brominated DBPs. Granulated activated charcoal filters remove almost all THMs, other DBPs, and VOCs such as trichloroethylene; the filters must be replaced frequently, as their efficiency drops sharply when they become saturated. Drinking water standards for DBPs and other chemical contaminants are presented in Table 12–3. There is no drinking water standard for MX at present, but the proposed virtual safe dose for MX genotoxicity is 5 ng/kg/day and the proposed tolerable daily intake for nongenotoxic effects is 40 ng/kg/day (Hirose et al., 1999).

Other Chemical Contaminants

Approximately 85% of all U.S. drinking water systems have at least one potential source of contamination within 2 miles of their water intake or well, but only about 10% of water suppliers have implemented protective measures ranging from land use ordinances to public education. Hazardous waste disposal and leakage from storage tanks are major causes of groundwater contamination and potential threats to the health of persons dependent on well water; for example, disposal of trichloroethylene and leakage from storage tanks explain its frequent occurrence in groundwater samples. The ATSDR was established in 1980 under CERCLA (also known as the Superfund Act) to identify and remediate the estimated 40,000 uncontrolled hazardous waste sites in the United States. Trichoro-

TABLE 12–3. Drinking Water Guidelines and Standards for Microorganisms and
Chemical Contaminants

Contaminant	EPA Standard	Contaminant	EPA Standard
Microorganisms		*Selected other organic chemicals[c]*	
Cryptosporidium, Giardia *lamblia*, heterotrophic plate count, *Legionella,* turbidity, enteric viruses	TT[a]	Benzene	5 μg/L
		1,2-Dichloroethane	5 μg/L
		Dichloromethane	5 μg/L
		Ethylbenzene	0.7 mg/L
Total coliforms	5.0%[b]	Tetrachloroethylene	5 μg/L
		Toluene	1 mg/L
Disinfectants and DBPs		1,1,1-Trichloroethane	0.2 mg/L
		Trichloroethylene	5 μg/L
Bromate	10 μg/L	Vinyl chloride	2 μg/L
Chloramine (as chlorine) (maximum residual disinfectant level) (MRDL)	4 mg/L	Xylenes (total)	10 mg/L
		Inorganic chemicals	
Chlorine (MRDL)	4 mg/L		
Chlorine dioxide (MRDL)	0.8 mg/L	Nitrate	10 mg/L
Chlorite	1.0 mg/L	Nitrite	1 mg/L
Haloacetic acids	60 μg/L		
Total THMs	80 μg/L		

Source: U.S. Environmental Protection Agency (2001a).

[a]TT = treatment technique, that is, a required process intended to reduce the level of a contaminant in drinking water; for further information on application of this standard see U.S. Environmental Protection Agency (2001a).

[b]No more than 5% of samples can be total coliform-positive in a month (for systems that collect fewer than 40 routine samples per month, no more than 1 sample can be total coliform-positive); every sample that has total coliforms must be analyzed for fecal coliforms, and no fecal coliforms or E. coli may be present.

[c]Frequently detected non-THM VOCs in Canadian and U.S. water supplies.

See other chapters for standards for metals, pesticides, and radionuclides in drinking water.

ethylene, lead, tetrachloroethylene, benzene, and chromium were the most frequently detected substances in water near the 1300 National Priorities List sites.

To protect source waters from chemical contamination, the EPA has planned a strategy to (1) ensure strong and useful source water assessments for all public water supplies, (2) target relevant state and federal programs to address source water contamination prevention priorities, (3) increase awareness, education, and involvement by private industry, government, and the public, (4) foster local control and capacity, and (5) document and report on risks identified and progress made on reducing those risks. Even if this strategy is implemented, there will be major challenges including the need to protect persons dependent on private wells and small water systems (U.S. Environmental Protection Agency, 2001d).

CONCLUSIONS

Unresolved Issues and Knowledge Gaps

- Disinfection by-products
  - Developmental effects—there is limited evidence that THMs (or related DBPs) may cause spontaneous abortions, stillbirths, IUGR, and certain birth defects (neural tube, urinary tract); spontaneous abortions and stillbirths may be more closely related to bromodichloromethane than total THMs.
  - Cancer

    Although THMs were associated with childhood leukemia among children with certain polymorphisms, there is inadequate evidence for the role of DBPs in childhood cancer.

    There is limited evidence that DBPs may cause certain adult cancers (especially bladder cancer).
- Non-THM VOCs and nitrate/nitrite
  - Developmental effects

    There is inadequate evidence to assess the role of drinking water nitrate/nitrite in neural tube defects.

    There is inadequate evidence to assess the role of trichloroethylene and related VOCs in birth defects (cardiac, neural tube) and childhood leukemia.
  - Drinking water (especially farm well water) containing high nitrate levels can cause infantile methemoglobinemia; it is not clear if the causal agent is nitrate per se or waterborne infectious agents.

Risk Management

- Prevention
  - Protection of source waters, prefiltration of raw water, and use of activated charcoal (at the source or the point of use) may be necessary to simultaneously achieve adequate disinfection and minimal DBP levels in chlorinated surface tap water.
  - Control of hazardous waste disposal is needed to prevent contamination of groundwater by VOCs and other hazardous chemicals.

- Monitoring—periodic measurement of DBP and other chemical contaminant levels is needed to evaluate progress in meeting existing drinking water standards and to identify unmet needs.

II. WATERBORNE INFECTIONS

An adequate supply of safe drinking water is an elusive goal in many parts of the world, particularly among economically disadvantaged groups. Each year, about 11 million children die worldwide, primarily from pneumonia, diarrhea, measles, malaria, and malnutrition. Diarrhea causes about 2 million childhood deaths annually in developing countries, mostly because of fecally contaminated water used for drinking and washing, and is an important cause of malnutrition (World Health Organization, 1998). Major causes of childhood diarrhea in developing countries include rotavirus, *Shigella dysenteriae*, *Campylobacter jejuni*, *Cryptosporidium parvum*, *Vibrio cholerae*, and various *Salmonella* serotypes. Children in developing countries also have high illness and death rates because of water-related parasitic infections, such as, *Schistosoma* infection from bathing or wading in contaminated water (Pruss et al., 2002). The continuing threat of waterborne infections to public health even in economically privileged countries was dramatically illustrated by the massive 1993 outbreak of *C. parvum* in Milwaukee that affected over 400,000 people. Unprotected water sources and absent or inadequate drinking water disinfection processes contribute to continuing outbreaks of *Giardia lamblia* and *Shigella sonnei* and sporadic cases of *E. coli 0157:H7* and other agents.

Waterborne pathogens originating in human or animal feces primarily affect the gastrointestinal system, with outcomes that vary from unapparent infections to life-threatening bloody diarrhea, dehydration, and liver or kidney failure. Toddlers and young children are exposed to enteric pathogens by ingesting contaminated water and through hand–mouth behavior while playing with other children or in fecally contaminated areas; older children have lower risks because of acquired immunity and less hand–mouth behavior. Foods exposed to contaminated water can also cause gastrointestinal infections; for example, formula-fed infants are at much greater risk than breast-fed infants in regions with microbiologically contaminated drinking water. This part of the chapter briefly focuses mainly on the major microbial threats to children in developed countries; see other sources for further information (Detels et al., 1997).

BACTERIA

Globally, about 50% of the fatal cases of childhood diarrhea episodes annually are caused by enteric pathogens including *Shigella, V. cholerae, Campylobacter, Salmonella,* and *E. coli* (Centers for Disease Control and Prevention, 2001a) (Table 12–4).

Shigella Species

Shigella, the most important global cause of epidemic dysentery (diarrhea containing blood), is spread by contaminated water and food and person-to-person contact. *S. sonnei* is the most common serotype in developed countries while *S. boydii, S. dysenteriae,* and *S. flexneri* cause most cases in developing countries. At-risk populations include low-income groups dependent on water supplies that are inadequately disinfected, such as, indigenous groups subject to household crowding, lack of piped water, and inadequate sewage disposal. About 14,000 confirmed cases of shigellosis are reported annually in the United States, and the true number may be twentyfold higher (Centers for Disease Control and Prevention 2000). Young children are at greatest risk, especially those in child-care centers. After infection with *S. flexneri*, persons with the genetic marker HLA-B27 may develop Reiter's syndrome, characterized by joint pain, eye irritation, painful urination, and, occasionally, chronic arthritis.

Escherichia coli

Enterotoxigenic *E. coli* is a common cause of diarrhea among travelers and young children in developing countries. The first evidence that *E. coli* could cause serious illness in otherwise healthy people came from an investigation in Oregon and Michigan showing a strong association between consumption of undercooked hamburgers from the same fast-food restaurant chain and bloody diarrhea caused by *E. coli O157:H7*. *Escherichia coli O157:H7* produces Shiga-like toxins that damage renal tubular epithelial and endothelial cells; it usually causes mild diarrhea but can cause life-threatening hemorrhagic colitis and hemolytic uremic syndrome and is an important cause of acute renal failure in children. Animals, especially cattle, are the main reservoirs of *E. coli O157:H7*, and the principal source of human infection is undercooked contaminated meat; other sources include unpasteurized milk and contaminated water. Outbreaks of bloody diarrhea caused by *E. coli O157:H7* were first linked to contaminated water supplies in Missouri and Japan; the latter incident in-

TABLE 12–4. Potential Waterborne Infection Threats for Children[a]

Infectious Agent	Occurrence	Reported Annual Cases, USA, 1999[b] All Ages (Age < 15 Years)	Reservoir	Mode of Transmission
Shigella—S. dysenteriae, S. flexneri, S. boydii, S. sonnei	Worldwide; most cases and deaths occur among children aged <10 years	17,521 (9,656)	Humans	Direct or indirect fecal-oral from case or carrier, water, milk
Vibrio cholerae	Sporadic cases in developed countries, endemic areas, global pandemic (Asia, Africa, and Latin America) during the past 40 years	6 (2)	Humans, association with copepods and other zooplankton	Ingestion of fecal-contaminated water, contaminated foods, raw or undercooked seafoods naturally contaminated from polluted waters
Salmonella typhi	Sporadic cases in developed countries, about 16 million cases and 600,000 deaths globally	346 (121)	Humans	Fecal-contaminated water or food
Enterohemorrhagic Escherichia coli O157:H7	Children are at greatest risk; acute renal failure occurs in 2–7% of cases	4,513 (1,806)	Cattle	Meat, other foods, drinking water, swimming in contaminated water, person-to-person
Enterotoxigenic Escherichia coli	Travelers' diarrhea, young children in developing countries	79,000 (est.)	Humans, animals	Fecal-contaminated food or water
Helicobacter pylori	Widespread globally; prevalence increases with age; likely the most common chronic infection in humans; causes gastritis and stomach cancer	NA	Humans	Suspected oral-oral or fecal-oral or contaminated water

Organism	Distribution	Cases (deaths)	Reservoir	Transmission
Cryptosporidium parvum	Worldwide but prevalence higher in developing countries; outbreaks in day-care centers; waterborne outbreak in Milwaukee in 1993 affected about 400,000 people	2,361 (821)	Humans, animals	Fecal-oral including ingestion of contaminated drinking or recreational water, person-to-person, food
Entamoeba histolytica	Ubiquitous organism; infection rare before age 5 years	NA	Humans	Fecal-oral including ingestion of contaminated water and food, person-to-person
Giardia intestinalis (*G. lamblia*)	Worldwide but prevalence higher in developing countries; risk higher for children than for adults	NA	Humans, animals	Fecal-oral including ingestion of contaminated drinking or recreational water or food, person-to-person
Toxoplasma gondii	Worldwide; prevalence of infection quite high even in developed countries	NA	Cats, other felines	Transplacental if mother first infected <6 months before conception or during gestation; ingestion of contaminated meat, soil/sand, or water[c]
Cyclospora cayetanensis	Worldwide; outbreaks during recent years in the United States and Canada	56 (10)	Unknown	Fecal-oral including ingestion of contaminated food or water
Rotavirus	Most common cause of severe diarrhea among children aged <5 years worldwide; all children infected by age 3–4 years	55,000 (est.)	Humans	Fecal-oral including ingestion of contaminated water or food and contact with contaminated surfaces

(continued)

TABLE 12–4. Potential Waterborne Infection Threats for Children[a] (continued)

Infectious Agent	Occurrence	Reported Annual Cases, USA, 1999[b] All Ages (Age < 15 Years)	Reservoir	Mode of Transmission
Hepatitis A	Worldwide; children at risk, e.g., in day-care centers	17,047 (4,519)	Humans, other primates	Fecal-oral including person-to-person and ingestion of contaminated food or water
Adenoviruses	Worldwide; adenoviruses 40 and 41 cause gastroenteritis in children	NA	Humans	Fecal-oral including person-to-person and ingestion of contaminated drinking or recreational water
Norwalk and related caliciviruses	Sporadic and epidemic cases	181,000 (est.)	Humans	Ingestion of contaminated oysters or water

[a]Centers for Disease Control and Prevention (2000, 2001b).

[b]Centers for Disease Control and Prevention (2001d).

[c]Mullens (1996).

NA, not available.

volved hemorrhagic colitis and hemolytic uremic syndrome among children in a day-care school. Other water-related risk factors include swimming and consumption of foods such as lettuce exposed to contaminated irrigation water.

Helicobacter pylori

About half of the world's population has been infected with *H. pylori*, but infection rates vary widely by geographic region and socioeconomic status. Prevalence of infection often approaches 75% by age 10 years in developing countries compared to less than 10% even among adults in developed countries. *Helicobacter pylori* likely contributes to the syndrome of diarrhea, malnutrition, and growth failure of children in developing countries by suppressing the stomach's acid barrier and is an important cause of gastritis, peptic ulcers, and stomach cancer during adulthood. A longitudinal study of Japanese persons with gastrointestinal ulcers and related conditions showed that stomach cancer developed in 3% of those infected with *H. pylori* and in none of the uninfected persons (Uemura et al., 2001).

Children in the developing world acquire *H. pylori* soon after birth, and although the mode and route of transmission remain uncertain, it appears that infection may be acquired mainly from other family members or close contacts. Evidence supports both fecal-oral and oral-oral (through vomitus or possibly saliva) pathways. Risk factors for infection include drinking water from nonmunicipal water sources, inadequate sanitation, low social class, and high-density living conditions. *Helicobacter pylori* has been detected in water, soil, flies, cow feces, and most surface and shallow groundwater samples in a U.S. survey. There is little relation between the occurrence of total coliforms or *E. coli* in water and the presence of *H. pylori*, suggesting that routine screening of water supplies for traditional indicator organisms may fail to protect consumers from this organism.

Other Bacteria

Since the early 1800s, cholera has spread periodically to other parts of the world in pandemic waves from endemic areas in Southeast Asia. The most recent pandemic began in 1961 in Indonesia and spread rapidly to other countries in Asia, Europe, Africa, and Latin America. Peru, Guatemala, and other Latin American countries reported almost 1 million cases to the Pan American Health Organization during 1991–1993. Cholera is spread mainly through contaminated drinking water and food including consumption of raw or undercooked shellfish. Algal blooms may have supported the growth of *V. cholerae* in marine and fresh waters in Peru and contamination of fish, mollusks, and crustacea. Typhoid fever, a life-threatening illness, affects over 10 million persons annually in the developing world, with case-fatality rates being highest among infants and the elderly.

Cyanobacterial Toxins

Cyanobacteria (blue-green algae) produce several toxins that have adverse effects in experimental animals ranging from birth defects to neurotoxicity and liver cancer. Proliferation of cyanobacteria in a newly flooded reservoir area above the Itaparica dam in Brazil was the apparent cause of about 2000 gastroenteritis cases, including 88 deaths, mostly among children. Cyanobacteria levels in drinking water consumed by pregnant women were inconsistently related to low birth weight, prematurity, and birth defects in an ecologic study.

PROTOZOA

Protozoal infections pose threats even in developed countries because these organisms are shed from infected hosts in feces as oocysts with thick walls that enable them to resist chlorination. Disinfection of water contaminated by protozoa generally requires efficient filtration that is not always available.

Cryptosporidium parvum

There are no vaccines or effective treatments for *C. parvum*, a microbe responsible for up to 20% of childhood diarrhea in developing countries. Most cases are not life-threatening, but children with immune deficiency may develop serious, potentially fatal infections (e.g., children undergoing chemotherapy for cancer or organ transplantation). About 400,000 people developed acute watery diarrhea due to *C. parvum* in Milwaukee in early 1993 because one of the city's water treatment plant filtration systems failed to remove *Cryptosporidium* oocysts. Investigation showed that emergency room visits and hospital admissions for gastroenteritis before the outbreak were strongly associated with turbidity, with lag periods of about 8 days among children.

There have been at least 20 smaller cryptosporidiosis waterborne outbreaks in the United Kingdom and North America since the Milwaukee epidemic. Surveillance of *C. parvum* infections in seven states during

1997–1998 revealed over 1000 laboratory-confirmed cases including a seasonal peak in late summer among children aged 0–14 years (Dietz et al., 2000). Outbreaks have occurred after swimming in contaminated pools, suggesting that the summer peak may relate in part to recreational exposure to contaminated water. Children are at risk of infection in swimming pools because *C. parvum*

- Can survive the usual chlorine levels for several days
- Is not removed by conventional pool water filters
- Has a low infective dose

A single fecal accident can contaminate an entire pool to such a degree that a few mouthfuls of water can cause infection (Centers for Disease Control and Prevention, 2001c). *Cryptosporidium parvum* oocysts in human and animal feces can enter surface waters directly or through wastewater, leaky septic tanks, and runoff and have been detected in shellfish intended for human consumption. Calves appear to be a major reservoir, shedding oocysts for up to 2 weeks; a mixture of human and bovine *C. parvum* genotypes were detected in about half of raw surface water samples from several areas in the United States (Xiao et al., 2001).

Giardia intestinalis

Giardia intestinalis (also known as *G. lamblia*) is a ubiquitous enteric parasite affecting humans and a range of wild and domestic mammals, particularly dogs and dairy cattle. It is a globally important cause of waterborne diarrheal disease and the most common protozoan infection of the human small intestine, causing diarrhea particularly in children, for example, in day-care centers. Dormant *Giardia* cysts persist for months in cold fresh water, and ingestion of ten cysts can initiate infection.

Toxoplasma gondii

The largest recorded human toxoplasmosis outbreak, and the only one caused by a contaminated municipal water supply, occurred in Victoria, Canada, during 1994–1995. Ultimately, 112 serologically confirmed cases, including 37 pregnant women and 12 infants with *T. gondii* retinitis, were identified. There was no association with domestic cats, but mapping of cases and case-control studies showed that the incidence rate was highest for persons living or working in an area served by one of the city's water distribution systems. Domestic cats, cougars, and deer mice living in the watershed of a surface water reservoir showed serologic evidence of

T. gondii infection, and cougars were found to shed *T. gondii* oocysts. The municipal water system used unfiltered, chloraminated surface water and was the likely source of this community-wide outbreak of toxoplasmosis.

Cyclospora cayetanensis

Surveillance and investigations of cyclosporiasis in Guatemala and Peru have shown that prevalence rates were highest for young children and that cases were associated with drinking untreated water. Investigation of 96 cyclosporiasis outbreaks in the United States and Canada during 1996–1997 (totaling over 2000 cases) showed strong associations with consumption of fresh Guatemalan raspberries. The mode of contamination of the raspberries remains unknown, but *C. cayetanensis* oocysts have been detected in wastewater, a commodity used for irrigation in some regions; also, preharvest pesticide applications used on raspberries may have been diluted with contaminated water.

VIRUSES

Fecal-contaminated drinking water is an important source of the more than 100 different viruses that can infect the gastrointestinal tract.

Rotavirus

Rotavirus mainly affects infants aged 6–24 months and is the most common cause of infantile watery diarrhea worldwide, with potentially lethal dehydration occurring in almost 1% of affected infants. In developing countries, rotavirus infections account for about 6% of all diarrheal episodes and 20% of diarrhea-associated deaths of young children. In the United States, virtually all children have been infected by age 4 years. Reviews of childhood diarrhea in Australia, the United States, and Canada showed that rotavirus was the leading identified pathogen (up to half of all children aged 12–23 months). The virus particle is stable and can persist in the environment, including potable and recreational waters, and can be concentrated by shellfish; waterborne outbreaks have been reported.

Enteric Adenoviruses

Although much less common than rotaviruses, enteric adenoviruses (especially Ad40 and Ad41) are important causes of infantile watery diarrhea globally, accounting for 3%–12% of cases. Water is an important route of enteric adenovirus infection.

Hepatitis Viruses

Hepatitis A and E viruses transmitted via contaminated water, often through food vehicles, cause environment-related hepatitis. Hepatitis A virus infects all age groups, causing an estimated 1.4 million cases globally, while the less well-studied hepatitis E virus is found mainly in the developing world, often causing severe childhood infections. Assessment of hepatitis A control programs has relied mainly on cross-sectional surveys of local populations. Prevalence rates of anti-hepatitis A antibody among children aged 6–10 years in six Latin American countries varied from 30% in Chile to 70%–80% in Mexico and the Dominican Republic (Tanaka, 2000). Until about 1980, up to 90% of children aged 10–15 years in Southeast Asia were anti-hepatitis A antibody-positive; by the early 1990s, the prevalence had declined substantially in several regions, for example, from 31% in 1987 to 13% in 1996 among children aged 10–19 years in Bangkok. Hepatitis E infection often occurs in relation to the use of surface water for drinking, cooking, personal washing, and human excreta disposal. Many large outbreaks of hepatitis E have occurred after heavy rains and flooding that caused fecal contamination of surface waters and shallow wells.

Other Viruses

Norwalk and Norwalk-like viruses and related caliciviruses frequently cause gastroenteritis epidemics in developing countries and occasionally in economically advantaged countries. In a Finnish community, there were 1500–3000 cases in 1994 caused by a contaminated well, the main infectious agent being a calicivirus. Molecular diagnostic methods have shown that caliciviruses are the most common cause of acute gastroenteritis outbreaks in the United States and may be a common cause of sporadic cases among children and adults. Astrovirus is a significant cause of acute diarrhea among children, with transmission thought to involve fecal-oral spread from water or food sources. About 3% of hospitalized pediatric gastroenteritis cases in Australia were attributed to astrovirus, and most children had serologic evidence of previous infection by age 6 years. Childhood diarrhea sometimes involves coinfection with astrovirus, rotavirus, and caliciviruses.

RISK MANAGEMENT

The main source of human pathogens in drinking or recreational waters is feces of human or animal origin. Even in developed countries, problems arise when massive microbial contamination overwhelms disinfection processes. Rainfall or flooding enables the spread of *E. coli* O157:H7 and other enteric pathogens in animal feces into runoff and leachate from contaminated soils. For example, over 1300 cases of gastroenteritis, including infections with *E. coli* O157:H7 and *Campylobacter* species, occurred in an Ontario town in 2000 due to heavy rain, farm runoff, and contamination of at least one well (Health Canada, 2000).

Use of water free of human pathogens in food preparation, ingestion, and personal hygiene is essential for personal and public health. Safe disposal of human feces, protection of water supplies from microbial contamination, adequate water disinfection, and personal hygiene continue to be challenges in low-income populations globally. Although watershed management is recognized as an important preventive strategy, water supplies that can be safely used with no disinfection are relatively rare; even in relatively pristine environments, surface water may be contaminated with animal excreta containing human pathogens. High population density and poverty combine to favor microbial contamination of water and inadequate or nonexistent water treatment technologies; simple measures such as boiling water for ingestion are problematic in many impoverished regions. Even where available, conventional sewage and water treatment methods are relatively inefficient in the removal and inactivation of most enteric viruses and several protozoa.

Water treatment options aimed specifically at disinfection range from boiling water to complex water treatment systems in large urban centers; the reader is referred to other sources for more detailed information on this topic (Craun et al., 2001). The effectiveness of water treatment facilities is especially important for surface or near-surface waters subject to microbial contamination; for large populations, this generally requires relatively expensive technology that combines filtration and disinfection processes. Proposed regulations to control waterborne *C. parvum* will require billions of dollars to improve water-treatment facilities (particularly filtration) in the United States. It is important to note, however, that methods to reduce microbial contamination are similar to and compatible with those aimed at reducing DBP levels.

Waterborne disease surveillance is an important component of communicable disease control programs. In the absence of timely surveillance, pharmacists were the first to notice the Milwaukee outbreak after their antidiarrheal remedies were sold out. After the outbreak, analysis of cryptosporidiosis cases in Milwaukee during 1993 revealed a smaller outbreak about 3 weeks before the major epidemic. Effective surveillance might have detected this early warning and triggered actions to prevent the major epidemic. Drinking water standards for microorganisms are presented in Table 12–3.

Conclusions

Proven Health Outcomes

• Waterborne infectious agents are the major cause of childhood diarrheal diseases globally, including an estimated 2 million annual childhood deaths mainly in developing countries
• *Escherichia coli 0157:H7,* a major cause of acute renal failure in children, can be transmitted through contaminated drinking water

Unresolved Issues and Knowledge Gaps

• Water appears to be a source of *H. pylori* infection during childhood; this organism causes chronic gastrointestinal infection and an increased risk of peptic ulcers and stomach cancer during adulthood. Routine screening of water supplies for *E. coli* or total coliforms may not protect consumers from this organism.
• There is inadequate evidence to assess the potential role of waterborne infections in infantile methemoglobinemia.

Risk Management Issues

• Prevention—filtration is needed to reduce the hazards of both chlorine-resistant microbes (e.g., *C. parvum*) and DBPs.
• Monitoring—frequent measurements of microbial concentrations in drinking water are needed for early detection of breakdowns in disinfection practices and to evaluate progress in meeting drinking water standards.

References

Agency for Toxic Substances and Disease Registry. (2001). 2001 CERCLA priority list of hazardous substances. Located at http://www.atsdr.cdc.gov/clist.html

Arbuckle TE, Hrudey SE, Krasner SW, Nuckols JR, Richardson SD, Singer P, Mendola P, Dodds L, Weisel C, Ashley DL, Froese KL, Pegram RA, and others. (2002). Assessing exposure in epidemiologic studies to disinfection by-products in drinking water: report from an international workshop. Environ Health Perspect 110(Suppl 1):53–60.

Arbuckle TE, Sherman GJ, Corey PN, Walters D, Lo B. (1988). Water nitrates and CNS birth defects: a population-based case-control study. Arch Environ Health 43:162–7.

Aschengrau A, Zierler S, Cohen A. (1993). Quality of community drinking water and the occurrence of late adverse pregnancy outcomes. Arch Environ Health 48:105–13.

Bove FJ, Fulcomer MC, Klotz JB, Esmart J, Dufficy EM, Savrin JE. (1995). Public drinking water contamination and birth outcomes. Am J Epidemiol 141:850–62.

Bove F, Shim Y, Zeitz P. (2002). Drinking water contaminants and adverse pregnancy outcomes: a review. Environ Health Perspect 110(Suppl 1):61–74.

Bukowski J, Somers G, Bryanton J. (2001). Agricultural contamination of groundwater as a possible risk factor for growth restriction or prematurity. J Occup Environ Med 43:377–83.

Centers for Disease Control and Prevention. (2000). Division of Bacterial and Mycotic Diseases. Disease information. Located at http://www.cdc.gov/ncidod/dbmd/diseaseinfo/default.htm

Centers for Disease Control and Prevention. (2001a). Bacterial waterborne diseases. Atlanta: Centers for Disease Control and Prevention.

Centers for Disease Control and Prevention. (2001b). Parasitic disease information. Located at http://www.cdc.gov/ncidod/dpd/parasites/listing.htm

Centers for Disease Control and Prevention. (2001c). Protracted outbreaks of cryptosporidiosis associated with swimming pool use—Ohio and Nebraska, 2000. MMWR 50:406–10.

Centers for Disease Control and Prevention. (2001d). Summary of notifiable diseases, United States, 1999. MMWR 48 (No. 53):1–18.

Cohn P, Klotz J, Bove F, Berkowitz M, Fagliano J. (1994). Drinking water contamination and the incidence of leukemia and non-Hodgkin's lymphoma. Environ Health Perspect 102:556–61.

Craun GF, Hauchman FS, Robinson DE. (2001). Microbial pathogens and disinfection by-products in drinking water: health effects and management of risks. Washington, DC: International Life Science Institute.

Croen LA, Shaw GM, Sanbonmatsu L, Selvin S, Buffler PA. (1997). Maternal residential proximity to hazardous waste sites and risk for selected congenital malformations. Epidemiology 8:347–54.

Croen LA, Todoroff K, Shaw GM. (2001). Maternal exposure to nitrate from drinking water and diet and risk for neural tube defects. Am J Epidemiol 153:325–31.

Cutler JJ, Parker GS, Rosen S, Prenney B, Healey R , Caldwell GG. (1986). Childhood leukemia in Woburn, Massachusetts. Public Health Rep 101:201–5.

Detels R, Holland W, McEwen J, Omenn GS. (1997). Oxford textbook of public health. New York: Oxford University Press.

Dietz V, Vugia D, Nelson R, Wicklund J, Nadle J , McCombs KG, Reddy S. (2000). Active, multisite, laboratory-based surveillance for *Cryptosporidium parvum*. Am J Trop Med Hyg 62:368–72.

Dodds L, King W, Woolcott C, Pole J. (1999). Trihalomethanes in public water supplies and adverse birth outcomes. Epidemiology 10:233–7.

Dodds L, King WD. (2001). Relation between trihalomethane compounds and birth defects. Occup Environ Med 58:443–6.

Dolk H, Vrijheid M, Armstrong B, Abramsky L, Bianchi F, Garne E, Nelen V, Robert E, Scott JE, Stone D, Tenconi R. (1998). Risk of congenital anomalies near hazardous-waste landfill sites in Europe: the EUROHAZCON study. Lancet 352:423–7.

Dorsch MM, Scragg RK, McMichael AJ, Baghurst PA, Dyer KF. (1984). Congenital malformations and maternal drinking water supply in rural South Australia: a case-control study. Am J Epidemiol 119:473–86.

Dow JL, Green T. (2000). Trichloroethylene induced vitamin B(12) and folate deficiency leads to increased formic acid excretion in the rat. Toxicology 146: 123–36.

Eskes TK. (2000). Homocysteine and human reproduction. Clin Exp Obstet Gynecol 27:157–67.

Gallagher MD, Nuckols JR, Stallones L, Savitz DA. (1998). Exposure to trihalomethanes and adverse pregnancy outcomes. Epidemiology 9:484–9.

Goldberg SJ, Lebowitz MD, Graver EJ, Hicks S. (1990). An association of human congenital cardiac malformations and drinking water contaminants. J Am Coll Cardiol 16:155–64.

Graves CG, Matanoski GM, Tardiff RG. (2001). Weight of evidence for an association between adverse reproductive and developmental effects and exposure to disinfection by-products: a critical review. Regul Toxicol Pharmacol 34:103–24.

Health Canada. (2000). Waterborne outbreak of gastroenteritis associated with a contaminated municipal water supply, Walkerton, Ontario, May–June 2000. Can Commun Dis Rep 26:170–3.

Hirose A, Nishikawa A, Kinae N, Hasegawa R. (1999). 3-Chloro-4-(dichloromethyl)-5-hydroxy-2(5H)-furanone (MX): toxicological properties and risk assessment in drinking water. Rev Environ Health 14:103–20.

Infante-Rivard C, Amre D, Sinnett D. (2002). *GSTT1* and *CYP2E1* polymorphisms and trihalomethanes in drinking water: effect on childhood leukemia. Environ Health Perspect 110:591–3.

Infante-Rivard C, Olson E, Jacques L, Ayotte P. (2001). Drinking water contaminants and childhood leukemia. Epidemiology 12:13–9.

International Agency for Research on Cancer. (1995). IARC monographs on the evaluation of carcinogenic risks to humans. Vol. 63. Dry cleaning, some chlorinated solvents and other industrial chemicals. Lyon, France: International Agency for Research on Cancer.

International Agency for Research on Cancer. (2002). Search IARC Agents. Located at http://monographs.iarc.fr/htdig/search.html.

Jaakkola JJ, Magnus P, Skrondal A, Hwang BF, Becher G, Dybing E. (2001). Foetal growth and duration of gestation relative to water chlorination. Occup Environ Med 58:437–42.

Kallen BA, Robert E. (2000). Drinking water chlorination and delivery outcome—a registry-based study in Sweden. Reprod Toxicol 14:303–9.

Kanitz S, Franco Y, Patrone V, Caltabellotta M, Raffo E, Riggi C, Timitilli D, Ravera G. (1996). Association between drinking water disinfection and somatic parameters at birth. Environ Health Perspect 104:516–20.

King WD, Dodds L, Allen AC. (2000). Relation between stillbirth and specific chlorination by-products in public water supplies. Environ Health Perspect 108: 883–6.

Klotz JB, Pyrch LA. (1999). Neural tube defects and drinking water disinfection by-products. Epidemiology 10:383–90.

Kramer MD, Lynch CF, Isacson P, Hanson JW. (1992). The association of waterborne chloroform with intrauterine growth retardation. Epidemiology 3: 407–13.

Lynberg M, Nuckols JR, Langlois P, Ashley D, Singer P, Mendola P, Wilkes C, Krapfl H, Miles E, Speight V, Lin B, Small L, and others. (2001). Assessing exposure to disinfection by-products in women of reproductive age living in Corpus Christi, Texas, and Cobb County, Georgia: descriptive results and methods. Environ Health Perspect 109:597–604.

Magnus P, Jaakkola JJ, Skrondal A, Alexander J, Becher G, Krogh T, Dybing E. (1999). Water chlorination and birth defects. Epidemiology 10:513–7.

Mueller BA, Newton K, Holly EA, Preston-Martin S. (2001). Residential water source and the risk of childhood brain tumors. Environ Health Perspect 109: 551–6.

Mullens A. (1996). "I think we have a problem in Victoria": MDs respond quickly to toxoplasmosis outbreak in BC. CMAJ 154:1721–4.

Pruss A, Kay D, Fewtrell L, Bartram J. (2002). Estimating the burden of disease from water, sanitation, and hygiene at a global level. Environ Health Perspect 110:537–42.

Reif JS, Hatch MC, Bracken M, Holmes LB, Schwetz BA, Singer PC. (1996). Reproductive and developmental effects of disinfection by-products in drinking water. Environ Health Perspect 104:1056–61.

Savitz DA, Andrews KW, Pastore LM. (1995). Drinking water and pregnancy outcome in central North Carolina: source, amount, and trihalomethane levels. Environ Health Perspect 103:592–6.

Sonnenfeld N, Hertz-Picciotto I, Kaye WE. (2001). Tetrachloroethylene in drinking water and birth outcomes at the U.S. Marine Corps Base at Camp Lejeune, North Carolina. Am J Epidemiol 154:902–8.

Tanaka J. (2000). Hepatitis A shifting epidemiology in Latin America. Vaccine 18(Suppl 1):S57–60.

Thompson DJ, Warner SD, Robinson VB. (1974). Teratology studies on orally administered chloroform in the rat and rabbit. Toxicol Appl Pharmacol 29:348–57.

U.S. Environmental Protection Agency. (1998). National primary drinking water regulations: disinfectants and disinfection byproducts; final rule. Fed Reg 63: 69389–476.

U.S. Environmental Protection Agency. (1999). A review of contaminant occurrence in public water systems (EPA 816-R-99-006). Washington, DC: U.S. Environmental Protection Agency.

U.S. Environmental Protection Agency. (2000). National treated water levels of total trihalomethanes for July–September 1998. Located at http://www.epa.gov/enviro/html/icr/national/report/tthm/5.html

U.S. Environmental Protection Agency. (2001a). Current drinking water standards. Located at http://www.epa.gov/safewater/mcl.html

U.S. Environmental Protection Agency. (2001b). IRIS substance list. Located at http://www.epa.gov/iris/subst/index.html

U.S. Environmental Protection Agency. (2001c). Public drinking water systems: facts and figures. Located at http://www.epa.gov/safewater/pws/factoids.html

U.S. Environmental Protection Agency. (2001d). National source water contamination prevention strategy. Seventh draft for discussion. Washington, DC: U.S. Environmental Protection Agency.

Uemura N, Okamoto S, Yamamoto S, Matsumura N, Yamaguchi S, Yamakido M, Taniyama K, Sasaki N, Schlemper RJ. (2001). *Helicobacter pylori* infection and the development of gastric cancer. N Engl J Med 345:784–9.

Vrijheid M. (2000). Health effects of residence near hazardous waste landfill sites: a review of epidemiologic literature. Environ Health Perspect 108(Suppl 1): 101–12.

Waller K, Swan SH, DeLorenze G, Hopkins B. (1998). Trihalomethanes in drinking water and spontaneous abortion. Epidemiology 9:134–40.

Wartenberg D, Reyner D, Scott CS. (2000). Trichloroethylene and cancer: epidemiologic evidence. Environ Health Perspect 108(Suppl 2):161–76.

World Health Organization. (1998). Fact sheet No 178. Reducing mortality from major killers of children. Geneva: World Health Organization.

Wright JM, Schwartz J, Vartiainen T, Maki-Paakkanen J, Altshul L, Harrington JJ, Dockery DW. (2002). 3-Chloro-4-(dichloromethyl)-5-hydroxy-2(5H)-furanone (MX) and mutagenic activity in Massachusetts drinking water. Environ Health Perspect 110:157–64.

Xiao L, Singh A, Limor J, Graczyk TK, Gradus S, Lal A. (2001). Molecular characterization of *Cryptosporidium* oocysts in samples of raw surface water and wastewater. Appl Environ Microbiol 67:1097–101.

Yang CY, Cheng BH, Tsai SS, Wu TN, Lin MC, Lin KC. (2000). Association between chlorination of drinking water and adverse pregnancy outcome in Taiwan. Environ Health Perspect 108:765–8.

13
Conclusion

Environmental Threats to Child Health

This section describes the burden of child health conditions and summarizes their known and suspected environmental risk factors as discussed in previous chapters. The purpose is to provide an overview of progress to date in identifying environmental threats to the fetus and child and to highlight areas where research and monitoring on environmental exposures and child health outcomes are needed. The summary tables (Tables 13–1 to 13–5) have important limitations:

- Critical evidence for several of the known causal factors came from studies of children exposed to contaminant levels much higher than those experienced today in the general population; there is considerable uncertainty about health risks at much lower exposure levels.
- With very few exceptions, existing knowledge does not permit estimation of attributable risks; thus, inclusion of risk factors for a given adverse health outcome does not mean that these factors cause all or even most of the cases.
- The relationships are limited to those for which exposure occurs prenatally or during childhood.

• The tables do not identify critical exposure pathways or timing (e.g., ingested vs. inhaled, prenatal vs. postnatal); for information on these and other details, see the subject-area chapters.

• The tables do not address nonenvironmental risk factors such as genetic traits, infections (other than waterborne infections), maternal prenatal alcohol and drug use, and parental or child diet; for information on these issues, see other sources.

Adverse Developmental Outcomes

Behavioral (tobacco, alcohol), pharmaceutical, and microbial factors are important risk factors for some adverse developmental outcomes but the causes of these conditions remain poorly defined. Based on sheer numbers, fetal deaths, low birth weight, and birth defects are major child health burdens (Table 13–1). Although about 1 million recognized fetal deaths (excluding therapeutic abortions) occur annually in the United States, about the same number of fetal deaths occur very soon after conception but are not clinically recognized. There are few proven environmental causes of fetal death in humans, at least at widely prevalent exposure levels; there is limited evidence implicating prenatal parental (usually maternal) exposure to lead, PCBs/dioxin-like compounds, pesticides, ETS, ionizing radiation, and THMs and suggestive but inadequate evidence for ambient air pollutants. Suspected environmental causes of IUGR or preterm birth include prenatal maternal exposure to lead, ETS (independent of prenatal maternal smoking), ambient air pollution, and THMs.

Birth defects comprise many distinct conditions with few known causes. First trimester exposure to high-dose ionizing radiation caused microcephaly (and mental retardation) among infants of Japanese atomic bomb survivors. Suspected environmental causes of birth defects include lead, pesticides, low-dose ionizing radiation, THMs, and methylmercury. There is inadequate evidence for possible links between birth defects and arsenic, TCDD, HAAs, power-frequency magnetic fields, certain drinking water contaminants (nitrate/nitrite, non-THM solvents), and ambient air pollution. Despite public and scientific concern about reports of declining sperm counts in young adult men and premature breast development in young girls and potential links to hormonally active environmental contaminants, no adequately designed epidemiologic studies have assessed such relationships. There is limited evidence that prenatal or early childhood exposure to lead or PCBs/dioxin-like compounds can cause growth deficits during childhood.

TABLE 13–1. Role of Prenatal Exposure to Environmental Agents in Adverse Developmental Outcomes

Outcome	Number of events per year (United States)	Environmental risk factors and level of epidemiologic evidence[a]		
		Sufficient	Limited	Inadequate
Fetal deaths (spontaneous abortions and stillbirths)	983,000[b]		Lead, PCBs/dioxin-like compounds, pesticides, prenatal maternal ETS exposure, parental ionizing radiation exposure, THMs (or related DBP's)	Arsenic, HAAs, maternal exposure to power-frequency magnetic fields, multiple outdoor air pollutants
Low birth weight (<2500 g)	301,000[c]	PCBs/dioxin-like compounds	Lead, pesticides, prenatal maternal ETS exposure, outdoor air pollution (CO, SO_2, PM), THMs (or related DBP's)	Arsenic, cadmium, pesticides, HAAs, ionizing radiation exposure, power frequency magnetic fields, nitrate in drinking water, non-THM VOCs in drinking water
Preterm delivery	467,000[c]		Lead, pesticides, prenatal maternal ETS exposure	HAAs
Total birth defects[d]	120,000[e]			Arsenic, TCDD, HAAs, power-frequency magnetic fields
Neural tube defects	2,500		Lead, herbicides, preconceptual parental or first trimester maternal ionizing radiation exposure, THMs (or related DBP's)	Nitrate/nitrite in drinking water, non-THM VOCs in drinking water, lead
Microcephaly[f]	2,500	Ionizing radiation (prenatal atomic bomb exposure)	Methylmercury	

Birth defect	Prevalence	Sufficient or limited evidence[a]	Inadequate evidence[a]
Cardiac defects	13,000	Lead, pesticides, preconceptual parental or first trimester maternal ionizing radiation exposure	Ambient air pollution (CO), THMs, non-THM VOCs in drinking water, lead
Urinary tract defects[g]	3,600	THMs (or related DBPs)	
Hypospadias (second and third degree)	1,000		
Cryptorchidism (undescended testicles)	3,900		Pesticides, HAAs
Oral clefts	6,700	Lead, pesticides	Ambient air pollution (CO), THMs, non-THM solvents in drinking water
Limb reduction defects	2,200	Pesticides	
Skeletal defects	NA		Cadmium
Reduced stature during childhood	NA	Lead, PCBs/dioxin-like compounds	

ETS = environmental tobacco smoke; TCDD = 2,3,7,8-tetrachlorodibenzo-p-dioxin; THMs = trihalomethanes.

[a]Sufficient evidence—based on peer-reviewed reports of expert groups or authoritative reviews that concluded that a causal relationship existed; limited evidence—includes relationships for which several epidemiologic studies, including at least one case-control or cohort study, showed fairly consistent associations and evidence of exposure–risk relationships after control for potential confounders; inadequate evidence—relationships for which epidemiologic studies were limited in number and quality (e.g., small studies, ecologic studies, limited control of potential confounders), had inconsistent results, or showed little or no evidence of exposure–risk relationships.

[b]Ventura et al. (1999).

[c]Ventura et al. (2001).

[d]Birth defect birth prevalence rates are from California unless otherwise indicated (California Birth Defects Monitoring Program (2002).

[e]Based on 3% of the approximately 4 million births annually in the United States.

[f]Microcephaly birth prevalence rate from U.S. Metropolitan Atlanta Congenital Defects Program (International Clearinghouse for Birth Defect Monitoring Systems, 1999).

[g]Urinary tract birth prevalence rate from Canadian Congenital Anomaly Surveillance System (International Clearinghouse for Birth Defect Monitoring Systems, 1999).

NA = not available

Cancer

There have been numerous well-designed epidemiologic studies of relationships between prenatal and childhood exposures and risks of childhood and young adult cancers. There is sufficient evidence for causal roles for prenatal or childhood ionizing radiation exposure in childhood leukemia, brain cancer, and thyroid cancer and in adult cancers including breast and thyroid cancers and leukemia (Table 13–2). The evidence for these relationships came mainly from groups with high-level exposure (atomic bomb, Chernobyl nuclear reactor accident, therapeutic radiation). The lifetime excess cancer risk from a given dose of ionizing radiation during childhood appears to be about double that for an equivalent exposure during adulthood. The attributable risk of environmental sources of ionizing radiation is unknown but likely to be quite small because of the low prevalence of high exposures. Intense sun exposure during childhood is a major cause of malignant melanoma and basal cell skin cancers that occur mainly during adulthood.

Limited epidemiologic evidence precludes firm conclusions about the potential causal roles of pesticides, paternal smoking/ETS, ionizing radiation (parental occupational exposure, radioactive fallout from atmospheric nuclear tests), certain parental occupational exposures, and power-frequency magnetic fields in childhood cancers. Polychlorinated biphenyls have been linked to adult cancers including breast and non-Hodgkin's lymphoma but the role of childhood PCB exposures is unknown.

Neurobehavioral Outcomes

Neurobehavioral problems among children range from subtle deficits detectable only through specialized testing to severely disabling conditions (Table 13–3). High-dose prenatal maternal exposures to methylmercury, PCBs/dioxin-like compounds, and ionizing radiation are known causes of severe neurobehavioral effects including motor, sensory, and cognitive deficits. Early childhood exposure to lead is a known cause of sensory, motor, and cognitive deficits, and there is suggestive/limited evidence for a causal role in attention deficit hyperactivity disorder. There is limited evidence that relatively low-level exposure in early childhood to methylmercury or PCBs/dioxin-like compounds from contaminated foods (especially fish) can cause cognitive and other neurobehavioral deficits. Occupational exposure of youth and young adults to OP and carbamate insecticides has been linked to persistent sensorimotor deficits.

TABLE 13-2. Role of Prenatal or Childhood Exposure to Environmental Agents in Childhood and Adult Cancers[a]

Outcome	Cases per year (United States)[c]	Environmental Risk Factors and Level of Epidemiologic Evidence[b]		
		Sufficient	Limited	Inadequate
Childhood cancers (Age 0–19 years)				
Leukemia	12,800			PCBs, other PHAHs, RF radiation, indoor air VOCs
	3,250	Ionizing radiation (prenatal diagnostic x-rays)	Pesticides, paternal smoking, childhood ionizing radiation exposure (diagnostic X-rays), radioactive fallout from nuclear testing, child exposure to power-frequency magnetic fields, paternal occupational exposure to solvents and paints	Cadmium, ambient air pollution (traffic density, benzene), paternal preconceptual ionizing radiation exposure, childhood environmental radiation exposure (radon, other), paternal exposure to power-frequency magnetic fields, radiofrequency radiation, indoor air VOCs, THMs non-THM VOCs in drinking water
Lymphomas	1,700		Pesticides, paternal smoking (? ETS or other mechanism), parental occupational exposure to solvents and other petroleum products	Ambient air pollution, ionizing radiation (prenatal diagnostic)
Brain	2,200		Pesticides, paternal smoking (? ETS or other mechanism), paternal occupational exposure to solvents and paints	Childhood environmental radiation exposure (radon, other), power-frequency magnetic or electric fields or radiofrequency radiation, paternal exposure to power-frequency magnetic fields, drinking water nitrite

(continued)

TABLE 13–2. Role of Prenatal or Childhood Exposure to Environmental Agents in Childhood and Adult Cancers[a] (continued)

Outcome	Cases per year (United States)[c]	Environmental Risk Factors and Level of Epidemiologic Evidence[b]		
		Sufficient	Limited	Inadequate
Wilms' tumor	500		Pesticides	Prenatal maternal ionizing radiation (diagnostic X-rays)
Germ cell tumors	900			
Thyroid tumors	350	Childhood ionizing radiation exposure		
Melanoma	325		Intense sun exposure (see also adult melanoma below)	
Ewing's sarcoma (bone)	200		Pesticides	Childhood environmental radiation exposure (radium in drinking water)
Adult cancers (Age ≥ 20)	1,285,000			Role of childhood exposure to PCBs and other PHAHs
Breast	205,000	Ionizing radiation during childhood (atomic bomb survivors, high-dose X-rays)		PCBs, ETS
Testicular	7,500			Cadmium, HAAs
Brain	17,000	Ionizing radiation during childhood (therapeutic radiation)		

Cancer	Cases[c]			
Thyroid	20,700	Ionizing radiation during childhood (therapeutic radiation)	Ionizing radiation during childhood (radioactive fallout from nuclear testing)	HAAs
Leukemia	30,800	Ionizing radiation during childhood (atomic bomb survivors)		
Non-Hodgkin's lymphoma	53,900			PCBs
Melanoma[d]	53,600	Sun exposure during childhood		
Kidney	31,800			Lead
Bladder	56,500			THMs (or related DBPs)
Lung	169,400		ETS during childhood	TCDD
Stomach	21,600	H. pylori (infection during childhood from contaminated drinking water is a probable source)		

Note: exposure refers to childhood exposures unless otherwise indicated.

[a]Limited to prenatal and childhood exposures.

[b]See relevant chapters for supporting epidemiologic evidence.

[c]Children: cases per year, U.S SEER program, 1990–1995 (SEER, 1999); adults: estimated cases, 2002, American Cancer Society, 2002.

[d]Basal cell carcinomas are far more common than melanoma but are not included in most cancer registries (or data are very incomplete).

TABLE 13–3. Role of Prenatal or Childhood Exposure to Environmental Agents in Childhood Neurobehavioral Conditions

| Outcome | Number of affected children (United States)[b] | Environmental Risk Factors and Level of Epidemiologic Evidence[a] | | |
		Sufficient	Limited	Inadequate
Cognitive deficits	760,000 (mental retardation)[c]	Lead, methylmercury, ionizing radiation, PCBs/dioxin-like compounds		Pesticides
Motor deficits	270,000 (complete or partial paralysis of limbs)[d]	Lead, methylmercury, elemental mercury	PCBs/dioxin-like compounds, certain organophosphate and carbamate pesticides	
Visual or hearing deficits	1,300,000 (visual or hearing impairment)[d]	Lead, methylmercury	Certain organophosphate and carbamate pesticides	
Cerebral palsy (congenital)	160,000[e]	Methylmercury		
Attention deficit hyperactivity disorder	360,000[c]		Lead	
Learning disabilities	200,000[e]	Ionizing radiation	Lead	

[a]See relevant chapters for supporting epidemiologic evidence.
[b]Estimated by multiplying prevalence rates times the number of persons age <18 years in United States (2000).
[c]Parent-reported, aged <18 years, United States, 1992–1994 (Halfon and Newacheck, 1999).
[d]United States, 1996, aged <18 years (Adams et al., 1999).
[e]Boyle et al. (1996).

Respiratory Diseases

The only known environmental cause of incident asthma is house-dust mite antigen (Table 13–4). Factors known to exacerbate asthma include cat, cockroach, and house-dust mite antigens, ETS (in preschool-age children), and ambient air pollution. Environmental tobacco smoke is a known cause of acute respiratory conditions (bronchiolitis, pneumonia) and middle ear infections, and a probable cause of incident asthma in preschool-age children. There is suggestive evidence that incident asthma can be caused by cockroach antigens, personal NO_2, and outdoor activities in high-ozone areas. Exacerbation of existing asthma has been linked to dog, rodent, fungal, and soybean antigens, and NO_2 or formaldehyde from indoor sources. There is inadequate evidence of a causal role for several indoor contaminants in incident asthma or as triggers of asthma episodes.

Other Diseases

ETS is a probable cause of SIDS independent of prenatal maternal smoking, a known cause (Table 13–5). Moderately high childhood lead exposure is a known cause of anemia. Other known causal relationships include TCDD and PCBs/dioxin-like compounds and chloracne, intense sun exposure and benign skin nevi (moles), acute high-dose exposure to pesticides, lead, or CO and symptoms and signs of acute poisoning, and fecally contaminated drinking water and gastrointestinal infections. Lead and various forms of mercury have also been linked to increased urinary protein excretion suggestive of renal tubular damage. Perinatal PCB exposure has been linked to increased risk of infections during infancy.

KNOWLEDGE DEVELOPMENT POLICY ISSUES

This section is restricted to knowledge gaps and the need for improved environmental health research programs and tracking systems. Policy needs related to environmental risk management are beyond the scope of this book.

Information Gaps

The information summarized above and material presented throughout this book point to several key information gaps that limit our ability to

TABLE 13.4. Role of Prenatal or Childhood Exposure to Environmental Agents in Childhood Respiratory and Related Diseases

Outcome	Prevalence or number of events per year (United States)[b]	Environmental Risk Factors and Level of Epidemiologic Evidence[a]		
		Sufficient	Limited	Inadequate
Asthma	4.4 million children aged <18 years	House-dust mite antigens	Prenatal and postnatal maternal smoking (in preschool-age children), cockroach antigen, personal air NO_2, outdoor activities in high-ozone areas	ETS (in school-age children), animal and fungal antigens, endotoxins, pollen, *Alternaria*, VOCs, formaldehyde, pesticides, plasticizers
Asthma episodes	14,000,000 school absence days for asthma among children aged 5–17 years	ETS in preschool-age children, cat, cockroach, and house-dust mite antigens, outdoor air pollutants (SO_2, ozone, PM_{10})	ETS (in school-age children), dog, rodent, fungal and soybean antigens, NO_2 from indoor sources, formaldehyde	Cow and horse antigens, insects other than cockroaches or house-dust mites, endotoxins, pollens, pesticides, VOCs, plasticizers
Acute respiratory conditions (mainly infections)	207 million restricted activity days per year among children aged <18 years	ETS, outdoor PM_{10}	Indoor air NO_2, outdoor air pollutants (SO_2, ozone, PM_{10})	
Idiopathic pulmonary hemosiderosis	NA		*Stachybotrys chartarum* (fungus)	
Middle ear infections	34 million restricted activity days per year among children aged <18 years	ETS		

[a]See relevant chapters for supporting epidemiologic evidence.
[b]United States, 1996 (Adams et al. 1999).

understand and prevent adverse health effects of environmental hazards, including knowledge of

- The role of prenatal and childhood exposures to environmental, genetic, and other factors in the etiology of adverse developmental outcomes and childhood and adult diseases
- The distribution of environmental contaminant exposure levels among reproductive-age persons, infants, and children in the general population
- Given the above two information gaps, and with some exceptions, it is not yet possible to quantify with confidence
  - The proportions of adverse pregnancy outcomes and childhood and adult diseases attributable to environmental contaminants
  - The benefits of interventions to reduce exposure levels
  - Progress in reducing environmental threats to child health

Policy Needs

To address the knowledge gaps described above, there is an urgent need for countries and international agencies to invest in population and laboratory research on the role of environmental hazards in fetal and child health and development, including (Bennett and Waters, 2000; Carroquino et al., 1998; Lucier and Schecter, 1998; Needham and Sexton, 2000; Pirkle et al., 1995; Suk et al., 1996; U.S. General Accounting Office, 2000; Warren and Shields, 1997; Weaver et al., 1998):

- Research infrastructure—scientists, laboratories, childhood cancer registries
- Large-scale epidemiologic research programs and projects that incorporate strong statistical power, exposure assessment (including the periconceptual period), biomarkers of exposure and susceptibility, and control of potential confounders
- Tracking systems—purpose-defined surveys and special studies to measure baselines and time trends for exposure to environmental contaminants and the occurrence of adverse health effects including structural and functional abnormalities and diseases
- The United States has taken promising steps in these directions (Centers for Disease Control and Prevention, 2001; U.S. Environmental Protection Agency, (2000a, 2002b). These should be maintained, and other countries and international agencies should take up the challenge.

TABLE 13-5. Role of Prenatal or Childhood Exposure to Environmental Agents in Other Childhood Conditions

Outcome	Number of events per year (United States)[b]	Environmental Risk Factors and Level of Epidemiologic Evidence[a]		
		Sufficient	Limited	Inadequate
Sudden infant death syndrome (SID)	2,600 deaths per year[b]	Prenatal maternal smoking	ETS (independent of prenatal maternal smoking)	
Anemia	NA	Lead		
Renal function abnormalities	NA	Lead, mercury (all three forms), fecally contaminated drinking water—E. coli 0157:H7	Cadmium	
Immune function (susceptibility to infections) during infancy	NA		PCBs/dioxin-like compounds	
Hypothyroidism (neonatal)	NA	NA		PCBs (prenatal hypothyroidism)
Premature menarche	NA	NA		HAAs
Reduced sperm quality	NA	NA		HAAs
Chloracne (severe acne-like skin condition)	NA	TCDD, PCBs/dioxin-like compounds		

Health condition	Estimated number			
Other nonmalignant skin abnormalities conditions	NA	PCBs/dioxin-like compounds (skin pigmentation), inorganic mercury (skin rash), sun exposure (nevi or "moles")		
Tooth abnormalities (hypomineralization)	NA		PCBs/dioxin-like compounds	
Poisonings	54,500[c]	Lead, arsenic, pesticides, CO		
Gastrointestinal viral infections, aged <18 years	20 million restricted activity days per year[d]	Fecally contaminated drinking water		
Infantile methemoglobinemia	NA			Nitrate in drinking water (especially farm wells)
Cataracts	NA			Sun exposure during childhood

[a]See relevant chapters for supporting epidemiologic evidence.

[b]United States, 1999 (National Center for Health Statistics, 2002).

[c]United States, 2000 (Litovitz et al., 2001).

[d]United States, 1996 (Adams et al., 1999).

EPILOGUE

Until recently, countries and international health agencies have generally assigned lower priority to addressing environmental threats to fetal and child health than to more immediate or obvious threats, particularly infectious diseases. Certainly, the dramatic increases in life expectancy observed during the twentieth century were mainly attributable to the control of childhood infectious diseases. History, however, has shown repeatedly the potential for serious adverse health effects after prenatal or childhood exposures to environmental toxicants such as lead and ionizing radiation.

Much of the evidence for the proven environmental health hazards described in this book comes from studies of pregnant women or children who were highly exposed accidentally or deliberately at a time when the health risks were incompletely understood. In several instances, exposure of children and/or pregnant women has continued even after demonstration of likely health risks. This drives home the need to avoid arrogance and to adopt a precautionary approach that protects children from exposure to hazards in the face of scientific uncertainty and opposition from vested interests.

In the past, epidemiologic studies had a limited ability to quantify the health risks of low-level environmental contaminant exposure. Recent advances in environmental exposure and genetic susceptibility assessment promise to enable substantially improved knowledge of health risks including exposure–risk relationships and gene–environment interactions. Assuming that this materializes, it will help ensure evidence-based public health decisions that improve child health protection within a sustainable economy.

This book will be supplemented by a website at the R. Samuel McLaughlin Centre for Population Health Risk Assessment, Institute of Population Health, University of Ottawa, Ottawa, Canada. The website will include supplementary tables and citations relevant to the topics covered in this book. The website address is http://www.mclaughlincentre.ca.

REFERENCES

Adams PF, Hendershot GE, Marano MA. (1999). Current estimates from the National Health Interview Survey. Vital Health Stat 10:212 p.
American Cancer Society. (2002). Facts and figures 2002. Located at http://www.cancer.org/
Bennett DA, Waters MD. (2000). Applying biomarker research. Environ Health Perspect 108:907–10.

Boyle CA, Yeargin-Allsopp M, Doernberg NS, Holmgreen P, Murphy CC, Schendel DE. (1996). Prevalence of selected developmental disabilities in children 3–10 years of age: the Metropolitan Atlanta Developmental Disabilities Surveillance Program, 1991. MMWR CDC Surveill Summ 45:1–14.

California Birth Defects Monitoring Program. (2002). Birth defects in California. Located at http://www.cbdmp.org/index.htm

Carroquino MJ, Galson SK, Licht J, Amler RW, Perera FP, Claxton LD, Landrigan PJ. (1998). The U.S. EPA conference on preventable causes of cancer in children: a research agenda. Environ Health Perspect 106(Suppl 3):867–73.

Centers for Disease Control and Prevention. (2001). National report on human exposure to environmental chemicals. Atlanta: Centers for Disease Control and Prevention.

Halfon N, Newacheck PW. (1999). Prevalence and impact of parent-reported disabling mental health conditions among U.S. children. J Am Acad Child Adolesc Psychiatry 38:600–9.

International Clearinghouse for Birth Defect Monitoring Systems. (1999). Annual report (1999). Rome: International Centre for Birth Defects.

Litovitz TL, Klein-Schwartz W, White S, Cobaugh DJ, Youniss J, Omslaer JC, Drab A, Benson BE. (2001). 2000 annual report of the American Association of Poison Control Centers Toxic Exposure Surveillance System. Am J Emerg Med 19:337–95.

Lucier GW, Schecter A. (1998). Human exposure assessment and the National Toxicology Program. Environ Health Perspect 106:623–27.

National Center for Health Statistics. (2002). Fast stats A to Z. Infant mortality. Located at http://www.cdc.gov/nchs/fastats/infmort.htm

Needham LL, Sexton K. (2000). Assessing children's exposure to hazardous environmental chemicals: an overview of selected research challenges and complexities. J Expo Anal Environ Epidemiol 10:611–29.

Pirkle JL, Sampson EJ, Needham LL, Patterson DG, Ashley DL. (1995). Using biological monitoring to assess human exposure to priority toxicants. Environ Health Perspect 103(Suppl 3):45–8.

SEER. (1999). Cancer Incidence and Survival among Children and Adolescents: United States SEER Program 1975–1995. National Cancer Institute, SEER Program (NIH Pub. No. 99-4649). Ries LAG, Smith MA, Gurney JG, Linet M, Tamra T, Young JL, Bunin GR (eds). Bethesda, MD.

SEER (Surveillance, Epidemiology, and End Results). (2002). Childhood cancer by site incidence, survival and mortality. Located at http://seer.cancer.gov/

Suk WA, Collman G, Damstra T. (1996). Human biomonitoring: research goals and needs. Environ Health Perspect 104(Suppl 3):479–83.

U.S. Environmental Protection Agency. (2002a). Centers for Children's Environmental Health and Disease Prevention Research. Located at http://es.epa.gov/ncer/centers/cecehdpr/01/.

U.S. Environmental Protection Agency. (2002b). The National Children's Study. Located at http://nationalchildrensstudy.gov/

U.S. General Accounting Office. (2000). Toxic chemicals. Long-term coordinated strategy needed to measure exposures in humans (GAO-HEHS-00-80). Washington, DC: U.S. General Accounting Office.

Ventura SJ, Martin JA, Curtin SC, Menacker F, Hamilton BE. (2001). Births: final data for 1999. Natl Vital Stat Rep 49:16–7.

Ventura SJ, Mosher WD, Curtin SC, Abma JC, Henshaw S. (1999). Highlights of trends in pregnancies and pregnancy rates by outcome: estimates for the United States, 1976–96. Natl Vital Stat Rep 47:1–9.

Warren AJ, Shields PG. (1997). Molecular epidemiology: carcinogen-DNA adducts and genetic susceptibility. Proc Soc Exp Biol Med 216:172–80.

Weaver VM, Buckley TJ, Groopman JD. (1998). Approaches to environmental exposure assessment in children. Environ Health Perspect 106(Suppl 3):827–32.

Index